Atlas of Anatomic
Correlations in CT and MRI

Atlas of Anatomic Correlations in CT and MRI

By Paul Gerhardt
and Walter Frommhold

329 Illustrations
Anatomic Illustrations by Karl Herzog
Translated by Horst N. Bertram

1988
Georg Thieme Verlag
Stuttgart · New York

Thieme Medical Publishers, Inc.
New York

Dr. med. Paul Gerhardt, Professor
Director of the Institute for Radiodiagnostics
Technical University of Munich
Ismaningerstr. 22
D-8000 München 80 FRG

Dr. med. Walter Frommhold, Dr. h. c., Professor
Director of the Department of Radiology
University of Tübingen
Röntgenweg 11
D-7400 Tübingen FRG

Dr. med. Horst N. Bertram
13 Juliada Drive
Lebanon, Pennsylvania 17042 USA

Karl Herzog
Friedrich-Dannenmann-Str. 45
D-7400 Tübingen FRG

Library of Congress Cataloging-in-Publication Data

Gerhardt, Paul
Atlas of anatomic correlations in CT and MRI / Paul Gerhardt and Walter Frommhold ; anatomic illustrations by Karl Herzog ; translated by Horst Bertram.
p. cm.
Includes bibliographies and index.
ISBN 0-86577-227-4 (Thieme Medical)
1. Anatomy, Human--Atlases. 2. Magnetic resonance imaging--Atlases. 3. Tomography--Atlases. I. Frommhold, Walter. II. Title.
[DNLM: 1. Anatomy--atlases. 2. Nuclear Magnetic Resonance--atlases. 3. Tomography, X-Ray Computed--atlases. QS 17 G368a] QM25.G47 1988
611'. 022'2--dc 19
DNLM/DLC
for Library of Congress 88-12369

Cover design by Renate Stockinger

Important Note: Medicine is an ever-changing science. Research and clinical experience are continually broadening our knowledge, in particular our knowledge of proper treatment and drug therapy. Insofar as this book mentions any dosage or application, readers may rest assured that the authors, editors and publishers have made every effort to ensure that such references are strictly in accordance with the state of knowledge at the time of production of the book. Nevertheless, every user is requested to examine carefully the manufacturer's leaflets accompanying each drug to check on his own responsibility whether the dosage schedules recommended therein or the contraindications stated by the manufacturers differ from the statements made in the present book. Such examination is particularly important with drugs that are either rarely used or have been newly released on the market.

Typesetting: Kittelberger GmbH, Reutlingen
(System: Digiset 40T30)
Printed in West-Germany by Grammlich, Pliezhausen

ISBN 3-13-662001-1 (Georg Thieme Verlag, Stuttgart)
ISBN 0-86577-227-4 (Thieme Medical Publishers, Inc., New York)

1 2 3 4 5 6

Preface

The beginnings of this Atlas go back many years.

In 1936 Professor Wetzel became Chairman of the Institute of Anatomy of the University of Tübingen. While still at the University of Würzburg he began preparing three-plane frozen sections of the human body, and with the help of the Institute's illustrators, transforming slide projections of the sections into large-scale drawings. In Tübingen, Karl Herzog, the University's illustrator, carried on with the production of the demonstration charts and later added the detailed anatomical nomenclature to them. The Institute of Anatomy in Tübingen was thus in possession of excellent demonstration material for teaching purposes. The drawings of anatomic sections through the male pelvis were done my Mr. Ernst Schnackig, a medical illustrator in Würzburg. The drawings, some of which have already been published in „Das Röntgenschichtsbild" by A. Gebauer (Thieme, Stuttgart, 1959), have been thoroughly revised and adapted to the latest anatomic nomenclature.

Following the death of Professor Wetzel in 1970, the charts themselves were officially turned over to the Anatomical Institute of the University of Tübingen, although the copyright for the drawings was retained by Professor Wetzel's widow, Mrs. Lore Wetzel.

The idea to use a selection of these excellent drawings as an Atlas for planning computerized radiotherapy of malignant tumors arose quickly after Karl Herzog had called our attention to certain illustrations suitable to this purpose.

During the years that followed the Atlas underwent several phases of development due to progress in imaging technology. Constant improvements in image quality made it necessary to replace even recent scans with those of better quality as they became available. This delayed the realization of our plans until the introduction of magnetic resonance imaging provided the final impulse to complete our project, with great assistance from all involved.

Our first and foremost thanks go to the late Mrs. Lore Wetzel who gave us immediate permission to use the drawings. It is her wish and ours, to thus preserve the memory of Professor Robert Wetzel.

We would also like to thank Mr. Karl Herzog, the now retired illustrator of the University, who helped develop the Atlas in its early stages and did the first anatomical legends.

We are indebted to the Philips Company, Hamburg, for their spontaneous willingness years ago to let us make our first magnetic resonance scans with their equipment in Best in the Netherlands, with the most valuable assistance of Mrs. A. Brouwer. Because of rapid technical progress many of these early pictures soon had to be replaced. A small portion of our most recent magnetic resonance studies was done on the Siemens 1.5 Tesla Magnetom of the Dept. of Radiology, University of Tübingen.

We would like to take this opportunity to also thank our medical colleagues of the Department of Radiodiagnostics of the University of Heidelberg, those of the Institute for Radiodiagnostics of the Clinicum of the Technical University in Munich, and those at the Department of Radiology of the University of Tübingen.

Repeated corrections were made to the anatomical drawings with the help of physicians from Heidelberg and Munich, especially Dr. Sabine Siess, Heidelberg, and Dr. Helga Gräfin von Einsiedel, Munich.

We owe another debt of gratitude to Professor H. P. Schmidt of Heidelberg, for his assistance with sections of the brain, to Mr. Kramer, Heidelberg and Mrs. Christine Garnebode, Munich, for their graphic work.

Grateful acknowledgement is due to Dr. Horst N. Bertram of Lebanon, Pennsylvania, USA, for the English translation.

Our final and special thanks are reserved for the Publishers, the Georg Thieme Verlag, Stuttgart, and particularly for Messrs. A. Menge and H. Doellert, who helped us to overcome all the difficulties and obstacles inherent to the production of this Atlas. Their harmonious cooperation contributed much to its succesful conclusion.

Paul Gerhardt
Walter Frommhold

Spring 1988

Table of Contents

Introduction

The development of Computerized Tomography and Nuclear Magnetic Resonance tomography has brought new anatomical dimensions to the field of diagnostic imaging. These new tomographic procedures have added axial sectioning to the usual way of seeing topographic details of the human body. This means that the physician who views these images, too, must have an understanding of seeing topographic anatomy in the third dimension.

We have therefore tried to create an Atlas which correlates axial, sagittal and coronal anatomical sections of the head and body with computerized and MR tomographic sections, and to provide the examining physician with a quick reference to compare topographic anatomy with sectional images.

Photographs of the brain in axial and coronal planes have been added to complement the anatomical drawings. All legends were brought up to the latest anatomical nomenclature, and were translated into English.

This now completed volume reflects the state of imaging technology at the time a major portion of these CT and MR tomographic illustrations were made. We are aware that after its publication the quality and detail of some images may still leave something to be desired.

The Atlas is divided into two major sections:

Section 1 contains, aside from whole body sections of general interest, sections of the cranial and adjacent cervical regions which are of interest mainly to the neuroradiologically oriented specialist.

Section 2 contains sections of the trunk, with the female and male pelvis presented separately.

With the exception of the brain we have not included any section level diagrams because the anatomic drawings and their assigned tomographic sections are of different origin and therefore do not correspond exactly. We have nevertheless been able to achieve a very close correlation between the anatomical drawings and their MR and CT scans.

The anatomical drawings are provided with reference lines connecting the anatomic structure to the English term. The corresponding Latin terminology is also listed on the same page. Reference lines with corresponding numbers have been added to the MR and CT scans. Structures not included in the anatomic drawings, but important to the scans, are distinguished by decimal numbers. These terms have also been included in the Latin legends.

The computer tomograms were made with different tomographic units. Due to technical differences not all images show the same resolution of detail. Where necessary oral and intravascular contrast media have been used for the enhancement of certain structures. We have not discussed specific examination techniques since the Atlas contains only normal human topographic anatomy.

CT reconstructions were obtained for some of the cranial scans, since they are frequently used in diagnostic evaluation.

Equipment with a magnetic field strength of 0.5 and 1.5 Tesla was used for MR tomography. As in the computerized tomograms differences in image quality were unavoidable.

Legends are generally brief, which for MR tomography means sampling parameters only. SE 600/30, for instance, means: Spin Echo Sequence of TR = 600 ms, TE = 30 ms. IR 1.900/400/30 means: Inversion Recovery Sequence of TR 1.900 ms, TI = 400 ms, TE = 30 ms.

Unless otherwise indicated multiple slice samplings were taken during MR tomography. We have not shown any of the possibilities of MR imaging differences through changes in the parameters.

We hope that this Atlas will be a useful tool for the reader. We will be most grateful for any suggestions the reader may have for improving future editions.

Coronal Sections of the Whole Body

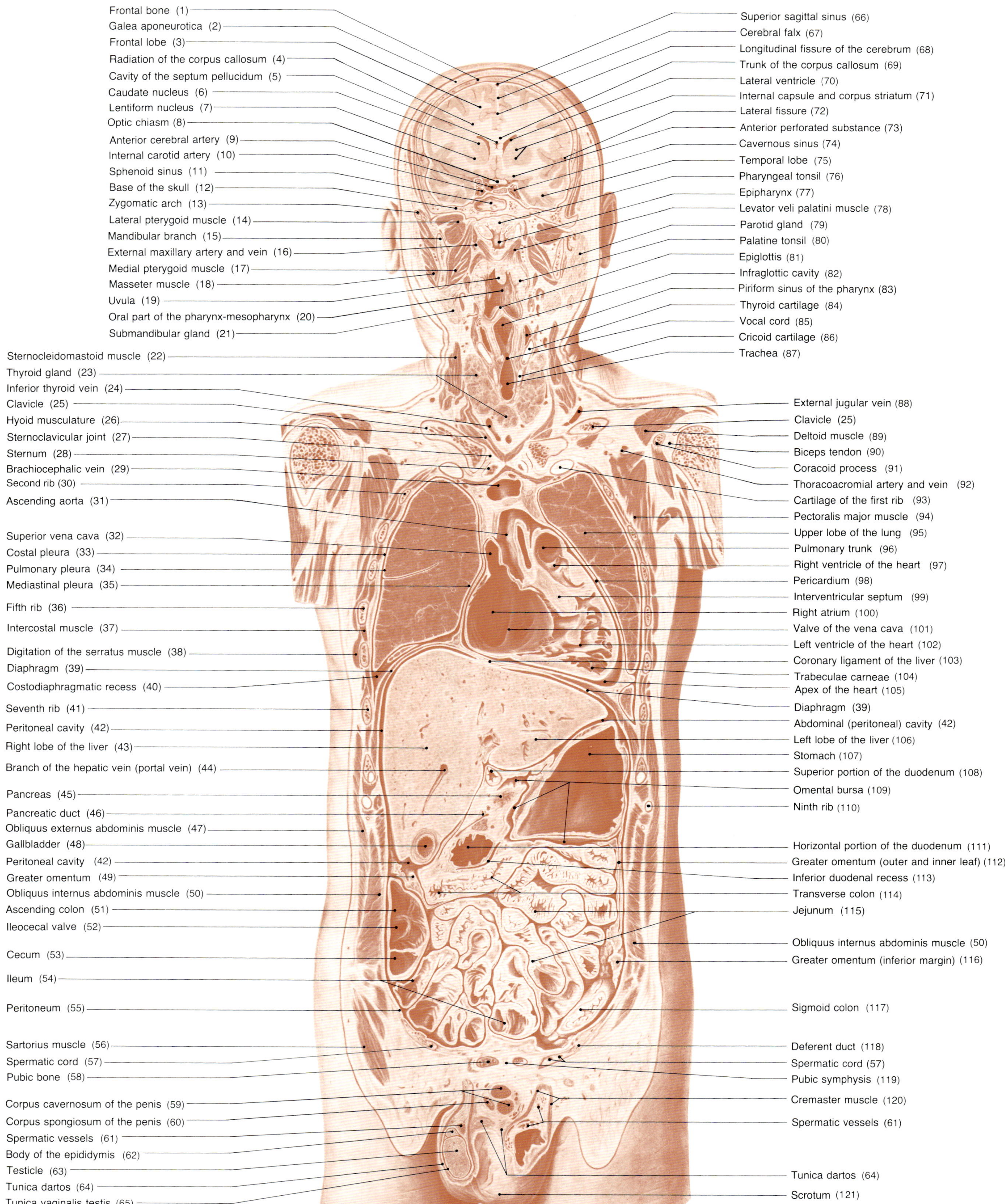

1 Os frontale
2 Galea aponeurotica
3 Lobus frontalis
4 Radiatio corporis callosi
5 Cavum septi pellucidi
6 Nucleus caudatus
7 Nucleus lentiformis
8 Chiasma opticum
9 A. cerebri anterior
10 A. carotis interna
11 Sinus sphenoidalis
12 Basis cranii
13 Arcus zygomaticus
14 M. pterygoideus lateralis
15 R. mandibulae
16 A. et V. maxillaris externa
17 M. pterygoideus medialis
18 M. masseter
19 Uvula
20 Pars oralis pharyngis – Mesopharynx
21 Glandula submandibularis
22 M. sternocleidomastoideus
23 Glandula thyreoidea
24 V. thyreoidea inferior
25 Clavicula
26 Mm. ossis hyoidei
27 Articulatio sternoclavicularis
28 Sternum
29 V. brachiocephalica
30 Pericardium
31 Aorta ascendens
32 V. cava superior
33 Pleura costalis
34 Pleura pulmonalis
35 Pleura mediastinalis
36 Costa V
37 M. intercostalis
38 M. serratus anterior
39 Diaphragma
40 Recessus costodiaphragmaticus
41 Costa VII
42 Cavum peritonaei
43 Lobus hepatis dexter
44 R. venae hepaticae (V. portae)
45 Pancreas
46 Ductus pancreaticus
47 M. obliquus externus abdominis
48 Vesica fellea
49 Omentum majus
50 M. obliquus internus abdominis
51 Colon ascendens
52 Valva ileocaecalis
53 Caecum
54 Ileum
55 Peritonaeum
55.1 M. glutaeus medius
55.2 M. iliopsoas
56 M. sartorius
56.1 M. rectus femoris
57 Funiculus spermaticus
58 Os pubis
59 Corpus cavernosum penis
60 Corpus spongiosum penis
61 Vasa spermatica
62 Corpus epididymidis
63 Testis
64 Tunica dartos
65 Tunica vaginalis testis
66 Sinus sagittalis superior
67 Falx cerebri
68 Fissura longitudinalis cerebri
69 Truncus corporis callosi
70 Ventriculus lateralis
71 Capsula interna et Corpus striatum
72 Fissura lateralis (Sylvii)
72.1 Ventriculus III
73 Substantia perforata inferior
74 Sinus cavernosus
75 Lobus temporalis
75.1 Caput mandibulae
76 Tonsilla pharyngea
77 Epipharynx
78 M. levator veli palatini
79 Glandula parotis
80 Tonsilla palatina
81 Epiglottis
82 Cavum infraglotticum
83 Sinus piriformis
84 Cartilago thyreoidea
85 Plica vocalis
86 Cartilago cricoidea
87 Trachea
88 V. jugularis externa
89 M. deltoideus
90 Tendo m. bicipitis
91 Processus coracoideus
92 A. et V. thoracoacromialis
93 Cartilago costae I
94 M. pectoralis major
95 Lobus superior pulmonis
96 Truncus pulmonalis
97 Ventriculus dexter cordis
98 Pericardium
99 Septum interventriculare
100 Atrium dextrum
101 Valvula venae cavae
102 Ventriculus sinister cordis
103 Lig. coronarium hepatis
104 Trabeculae carneae
105 Apex cordis
106 Lobus hepatis sinister
107 Ventriculus (Gaster)
107.1 M. rectus
108 Pars superior duodeni
109 Bursa omentalis
110 Costa IX
111 Pars horizontalis duodeni
112 Omentum majus
113 Recessus duodenalis inferior
114 Colon transversum
115 Jejunum
116 Omentum majus (Margo inferior)
117 Colon sigmoideum
118 Ductus deferens
119 Symphysis ossis pubis
120 M. cremaster
121 Scrotum

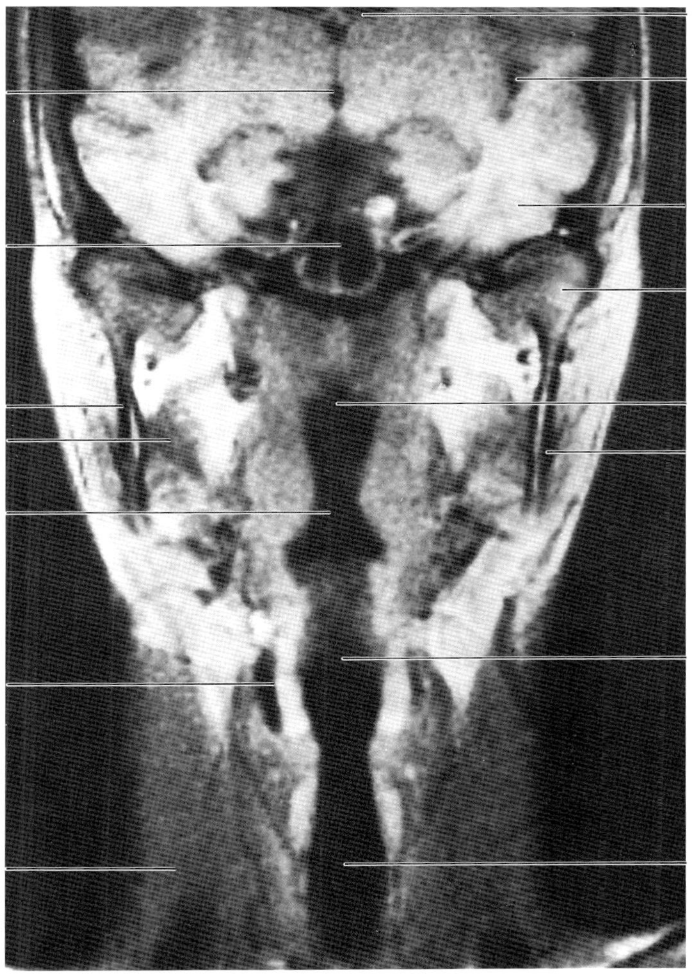

MRI, SE 600/30

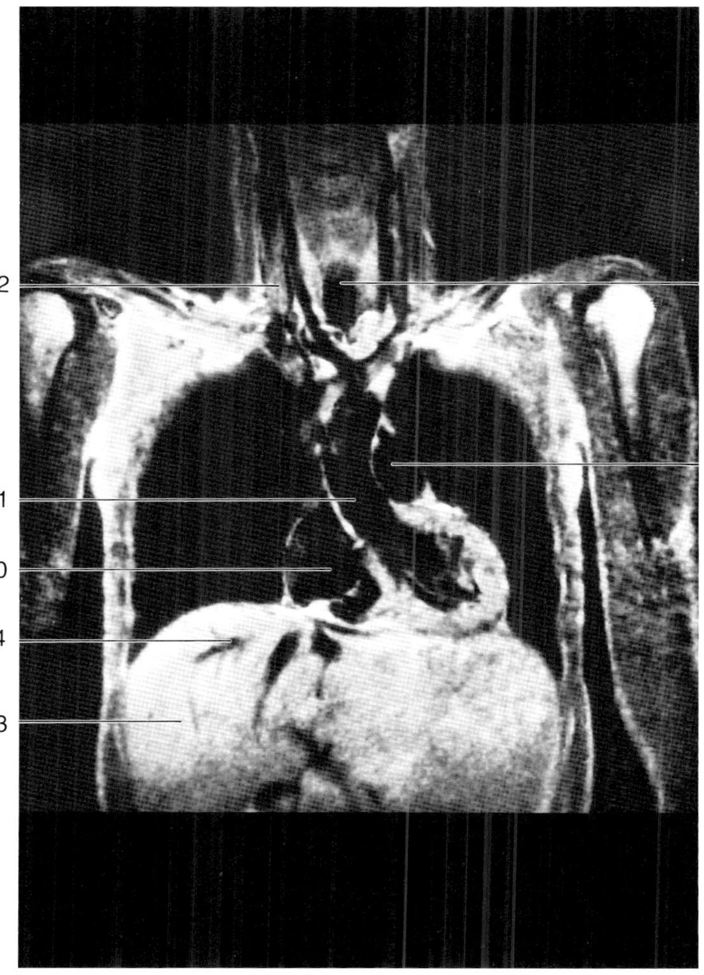

MRI, SE, ECG-triggered, $T_E = 30$

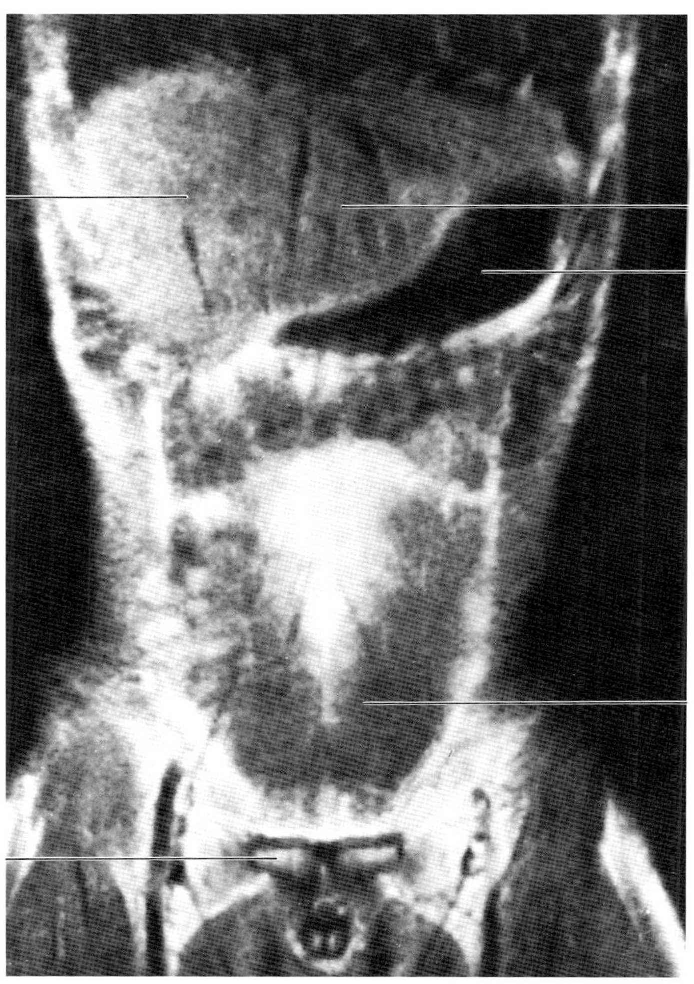

MRI, SE 600/30

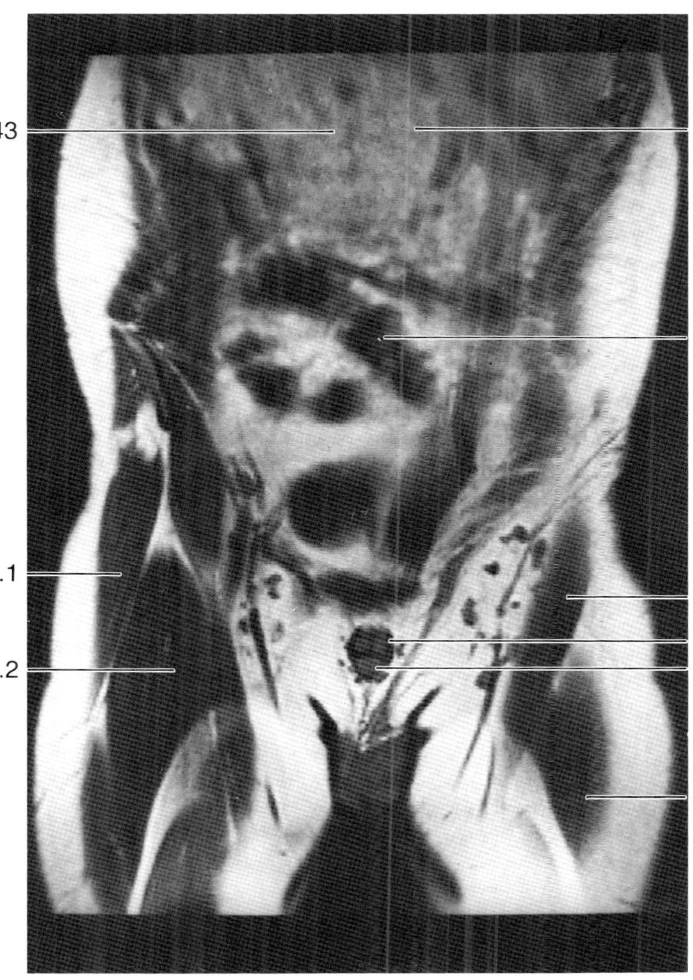

MRI, SE 800/22

11 Sphenoid sinus
15 Mandibular branch
17 Medial pterygoid muscle
18 Masseter muscle
20 Oral part of the pharynx – mesopharynx
22 Sternocleidomastoid muscle
31 Ascending aorta
43 Right lobe of the liver
44 Branch of the hepatic vein (portal vein)
55.1 Gluteus medius muscle
55.2 Iliopsoas muscle
56 Sartorius muscle
56.1 Rectus femoris muscle
58 Pubic bone
59 Corpus cavernosum of the penis
60 Corpus spongiosum of the penis
70 Lateral ventricle
72 Lateral sulcus (of Sylvius)
72.1 Third ventricle
75 Temporal lobe
75.1 Mandible (head)
77 Epipharynx – nasal part of the pharynx
82 Infraglottic cavity
83 Pyriform sinus of the pharynx
87 Trachea
96 Pulmonary trunk
100 Right atrium
106 Left lobe of the liver
107 Stomach
107.1 Rectus muscle
114 Transverse colon

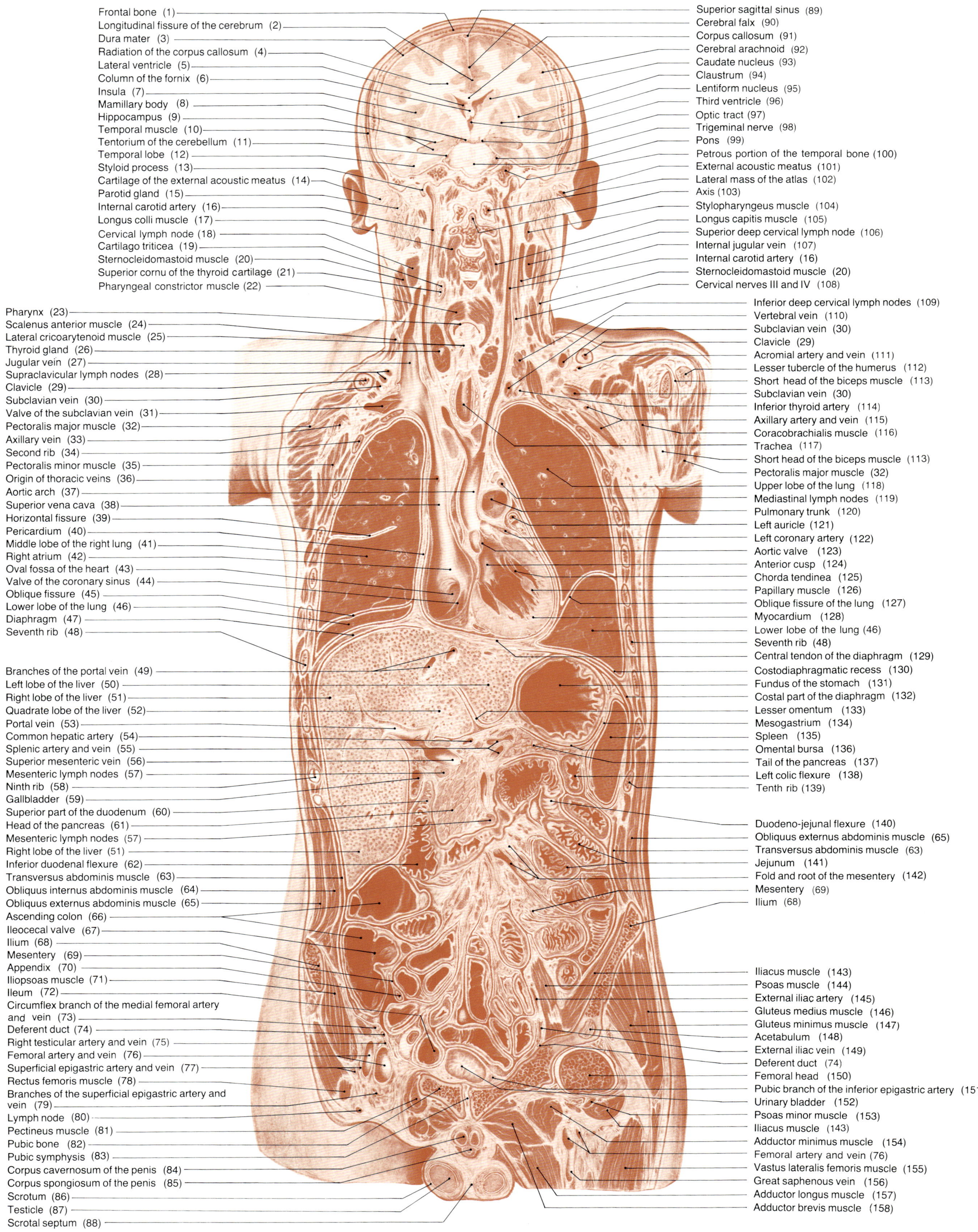

1 Os frontale
2 Fissura longitudinalis cerebri
3 Dura mater encephali
4 Radiatio corporis callosi
5 Ventriculus lateralis
6 Columna fornicis
7 Insula
8 Corpus mamillare et ventriculus lateralis
9 Hippocampus
10 M. temporalis
11 Tentorium cerebelli
12 Lobus temporalis
13 Processus styloideus
14 Cartilago meatus acustici externi
15 Glandula parotis
16 A. carotis interna
16.1 A. carotis communis
17 M. longus colli
18 Nodi lymphatici cervicales profundi
19 Cartilago triticea
20 M. sternocleidomastoideus
21 Cornu superius cartilaginis thyroideae
22 M. constrictor pharyngis
23 Pharnyx
24 M. scalenus anterior
25 M. cricoarytaenoideus lateralis
26 Glandula thyroidea
27 V. jugularis
28 Nodi lymphatici supraclaviculares
29 Clavicula
30 V. subclavia
31 Valvula v. subclaviae
32 M. pectoralis major
33 V. axillaris
34 Costa II
35 M. pectoralis minor
36 Vv. thoracicae
37 Arcus aortae
37.1 A. subclavia
37.2 Truncus brachiocephalicus
38 V. cava superior
39 Fissura horizontalis
40 Pericardium
41 Lobus medius pulmonis dextri
42 Atrium dextrum
43 Fossa ovalis cordis
44 Valvula sinus coronarii
45 Fissura obliqua
46 Lobus inferior pulmonis
47 Diaphragma
48 Costa VII
49 Rr. venae portae
50 Lobus hepatis sinister
51 Lobus hepatis dexter
52 Lobus quadratus
53 V. portae
54 A. hepatica communis
55 A. et V. lienalis
56 V. mesenterica superior
57 Nodi lymphatici mesenterici
58 Costa IX
59 Vesica fellea
60 Duodenum (Pars superior)
61 Caput pancreatis
62 Flexura duodeni inferior
63 M. transversus abdominis
64 M. obliquus internus abdominis
65 M. obliquus externus abdominis
66 Colon ascendens
67 Valva ileocaecalis
68 Os ilium
69 Mesenterium
70 Appendix vermiformis
71 M. iliopsoas
72 Ileum
73 A. et V. circumflexa femoris medialis
74 Ductus deferens
75 A. et V. testicularis
76 A. et V. femoralis
77 A. et V. epigastrica superficialis
78 M. rectus femoris
79 Rr. A. et V. epigastricae superficialis
80 Nodus lymphaticus
81 M. pectineus
82 Os pubis
83 Symphysis pubica
84 Corpus cavernosum penis
85 Corpus spongiosum penis
86 Scrotum
87 Testis
88 Septum scroti
89 Sinus sagittalis superior
90 Falx cerebri
91 Corpus callosum
92 Cavum subarachnoideale
93 Nucleus caudatus
94 Claustrum
95 Nucleus lentiformis
96 Ventriculus tertius
97 Tractus opticus
98 N. trigeminus
99 Pons
100 Pars petrosa ossis temporalis
101 Meatus acusticus externus
102 Massa lateralis atlantis
103 Dens axis
104 M. stylopharyngeus
105 M. longus capitis
106 Nodus lymphaticus cervicalis profundus superior
107 V. jugularis interna
108 Nn. cervicales III et IV
109 Nodi lymphatici cervicales profundi inferiores
110 V. vertebralis
111 A. et V. acromialis
112 Tuberculum minus humeri
113 Caput breve (M. biceps brachii)
114 A. thyroidea inferior
115 A. et V. axillaris
116 M. coracobrachialis
117 Trachea
118 Lobus superior pulmonis
119 Nodi lymphatici mediastinales
120 Truncus pulmonis
121 Auricula sinistra
122 A. coronaria sinistra
123 Valva aortae
123.1 Ventriculus sinister cordis
124 Cuspis anterior
125 Chorda tendinea
126 M. papillaris
127 Fissura obliqua pulmonis
128 Myocardium
129 Centrum tendineum
130 Recessus costodiaphragmaticus
131 Fundus ventriculi
132 Diaphragma, Pars costalis
133 Omentum minus
134 Mesogastrium
135 Lien
136 Bursa omentalis
137 Cauda pancreatis
138 Flexura coli sinistra
138.1 A. mesenterica superior
138.2 Colon descendens
139 Costa X
140 Flexura duodenojejunalis
141 Jejunum
142 Plica et Radix mesenterii
143 M. iliacus
144 M. psoas
145 A. iliaca externa
146 M. glutaeus medius
147 M. glutaeus minus
148 Acetabulum
149 V. iliaca externa
150 Caput femoris
151 R. pubicus arteriae epigastricae inferioris
152 Vesica urinaria
153 M. psoas minor
154 M. adductor minimus
155 M. vastus lateralis femoris
156 V. saphena magna
157 M. adductor longus
158 M. adductor brevis

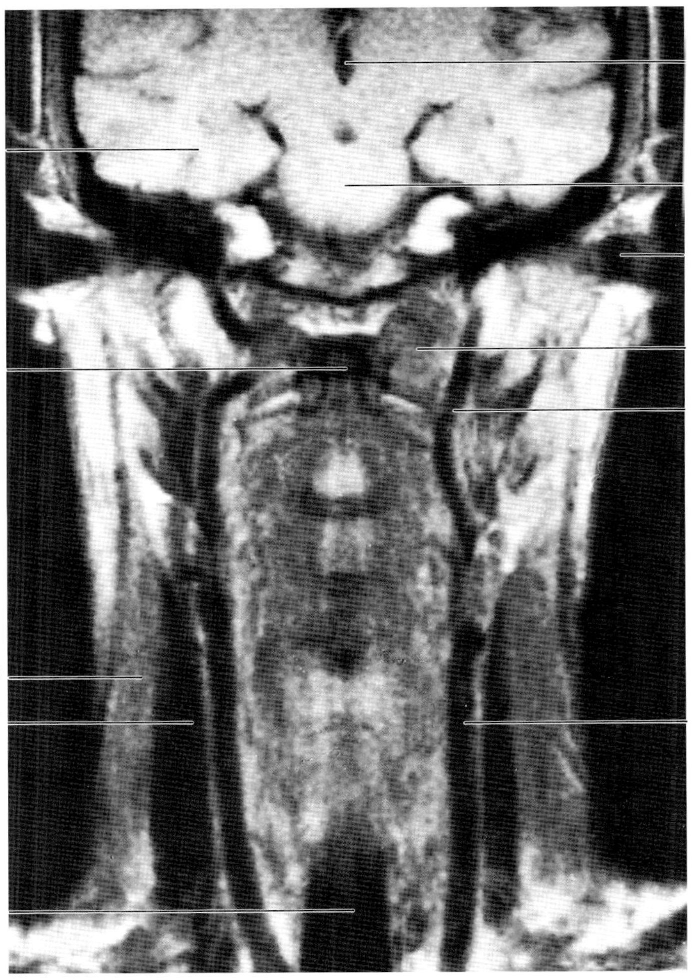

MRI, SE 600/30

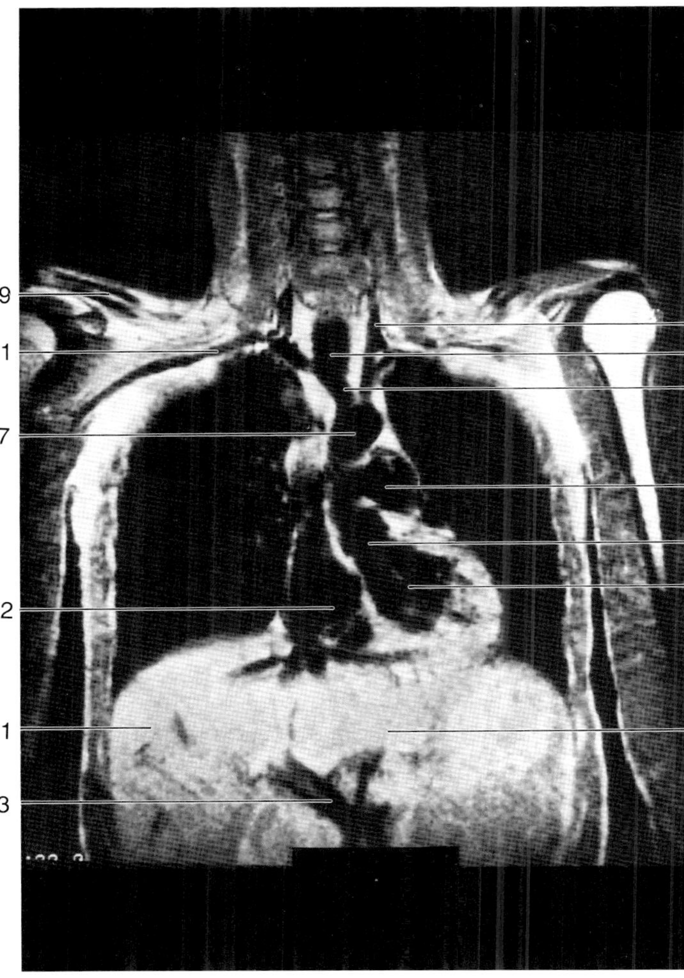

MRI, SE, ECG-triggered, $T_E = 30$

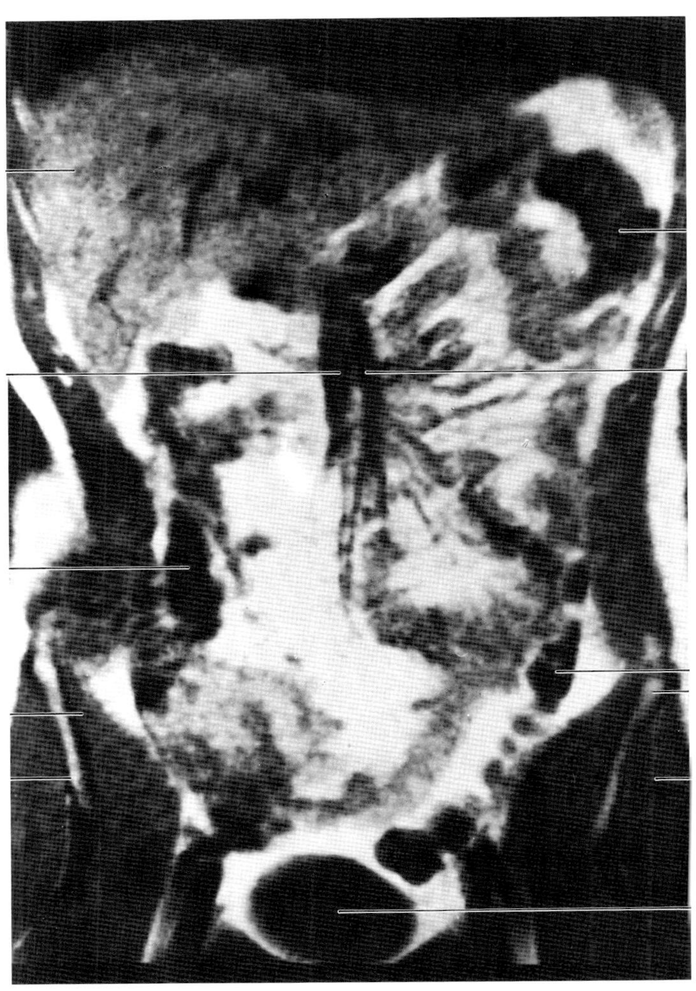

MRI, SE 600/30

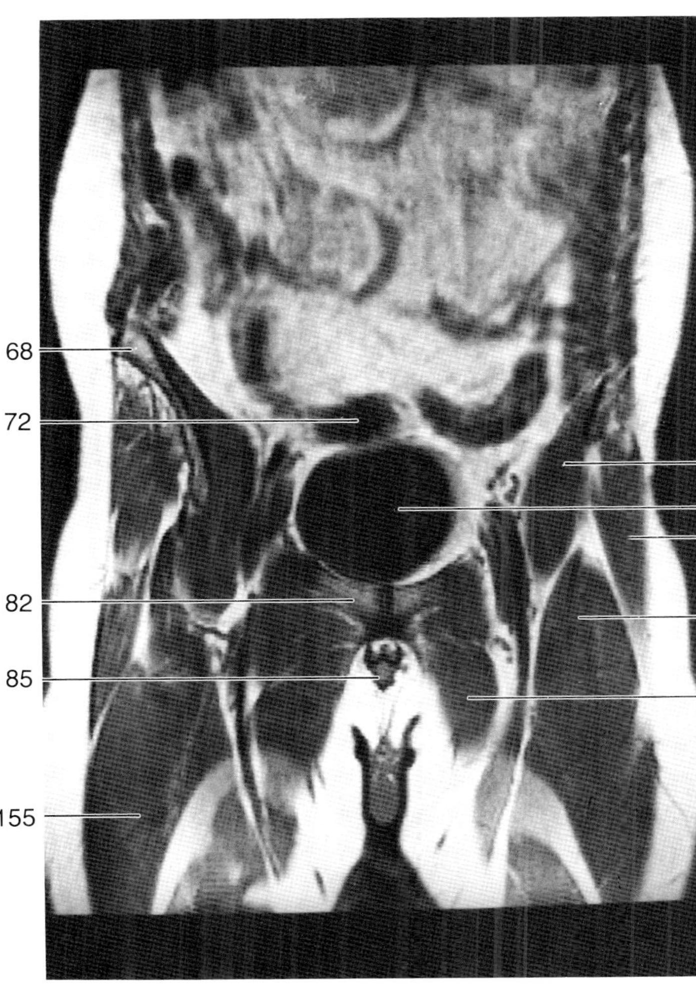

MRI, SE 800/22

12 Temporal lobe
16 Internal carotid artery
16.1 Common carotid artery
20 Sternocleidomastoid muscle
27 Jugular vein
29 Clavicle
37 Aortic arch
37.1 Subclavian artery
37.2 Brachiocephalic trunc
42 Right atrium
50 Left lobe of the liver
51 Right lobe of the liver
53 Portal vein
56 Superior mesenteric vein
66 Ascending colon
68 Ilium
72 Ileum
82 Pubic bone
85 Corpus spongiosum of the penis
96 Third ventricle
99 Pons
101 External acoustic meatus
102 Lateral mass of the atlas
103 Odontoid process of the axis
117 Trachea
120 Pulmonary trunk
123 Aortic valve
123.1 Left ventricle
138 Left colic flexure
138.1 Superior mesenteric artery
138.2 Descending colon
143 Iliacus muscle
146 Gluteus medius muscle
147 Gluteus minimus muscle
152 Urinary bladder
155 Vastus lateralis femoris muscle
158 Adductor brevis muscle

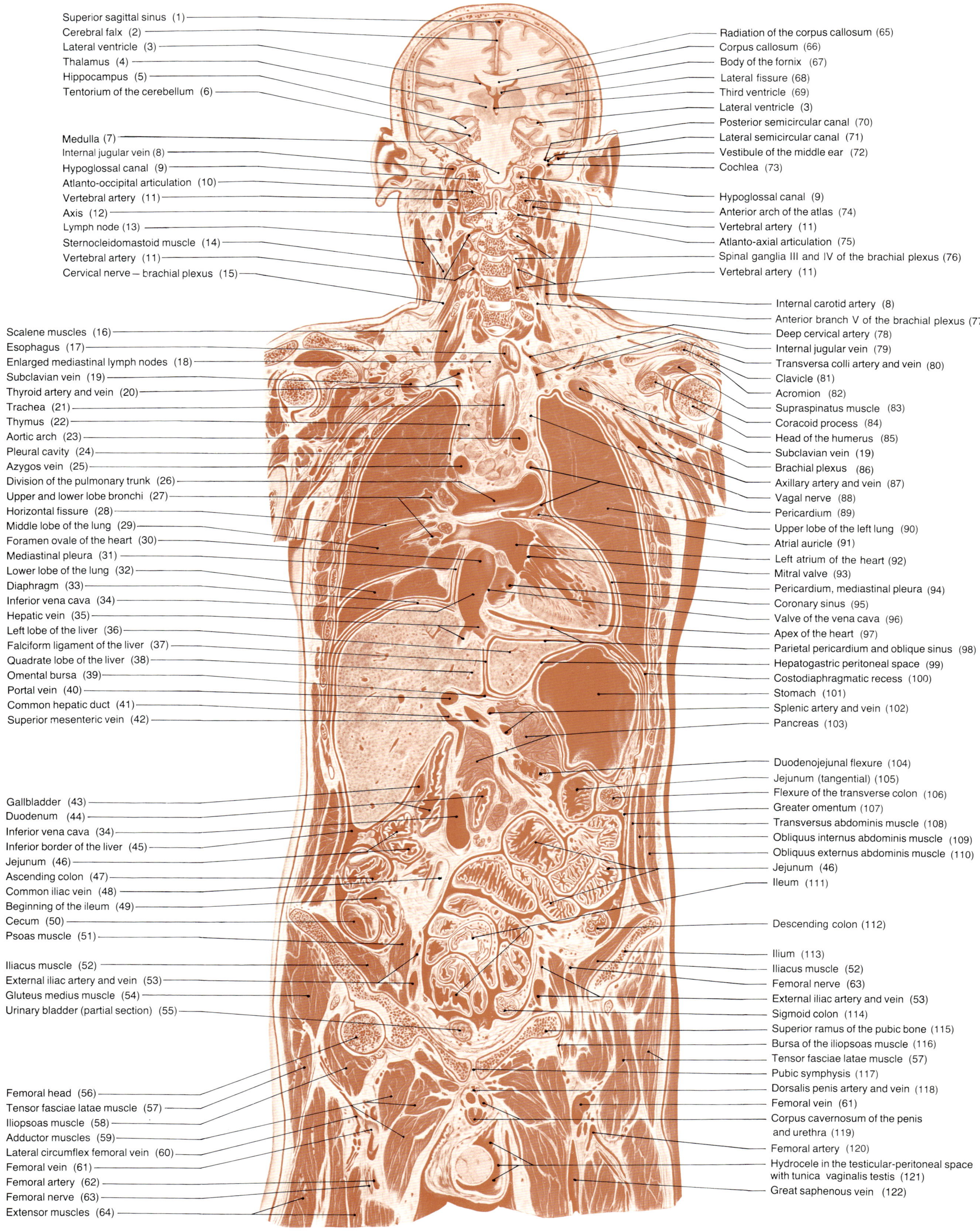

1 Sinus sagittalis superior
2 Falx cerebri
3 Ventriculus lateralis
4 Thalamus
5 Hippocampus
6 Tentorium cerebelli
7 Medulla
8 V. jugularis interna
9 Canalis hypoglossis
10 Articulatio atlantooccipitalis
10.1 Pedunculus cerebellaris
10.2 Pons
10.3 Atlas
10.4 Dens axis
11 A. vertebralis
12 Axis
13 Nodus lymphaticus
14 M. sternocleidomastoideus
15 N. cervicalis – Plexus brachialis
16 Mm. scaleni
17 Oesophagus
18 Nodi lymphatici mediastinales
19 V. subclavia
20 A. et V. thyroidea
21 Trachea
22 Thymus
23 Arcus aortae
24 Cavum pleurae
25 V. azygos
26 Bifurcatio trunci pulmonalis
27 Bronchus lobaris superior et inferior
28 Fissura horizontalis
29 Lobus medius pulmonis
30 Foramen ovale cordis
31 Pleura mediastinalis
32 Lobus inferior pulmonis
33 Diaphragma
34 V. cava inferior
35 V. hepatica
36 Lobus sinister hepatis
37 Lig. falciforme hepatis
38 Lobus quadratus hepatis
39 Bursa omentalis
40 V. portae
41 Ductus hepaticus communis
42 V. mesenterica superior
43 Vesica fellea
44 Duodenum
45 Margo inferior hepatis
46 Jejunum
47 Colon ascendens
48 V. iliaca communis
49 Ileum
50 Caecum
51 M. psoas
52 M. iliacus
53 A. et V. iliaca externa
54 M. glutaeus medius
55 Vesica urinaria
56 Caput femoris
57 M. tensor fasciae latae
58 M. iliopsoas
59 Mm. adductores
60 V. circumflexa femoris lateralis
61 V. femoralis
62 A. femoralis
63 N. femoralis
64 Mm. extensores
65 Radiatio corporis callosi
66 Corpus callosum
67 Corpus fornicis
68 Fissura lateralis (Sylvii)
69 Ventriculus III
70 Ductus semicircularis posterior
71 Ductus semicircularis lateralis
72 Cavum tympani (Vestibulum)
73 Cochlea
74 Arcus anterior
75 Articulatio atlantoaxialis
76 Ganglia spinalia III + IV plexus brachialis
77 R. anterior V plexus brachialis
78 A. cervicalis profunda
79 V. jugularis interna
80 A. et V. transversa colli
81 Clavicula
82 Acromion
83 M. supraspinatus
84 Processus coracoideus
85 Caput humeri
85.1 A. subclavia
85.2 A. axillaris
86 Plexus brachialis
87 A. et V. axillaris
88 N. vagus
89 Pericardium
90 Lobus superior pulmonis sinistri
91 Auricula atrii
92 Atrium cordis sinistrum
93 Valva mitralis
94 Pericardium, Pleura mediastinalis
95 Sinus coronarius
96 Valva v. cavae
97 Apex cordis
98 Pericardium parietale et planum inclinatum
99 Spatium peritoneale hepatogastricum
100 Recessus costodiaphragmaticus
101 Ventriculus (Gaster)
102 A. et V. lienalis
103 Pancreas
103.1 Aorta abdominalis
104 Flexura duodenojejunalis
105 Jejunum
106 Colon transversum (Flexura)
107 Omentum majus
108 M. transversus abdominis
109 M. obliquus internus abdominis
110 M. obliquus externus abdominis
111 Ileum
112 Colon descendens
113 Os ilium
114 Colon sigmoideum
115 R. superior ossis pubis
116 Bursa m. iliopsoas
117 Symphysis pubica
118 A. et V. dorsalis penis
119 Corpus cavernosum penis et urethra
120 A. femoralis
121 Hydrocele testis
122 V. saphena magna

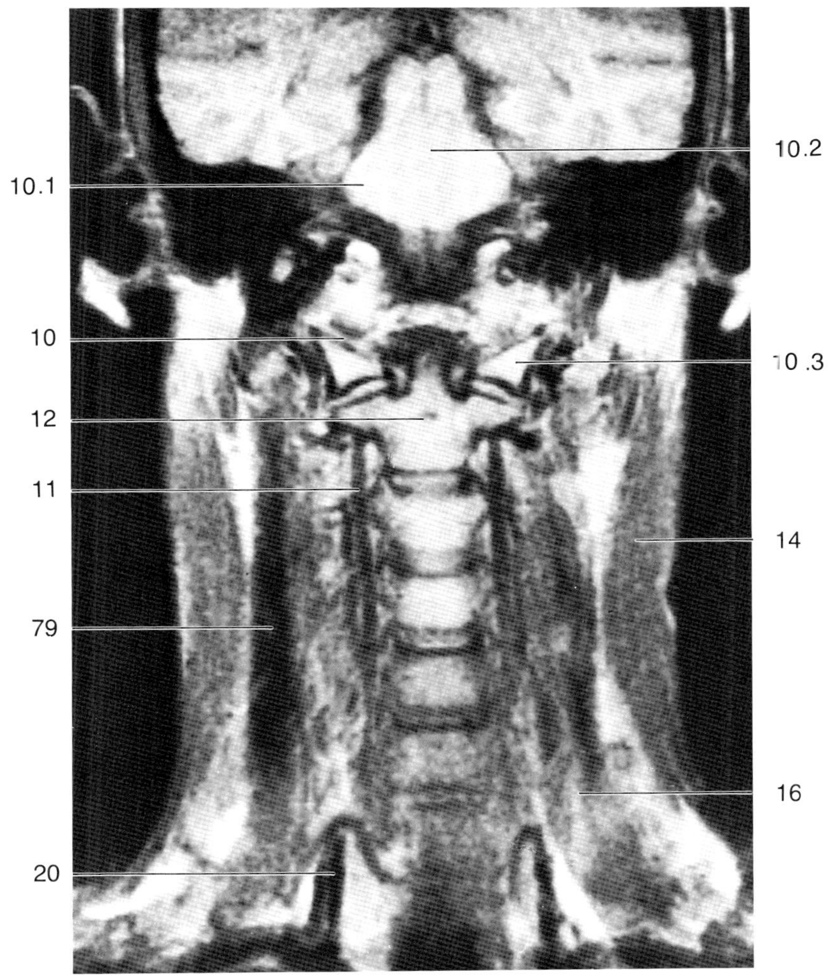

MRI, SE 600/30

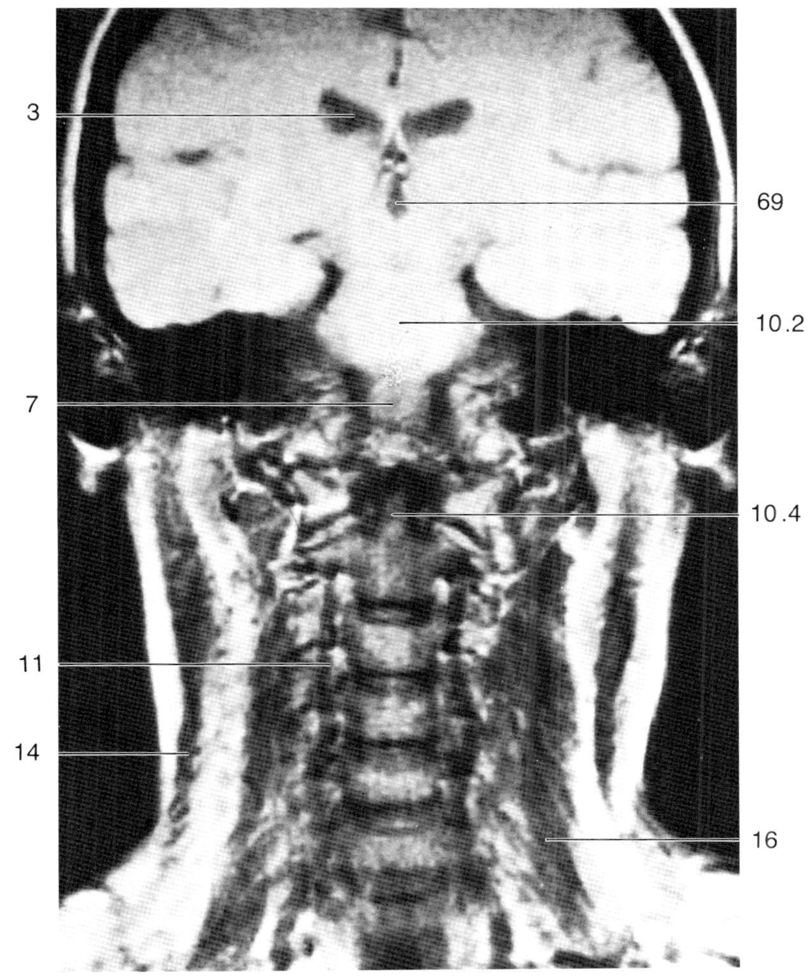

MRI, SE 600/30

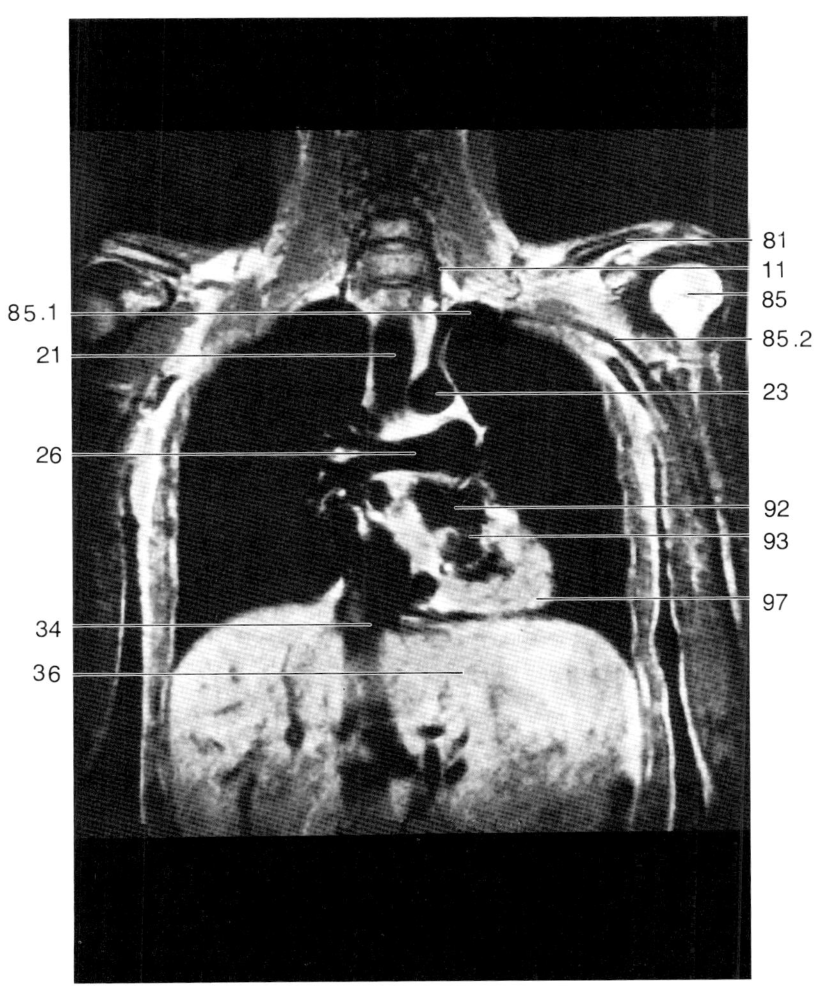

MRI, SE, ECG-triggered, $T_E = 30$

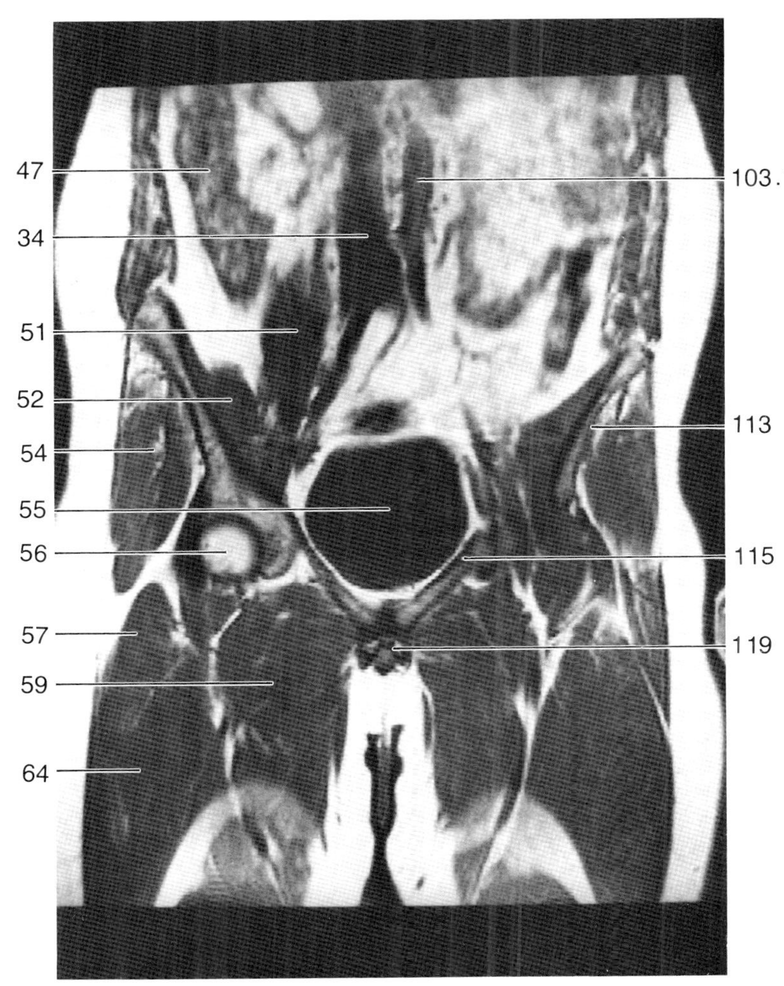

MRI, SE 800/22

3 Lateral ventricle
7 Metencephalon – crus cerebri
10 Atlanto-occipital articulation
10.1 Middle cerebellar peduncle
10.2 Pons
10.3 Atlas
10.4 Odontoid process
11 Vertebral artery
12 Axis
14 Sternocleidomastoid muscle
16 Scalene muscles
20 Thyroid artery and vein
21 Trachea
23 Aortic arch
26 Division of the pulmonary trunk
34 Inferior vena cava
36 Left lobe of the liver
47 Ascending colon
51 Psoas muscle
52 Iliacus muscle
54 Gluteus medius muscle
55 Urinary bladder
56 Femoral head
57 Tensor fasciae latae muscle
59 Adductor muscles
64 Extensor muscles
69 Third ventricle
79 Internal jugular vein
81 Clavicle
85 Head of the humerus
85.1 Subclavian artery
85.2 Axillary artery
92 Atrium of the heart
93 Mitral valve
97 Apex of the heart
103.1 Abdominal aorta
113 Ilium
115 Superior ramus of the pubic bone
119 Corpus cavernosum of the penis

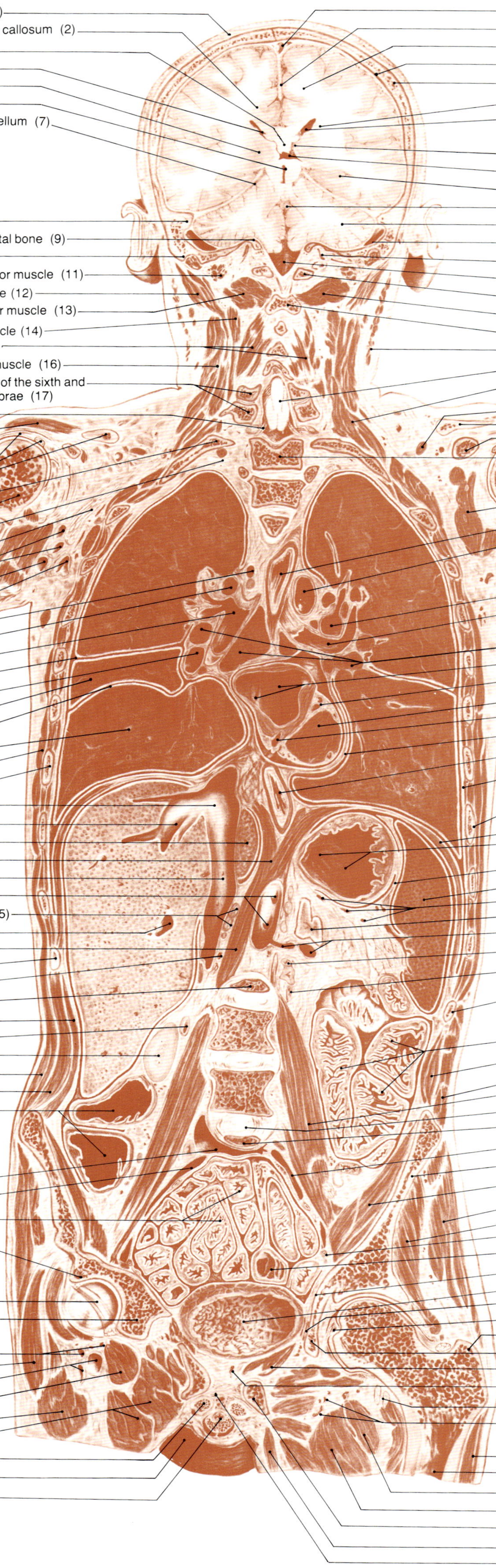

1 Galea aponeurotica
2 Radiatio corporis callosi
3 Corpus callosum
4 Fornix
5 Thalamus
6 Aquaeductus cerebri
7 Tentorium cerebelli
8 Pars petrosa pyramidis
9 Pars basalis ossis occipitalis
10 Processus mastoideus
11 M. obliquus capitis superior
12 M. splenius capitis
13 M. obliquus capitis inferior
13.1 Cornu posterius ventriculi lateralis
14 M. levator scapulae
15 M. multifidus
16 M. sternocleidomastoideus
17 Processus transversi vertebrarum thoracicarum VI et VII
18 Ganglion spinale, Radix ventralis
19 M. deltoideus
20 Capsula articularis, Tendo capitis longi m. bicipitis brachii
21 Clavicula
22 Costa I
23 Caput humeri
24 N. intercostalis I
25 Plexus brachialis
26 A. et V. brachialis
27 A. subscapularis
28 V. subscapularis
29 Nodi lymphatici mediastinales
30 Truncus pulmonalis
31 Bronchus principalis dexter
32 Cavum pleurae
33 V. pulmonalis
34 Lobus medius pulmonis
35 Fissura obliqua
36 Lobus inferior pulmonis
37 M. serratus anterior
38 Costa VII
39 V. hepatica
40 V. hepatica dextra
41 Lobus hepatis sinister
42 Diaphragma(Pars lumbalis)
43 V. cava inferior
44 Aorta abdominalis
45 Ganglion trunci sympathici lumbalis
46 R. v. portae
47 Crus mediale diaphragmatis
48 Costa X
49 V. phrenica inferior dextra
50 Vertebra lumbalis II
51 M. transversus abdominis
52 A. renalis dextra
53 Ren dexter
54 M. obliquus externus abdominis
55 M. obliquus internus abdominis
56 Colon ascendens
57 V. iliaca communis
58 A. iliaca communis
59 Jejunum
60 Acetabulum
60.1 Corpus uteri
60.2 Caput femoris
61 Lig. iliofemorale
62 Os pubis
63 Rr. A. et V. circumflexae femoris
64 M. rectus femoris
65 A. et V. femoralis
66 M. pectineus
67 M. vastus lateralis
68 Mm. adductores
69 Corpus cavernosum penis
70 Scrotum
71 Urethra
72 Sinus sagittalis superior
73 Falx cerebri
74 Praecuneus
75 Dura mater encephali
76 Os parietale
77 Cauda nuclei caudati
78 Ventriculus lateralis
79 Plexus chorioideus
80 Recessus pinealis
81 Hippocampus
82 Ventriculus IV
83 Cerebellum
83.1 Medulla
84 Sinus transversus
85 V. emissaria condylaris
86 Cisterna cerebellomedullaris
87 Atlas (Massa lateralis)
88 Massa lateralis atlantis
89 Processus spinosus axis
90 Funiculus posterior medullae spinalis
91 M. scalenus anterior
92 Nodi lymphatici
93 Processus coracoideus
94 Vertebra thoracica I
95 M. coracobrachialis
96 Oesophagus
97 Aorta thoracica
98 A. et V. subscapularis
99 Bronchus principalis sinister
100 M. triceps brachii
101 Nodi lymphatici bronchopulmonales
102 Atrium dextrum, Valvula v. cavae
103 A. et V. coronaria
104 Ventriculus sinister cordis
105 Sinus coronarius
106 Pericardium
107 Pleura
108 Costa VIII
109 Diaphragma, Pars costalis
110 Ventriculus et Cardia
111 Bursa omentalis
112 Lien
113 Aa. et Vv. gastricae breves
114 Glandula suprarenalis
115 A. et V. renalis
116 Extremitas superior renis sinistri
117 Ureter sinister
117.1 Colon descendens
118 Costa XI
119 M. psoas major
120 Discus intervertebralis
121 Vertebra lumbalis V
122 A. iliaca communis sinistra
123 Os ilium
123.1 Colon sigmoideum
124 M. iliacus
125 M. glutaeus maximus
126 M. glutaeus minimus
127 Ureter sinister
128 Ileum
129 N. obturatorius
130 Vesica urinaria
130.1 Prostata
131 A. et V. obturatoria
132 Lig. capitis femoris
133 Trochanter major
134 M. obturatorius internus
134.1 M. obturatorius externus
135 Urethra
136 Tendo musculi iliopsoae
137 Rr. A. et V. circumflexae femoris medialesis
138 Cavum medullare femoris
139 M. gracilis
140 Lig. transversum perinei

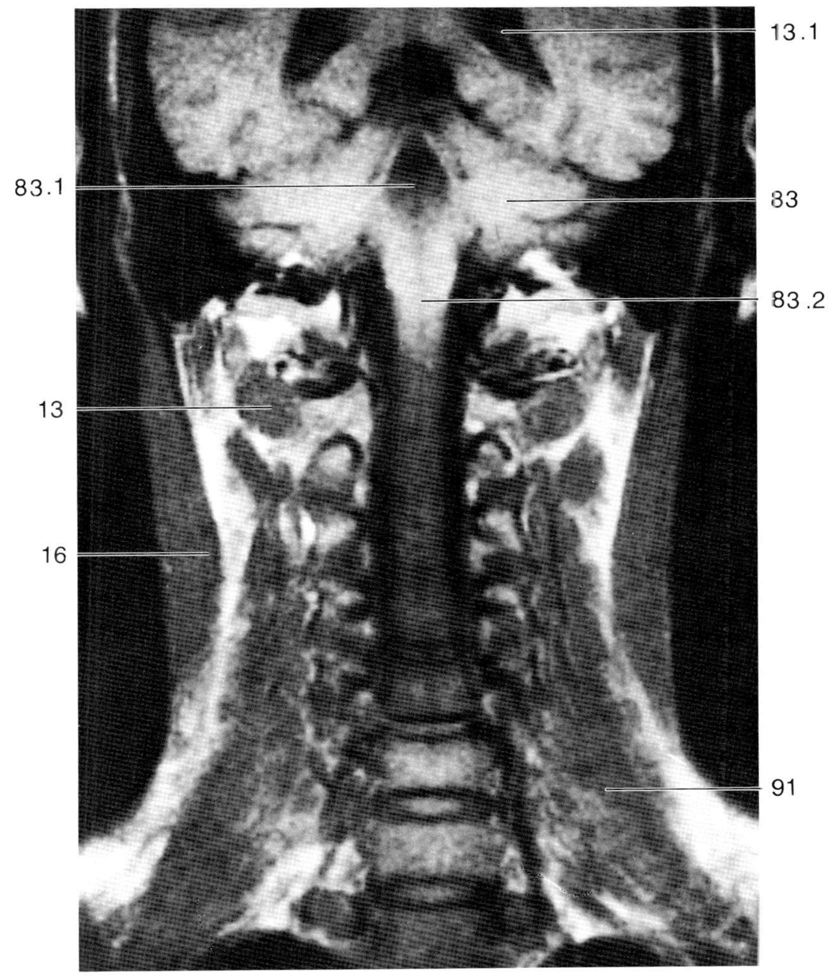

MRI, SE 600/30

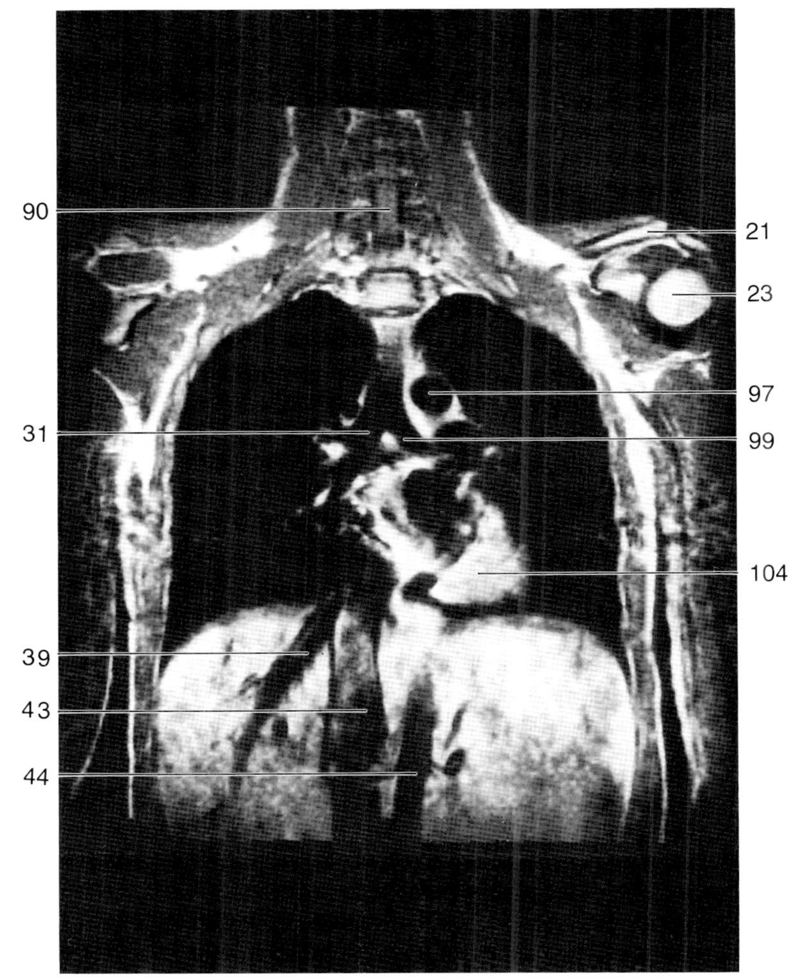

MRI, SE, ECG-triggered, $T_E = 30$

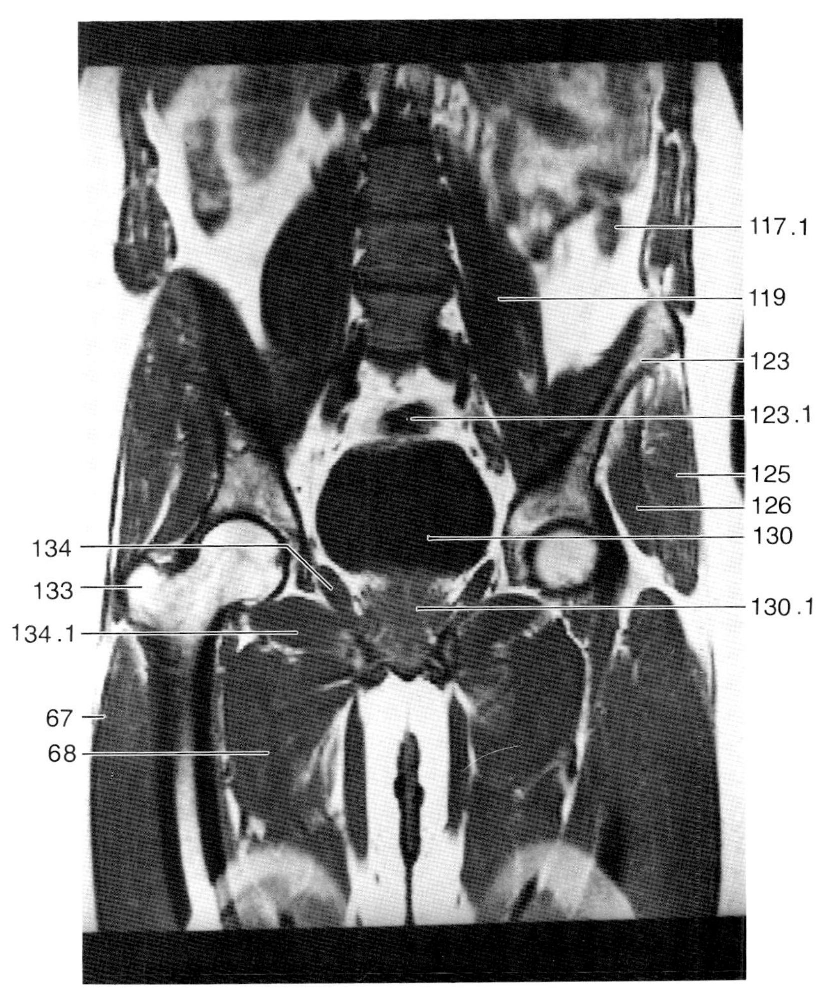

MRI, SE 800/22

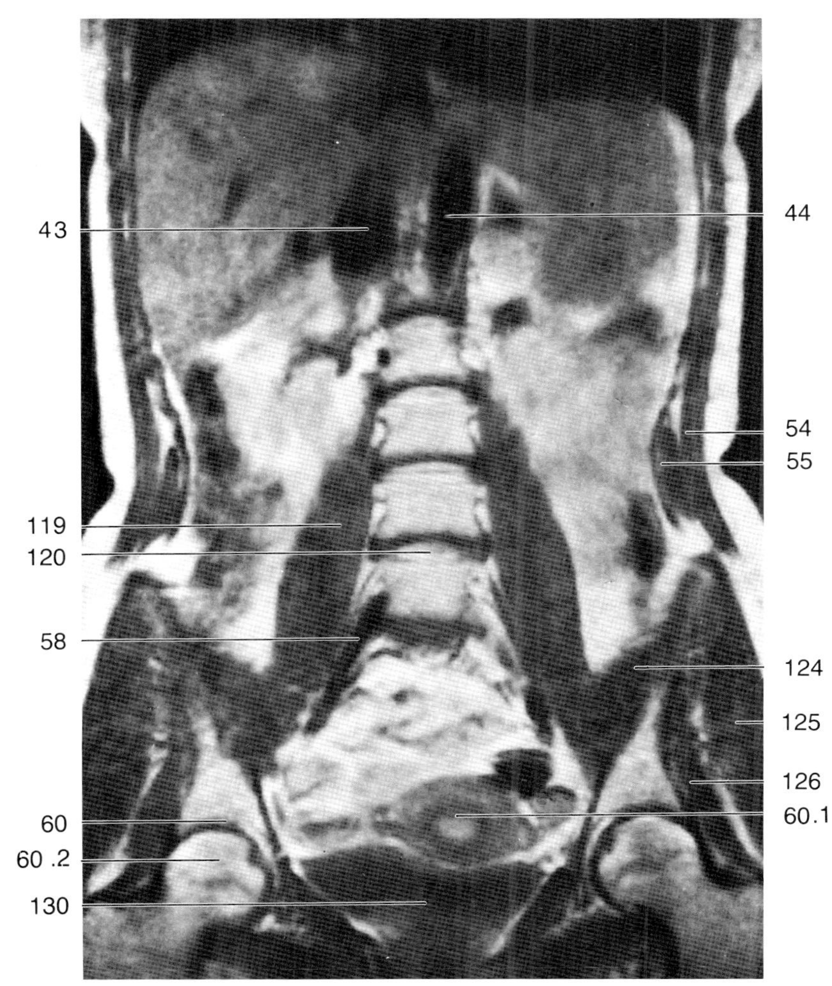

MRI, SE 600/30

13 Obliquus capitis inferior muscle
13.1 Posterior horn of the lateral ventricle
16 Sternocleidomastoid muscle
21 Clavicle
23 Head of the humerus
31 Right mainstem bronchus
39 Hepatic vein
43 Inferior vena cava
44 Abdominal aorta
54 Obliquus externus abdominis muscle
55 Obliquus internus abdominis muscle
58 Common iliac artery
60 Acetabulum
60.1 Corpus uteri
60.2 Femoral head
67 Vastus lateralis muscle
68 Adductor muscles
83 Cerebellum
83.1 Rhomboid fossa
83.2 Medulla
90 Posterior funiculus of the spinal cord
91 Scalenus anterior muscle
97 Thoracic aorta
99 Left mainstem bronchus
104 Left ventricle of the heart
117.1 Descending colon
119 Psoas major muscle
120 Intervertebral disc
123 Ilium
123.1 Sigmoid colon
124 Iliacus muscle
125 Gluteus maximus muscle
126 Gluteus minimus muscle
130 Urinary bladder
130.1 Prostate
133 Greater trochanter
134 Internal obturator muscle
134.1 External obturator muscle

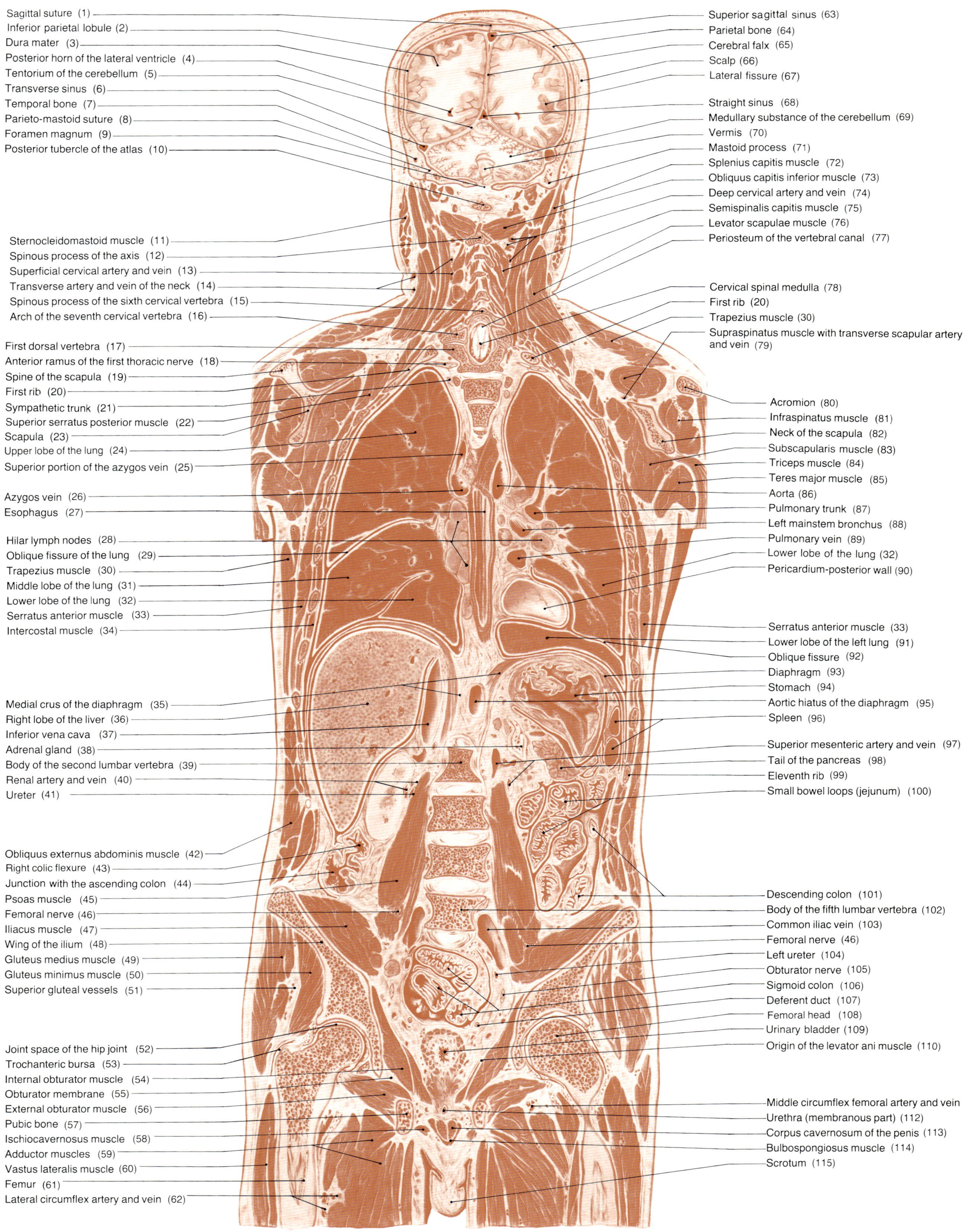

1 Sutura sagittalis
2 Lobulus parietalis inferior
3 Dura mater
4 Cornu posterius ventriculi lateralis
5 Tentorium cerebelli
6 Sinus transversus
7 Os temporale
8 Sutura parietomastoidea
9 Foramen magnum
10 Tuberculum posterius atlantis
11 M. sternocleidomastoideus
12 Processus spinosus
13 A. et V. cervicalis superficialis
14 A. et V. transversa colli
15 Processus spinosus vertebrae cervicis VI
16 Arcus vertebrae cervicis VII
17 Vertebra thoracica I
18 R. anterior n. thor. I
19 Spina scapulae
20 Costa I
21 Truncus sympathicus
22 M. serratus posterior superior
23 Scapula
23.1 Aorta descendens
24 Lobus superior pulmonis
25 Pars superior v. azygos
26 V. azygos
27 Oesophagus
28 Nodi lymphatici bronchopulmonales
29 Fissura obliqua pulmonis
30 M. trapezius
31 Lobus medius pulmonis
32 Lobus inferior pulmonis
33 M. serratus anterior
34 M. intercostalis
35 Crus mediale diaphragmatis
36 Lobus dexter hepatis
37 V. cava inferior
38 Glandula suprarenalis
39 Corpus vertebrae lumbalis II
40 A. et V. renalis
41 Ureter
42 M. obliquus externus abdominis
43 Flexura coli dextra
44 Colon ascendens
45 M. psoas
45.1 Ren dexter
46 N. femoralis
47 M. iliacus
48 Ala ossis ilii
49 M. glutaeus medius
50 M. glutaeus minimus
51 Vasa glutaea superiora
52 Cavum articulare coxae
53 Bursa trochanterica
54 M. obturatorius internus
55 Membrana obturatoria
56 M. obturatorius externus
57 Os pubis
58 M. ischiocavernosus
59 Mm. adductores
60 M. vastus lateralis
61 Femur
62 A. et V. circumflexa lateralis
63 Sinus sagittalis superior
64 Os parietale
65 Falx cerebri
66 Galea
67 Fissura lateralis
68 Sinus rectus
69 Corpus medullare cerebelli
70 Vermis
71 Processus mastoideus
72 M. splenius capitis
73 M. obliquus capitis inferior
74 A. et V. cervicalis profunda
75 M. semispinalis capitis
76 M. levator scapulae
77 Periostium canalis vertebralis
78 Medulla spinalis cervicis
79 M. supraspinatus, A. et V. transversa scapulae
80 Acromion
81 M. infraspinatus
82 Collum scapulae
83 M. suprascapularis
84 M. triceps brachii
85 M. teres major
86 Aorta, Aa. et Vv. intercostales
87 Truncus pulmonalis
88 Bronchus principalis sinister
89 V. pulmonalis
90 Pericardium, Pars posterior
91 Lobus inferior pulmonis sinistri
92 Fissura obliqua
93 Diaphragma
94 Ventriculus (Gaster)
95 Aorta, Hiatus aorticus
96 Lien
97 A. et V. mesenterica superior
98 Pancreas – Cauda
99 Costa XI
100 Jejunum
101 Colon descendens
102 Corpus vertebrae lumbalis V
103 V. iliaca communis
104 Ureter sinister
105 N. obturatorius
106 Colon sigmoideum
107 Ductus deferens
108 Caput femoris
109 Vesica urinaria
110 Origo m. levatoris ani
110.1 Prostata
111 A. et V. circumflexa femoris medialis
112 Urethra (Pars membranacea)
113 Corpus cavernosum penis
114 M. bulbospongiosus
115 Scrotum

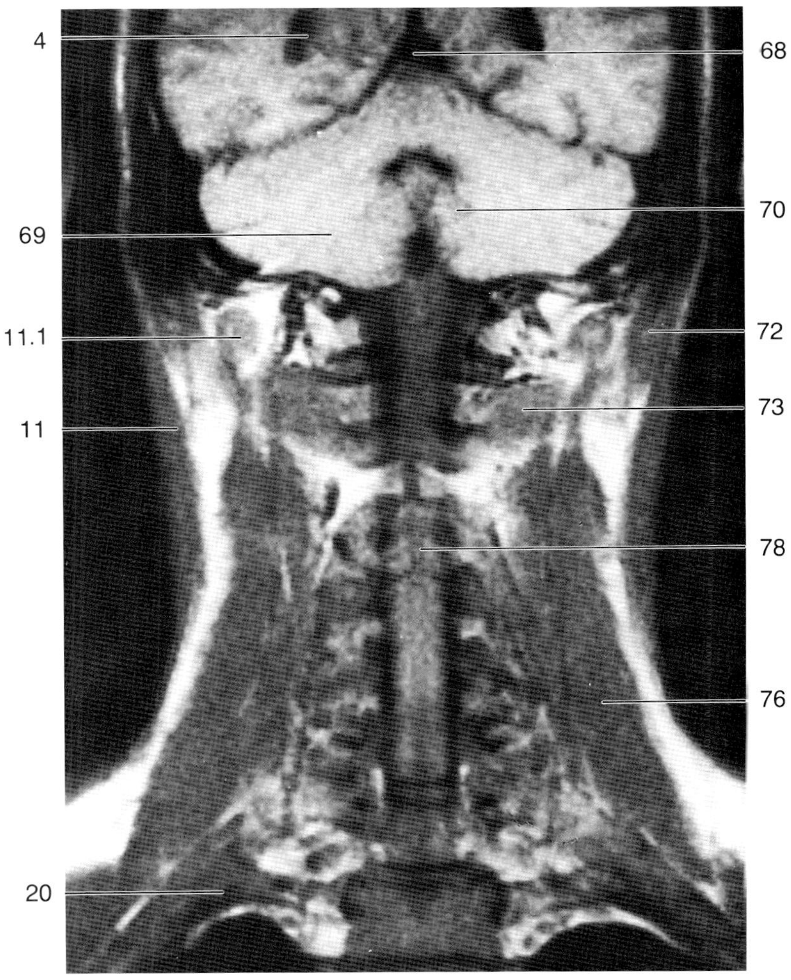

MRI, SE 600/30

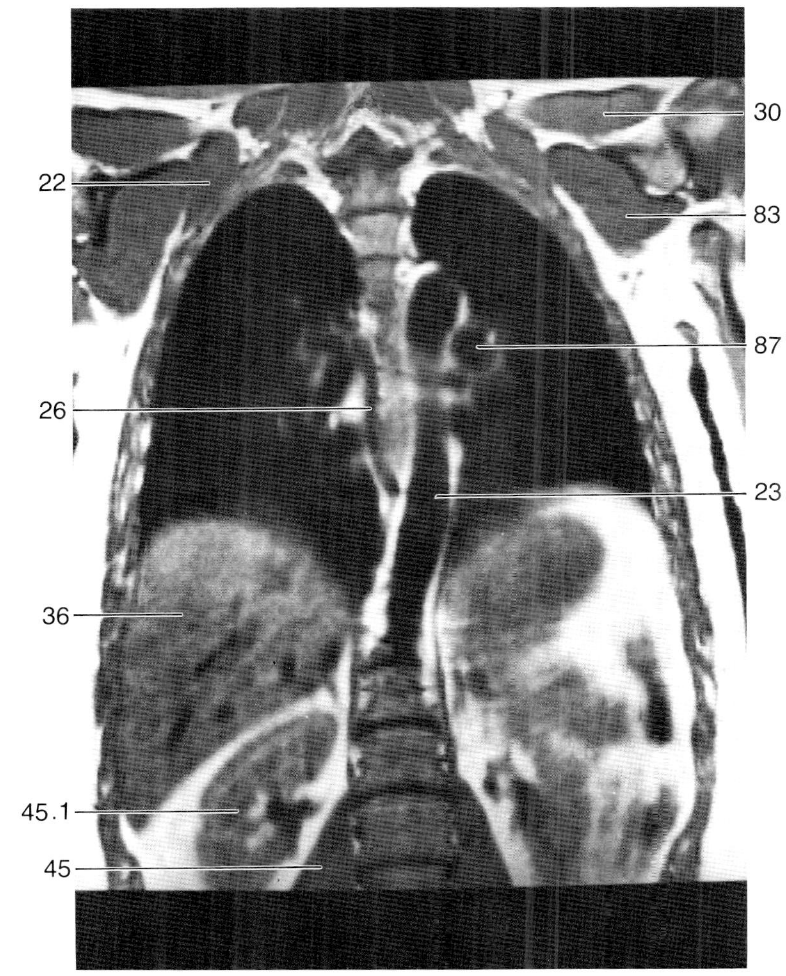

MRI, SE 1000/22

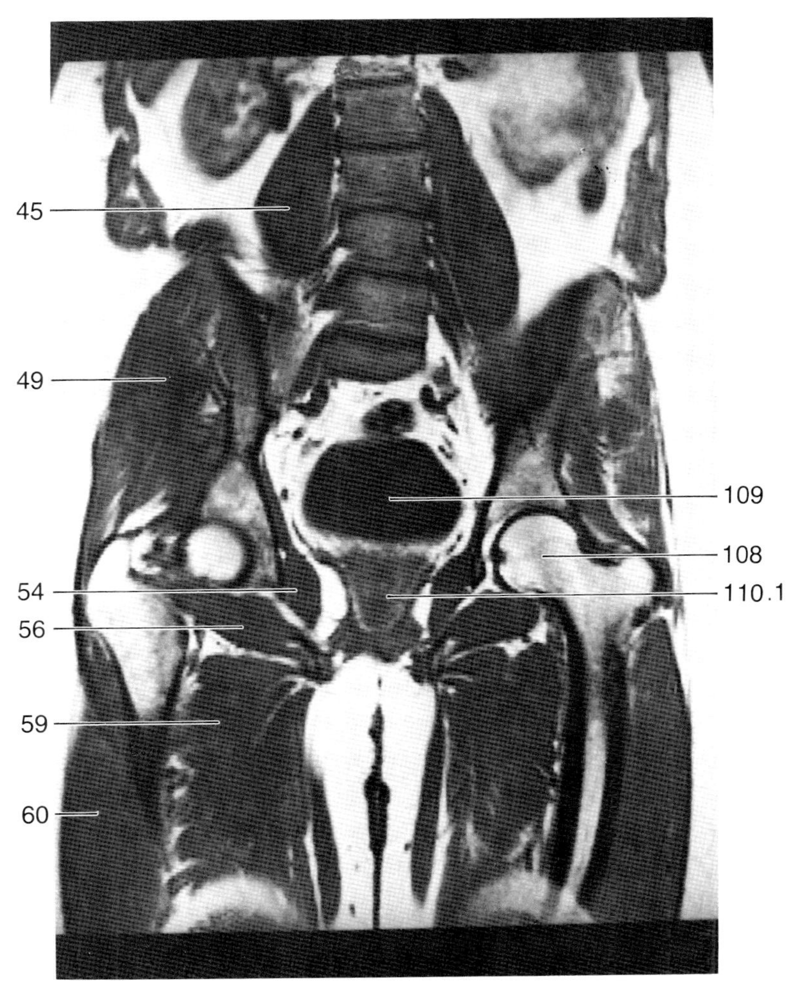

MRI, SE 800/22

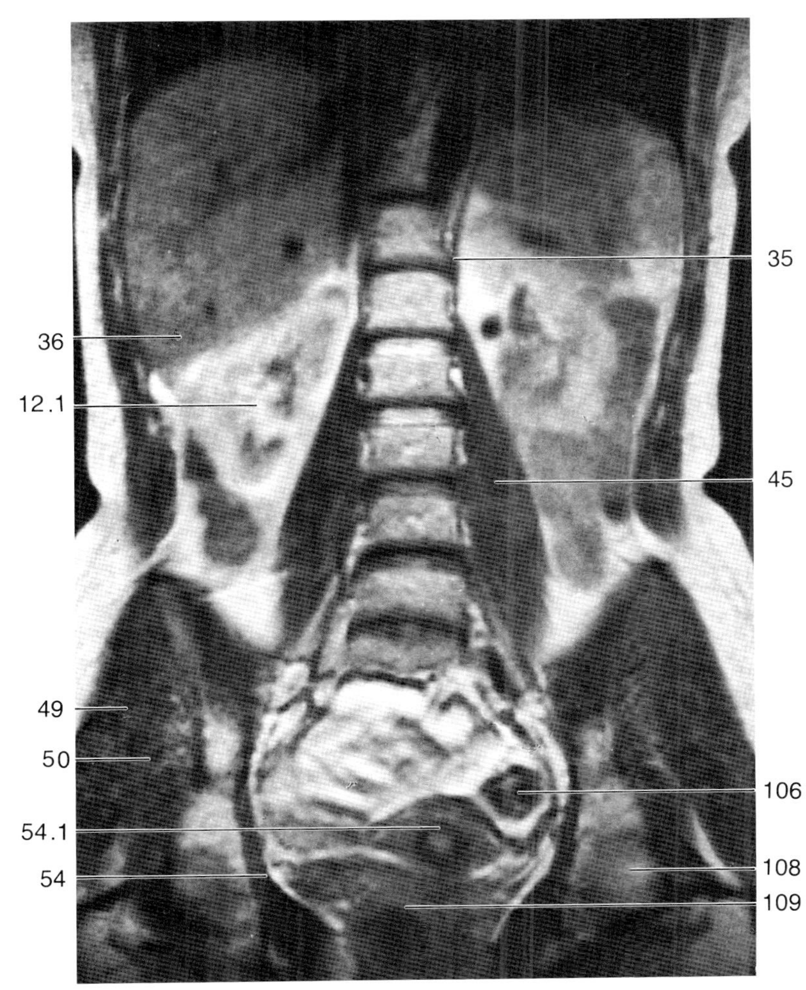

MRI, SE 600/30

4 Posterior horn of the lateral ventricle
11 Sternocleidomastoid muscle
11.1 Semispinalis capitis muscle
12.1 Right kidney
20 First rib
22 Superior serratus posterior muscle
23.1 Descending aorta
26 Azygos vein
30 Trapezius muscle
35 Medial crus of the diaphragm
36 Right lobe of the liver
45 Psoas muscle
45.1 Right kidney
49 Gluteus medius muscle
50 Gluteus minimus muscle
54 Internal obturator muscle
54.1 Corpus uteri
56 External obturator muscle
59 Adductor muscles
60 Vastus lateralis muscle
68 Straight sinus
69 Medullary substance of the cerebellum
70 Vermis
72 Splenius capitis muscle
73 Obliquus capitis inferior muscle
76 Sternocleidomastoid muscle
78 Cervical spinal medulla
83 Suprascapularis muscle
87 Pulmonary trunk
106 Sigmoid colon
108 Head of the femur
109 Urinary bladder
110.1 Prostate

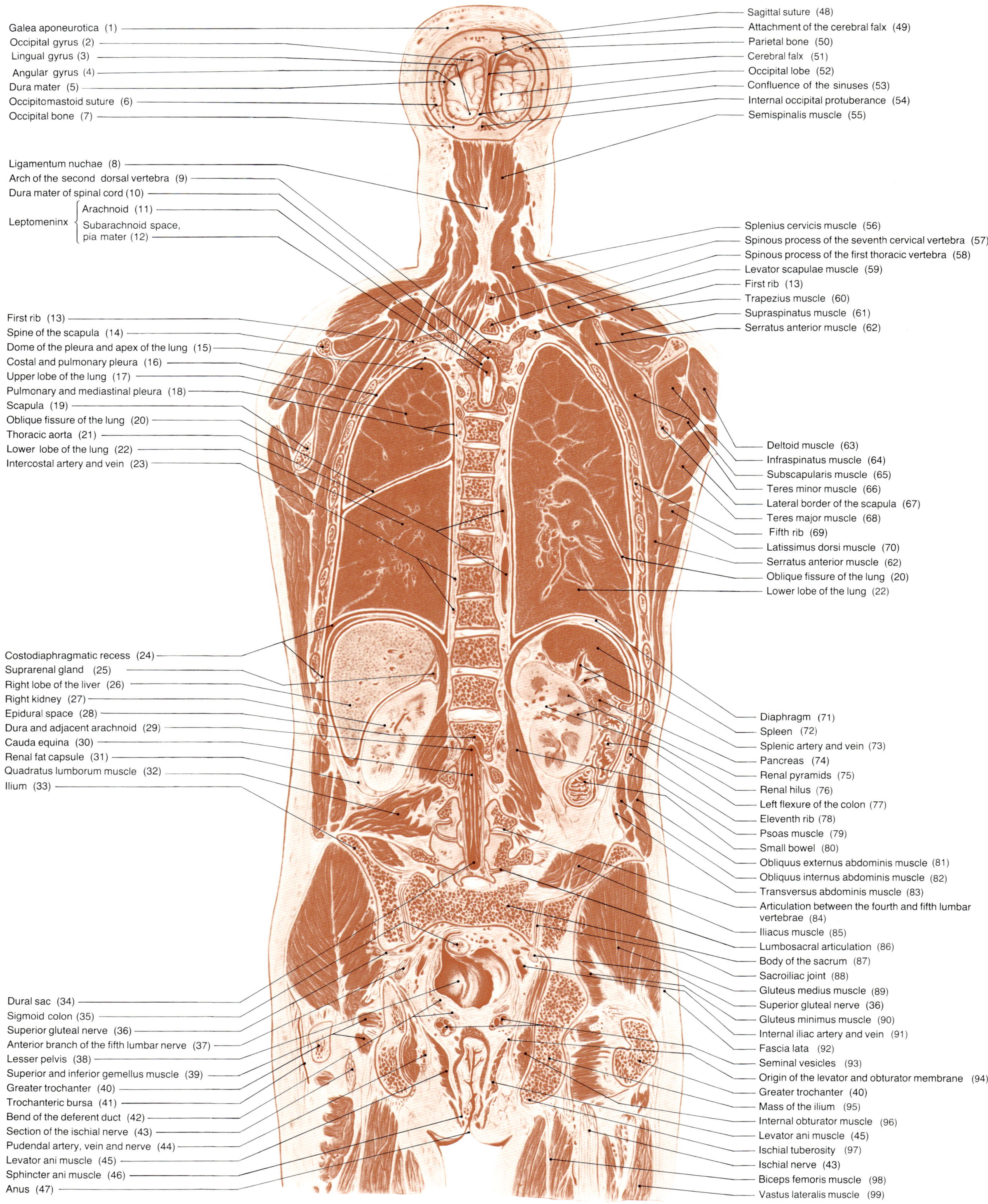

1 Galea aponeurotica
2 Gyrus occipitalis
3 Gyrus lingualis
4 Gyrus angularis
5 Dura mater
6 Sutura occipitomastoidea
7 Os occipitale
8 Lig. nuchae
9 Arcus vertebrae thoracalis
10 Dura mater spinalis
11 Arachnoidea
12 Spatium subarachnoidale et Pia mater
13 Costa I
14 Spina scapulae
15 Apex pulmonis
16 Pleura costalis et pulmonalis
17 Lobus superior pulmonis
18 Pleura pulmonalis et mediastinalis
19 Scapula
20 Fissura obliqua pulmonis
21 Aorta thoracica
22 Lobus inferior pulmonis
23 A. et V. intercostalis
24 Recessus costodiaphragmaticus
25 Glandula suprarenalis
26 Lobus dexter hepatis
27 Ren dexter
28 Spatium epidurale
29 Dura mater et Arachnoidea
30 Cauda equina
31 Capsula adiposa renis
32 M. quadratus lumborum
33 Os ilium
34 Spatium subdurale
35 Colon sigmoideum
36 N. glutaeus superior
37 R. anterior n. lumb. V
38 Pelvis minor
39 Mm. gemellus superior et inferior
40 Trochanter major
41 Bursa trochanterica
42 Ductus deferens
43 N. ischiadicus
44 A. et V. pudenda et N. pudendus
45 M. levator ani
46 M. sphincter ani
47 Anus
48 Sutura sagittalis
49 Origo falcis cerebri
50 Os parietale
51 Falx cerebri
52 Lobus occipitalis
53 Confluens sinuum
54 Protuberantia occipitalis interna
55 M. semispinalis
56 M. splenius cervicis
57 Processus spinosus vertebrae cervicalis VII
58 Processus spinosus vertebrae thoracalis I
59 M. levator scapulae
60 M. trapezius
61 M. supraspinatus
62 M. serratus anterior
63 M. deltoideus
64 M. infraspinatus
65 M. subscapularis
66 M. teres minor
67 Margo lateralis scapulae
68 M. teres major
69 Costa V
70 M. latissimus dorsi
71 Diaphragma
72 Lien
73 A. et V. lienalis
74 Pancreas
75 Pyramides renis
76 Hilus renalis
77 Flexura coli sinistra
78 Costa XI
79 M. psoas
80 Jejunum
81 M. obliquus externus abdominis
82 M. obliquus internus abdominis
83 M. transversus abdominis
84 Articulatio vertebrarum lumbalium IV et V
85 M. iliacus
86 Articulatio lumbosacralis
87 Corpus ossis sacri
88 Articulatio sacroiliaca
89 M. glutaeus medius
90 M. glutaeus minimus
91 A. et V. iliaca interna
92 Fascia lata
93 Vesiculae seminales
94 Origo m. levatoris et Membrana obturatoria
95 Massa ossis ilii
96 M. obturator internus
97 Tuber ischiadicum
98 M. biceps femoris
99 M. vastus lateralis

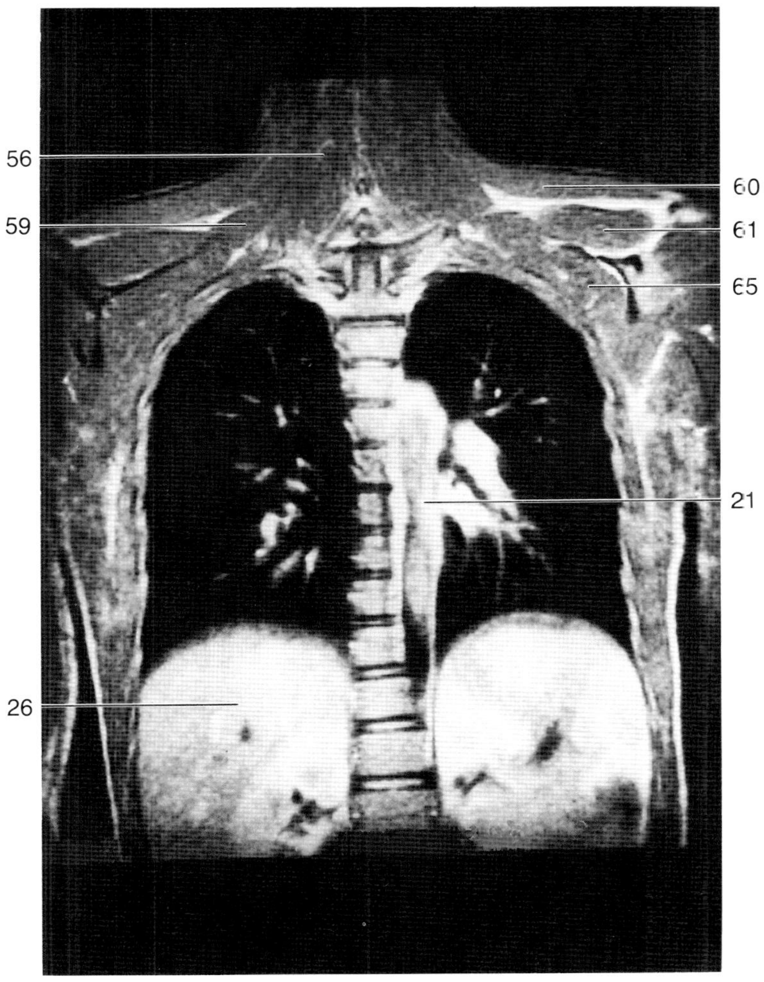

MRI, SE, ECG-triggered, $T_E = 30$

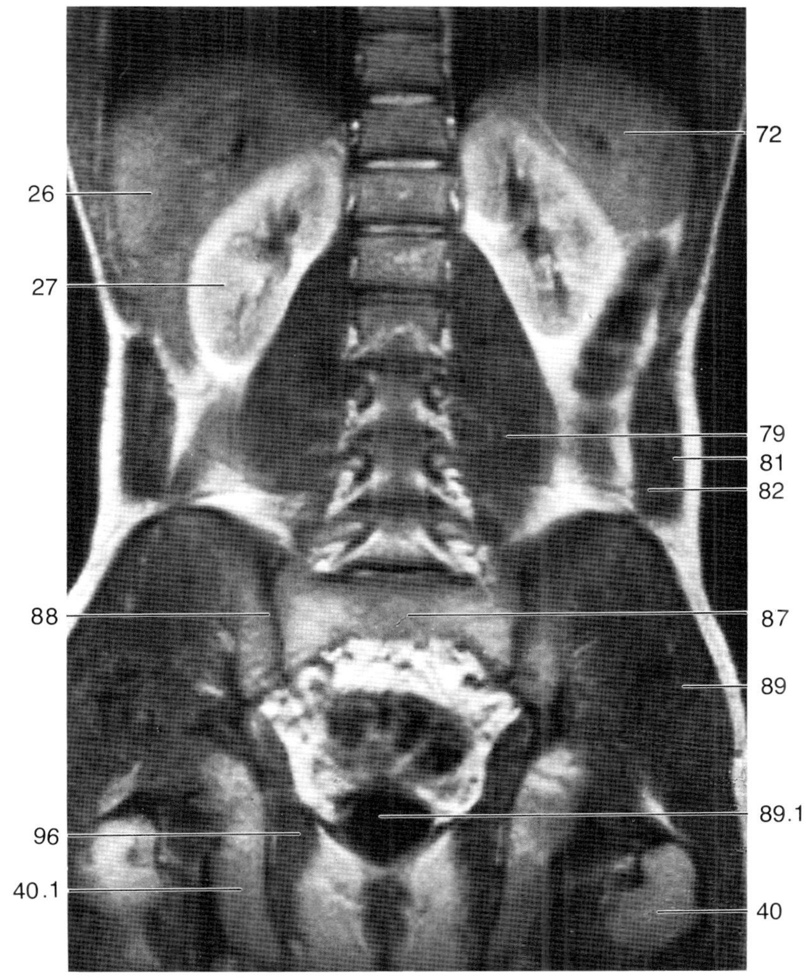

MRI, SE 600/30

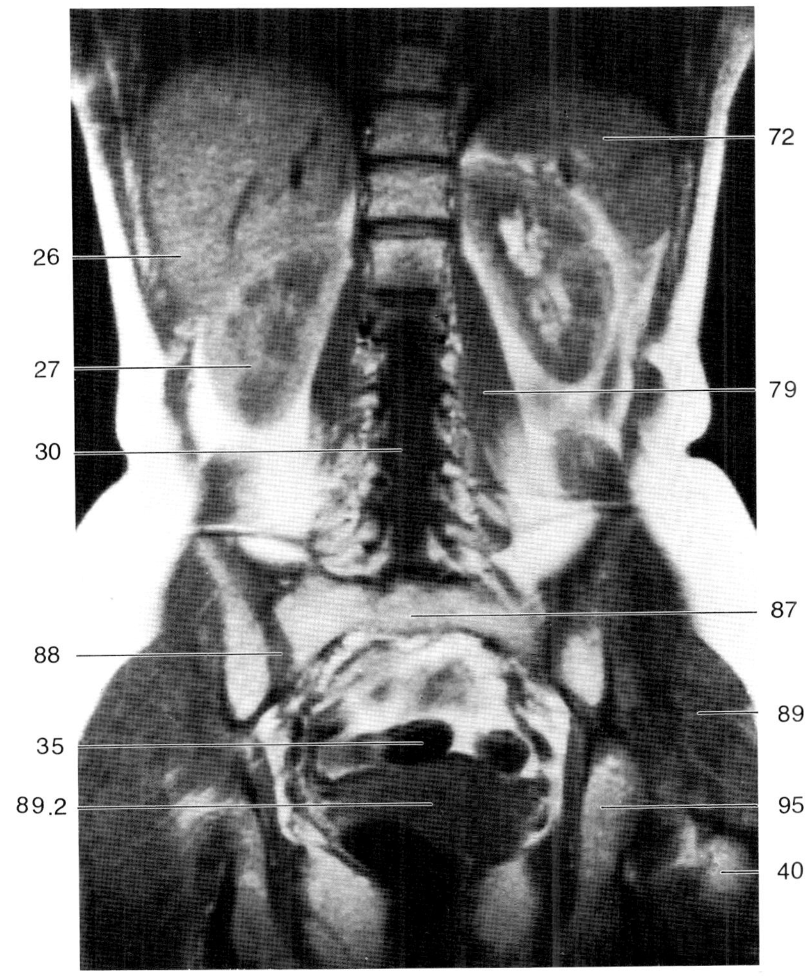

MRI, SE 600/30

21 Thoracic Aorta
26 Right lobe of the liver
27 Right kidney
30 Cauda equina
35 Rectum
40 Greater trochanter
40.1 Ischial bone
56 Splenius cervicis muscle
59 Levator scapulae muscle
60 Trapezius muscle
61 Supraspinatus muscle
65 Subscapularis muscle
72 Spleen
79 Psoas muscle
81 Obliquus externus abdominis muscle
82 Obliquus internus abdominis muscle
87 Body of the sacrum
88 Sacroiliac joint
89 Gluteus medius muscle
89.1 Rectum
89.2 Corpus uteri
95 Mass of the ilium
96 Internal obturator muscle

Sagittal Sections of the Whole Body

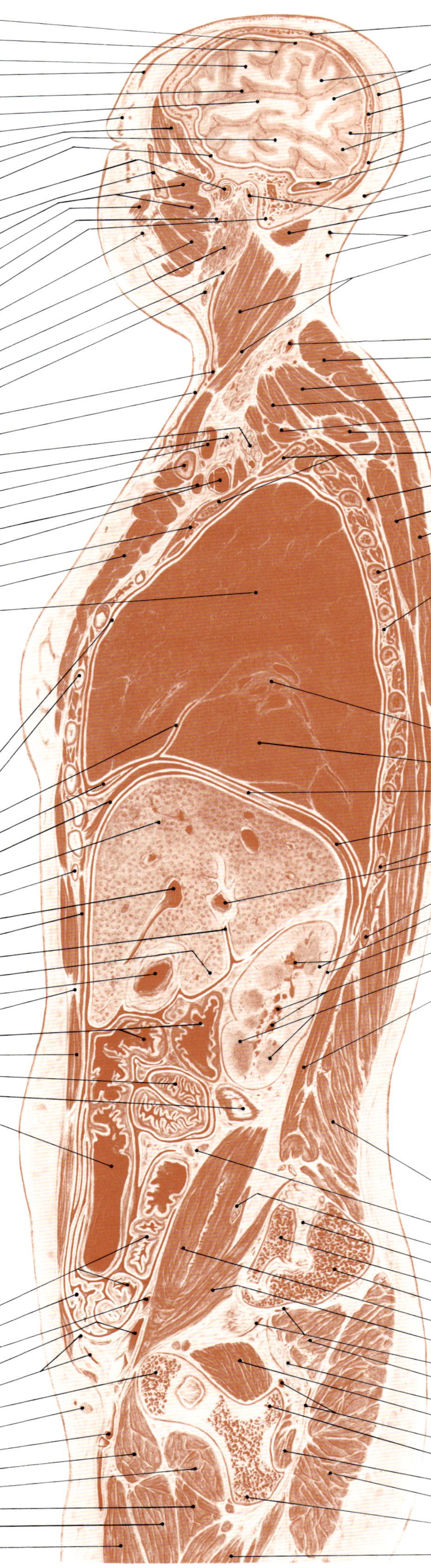

1 Gyrus postcentralis
2 Sulcus centralis
3 Gyrus praecentralis
4 Venter frontalis m. occipitalis
5 Fissura lateralis
6 Gyrus temporalis superior
7 M. orbicularis oculi
8 M. temporalis
9 Gyrus temporalis medius
10 Os temporale
10.1 Lobus temporalis
10.2 Cerebellum
11 Caput mandibulae
12 Maxilla
13 M. pterygoideus lateralis
14 M. levator anguli oris
15 A. maxillaris
16 Processus mastoideus
17 Ductus parotideus
18 M. pterygoideus medialis
19 Glandula parotis
20 V. retromandibularis
21 Nodus lymphaticus submandibularis
22 V. jugularis interna
23 Platysma
24 Plexus brachialis
25 Tendo m. omohyoidei
26 V. jugularis
27 Clavicula
28 M. subclavius
29 V. subclavia
30 M. pectoralis minor
31 M. pectoralis major
32 Lobus superior pulmonis
33 Cavum pleurae
34 Costa V
35 Fissura interlobaris
36 Lobus medius pulmonis dextri
37 Diaphragma, Pars costalis
38 Lobus hepatis dexter
39 Costa X
40 R. venae hepaticae
41 M. transversus abdominis
42 Porta hepatis
43 Lobus quadratus hepatis
44 Vesica fellea
45 Intersectiones tendineae
46 Flexura coli dextra
47 M. rectus abdominis
48 Jejunum
49 M. psoas minor
50 Colon ascendens
51 Ileum
52 Omentum majus
53 A. femoralis
54 V. femoralis
55 A. et V. epigastrica inferior
56 Caput femoris
57 V. pudenda externa
58 Confluens v. saphenae magnae et v. femoralis
59 M. iliopsoas
60 M. obturatorius externus
61 M. adductor brevis
62 M. pectineus
63 M. adductor longus
64 Os parietale
65 Lobus parietalis
66 Galea aponeurotica
67 Os occipitale
68 Gyri occipitales laterales
69 M. occipitalis
70 Sinus transversus
71 V. occipitalis
72 Meatus acusticus externus
73 M. splenius capitis
74 Vv. cervicales subcutaneae
75 M. sternocleidomastoideus
76 V. cervicalis profunda
77 M. trapezius
78 M. levator scapulae
79 M. scalenus posterior
80 M. scalenus medius
81 M. serratus anterior
82 Costa I
83 M. serratus posterior superior
84 M. rhomboideus major
85 A. et V. et N. intercostalis
86 Hilus pulmonis
87 Lobus inferior pulmonis dextri
88 Centrum tendineum
89 Crus laterale diaphragmatis
90 Costa XI
91 V. portae
92 Costa XII
93 Papilla renalis
94 Capsula renis
95 Calices renales
96 Pyramis renalis
97 M. quadratus lumborum
98 M. iliocostalis lumborum
99 Nodi lymphatici iliaci
100 N. femoralis
101 Ligg. sacroiliaca interossea
102 Os ilium
103 Os sacrum
104 M. psoas major
105 M. iliacus
106 V. glutaea superior
107 M. piriformis
108 Plexus sacralis
109 M. glutaeus medius
110 A. et V. pudenda interna
111 Trochanter major
112 M. quadratus femoris
113 M. glutaeus maximus
114 Femur
115 M. vastus intermedius

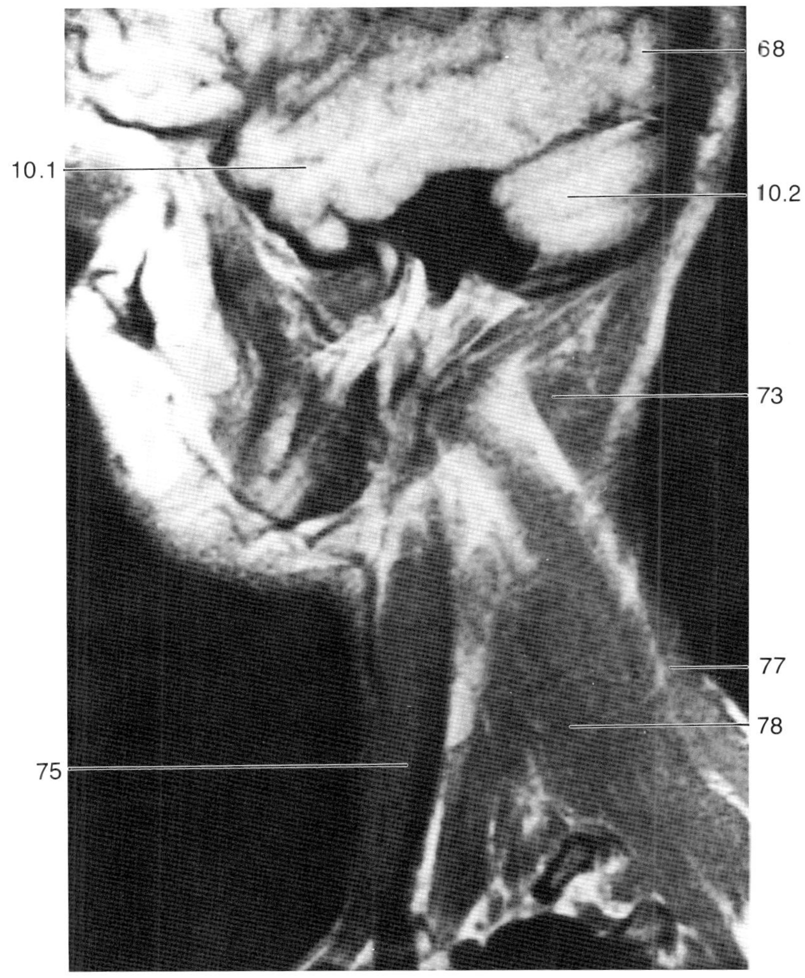

MRI, SE 600/30

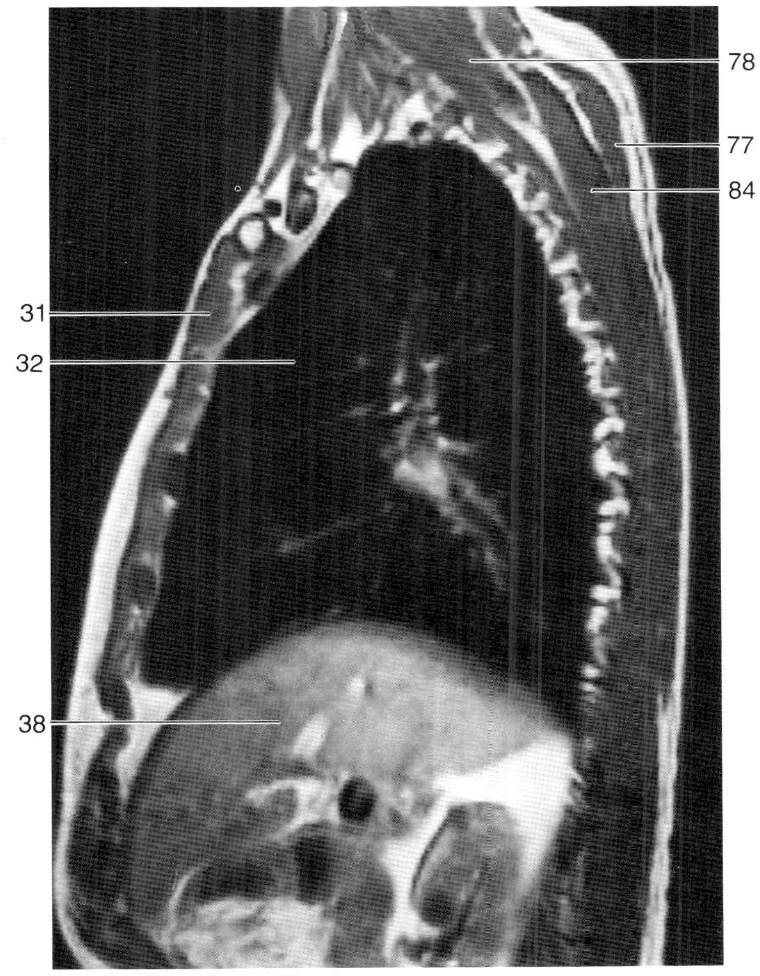

MRI, SE 970/22

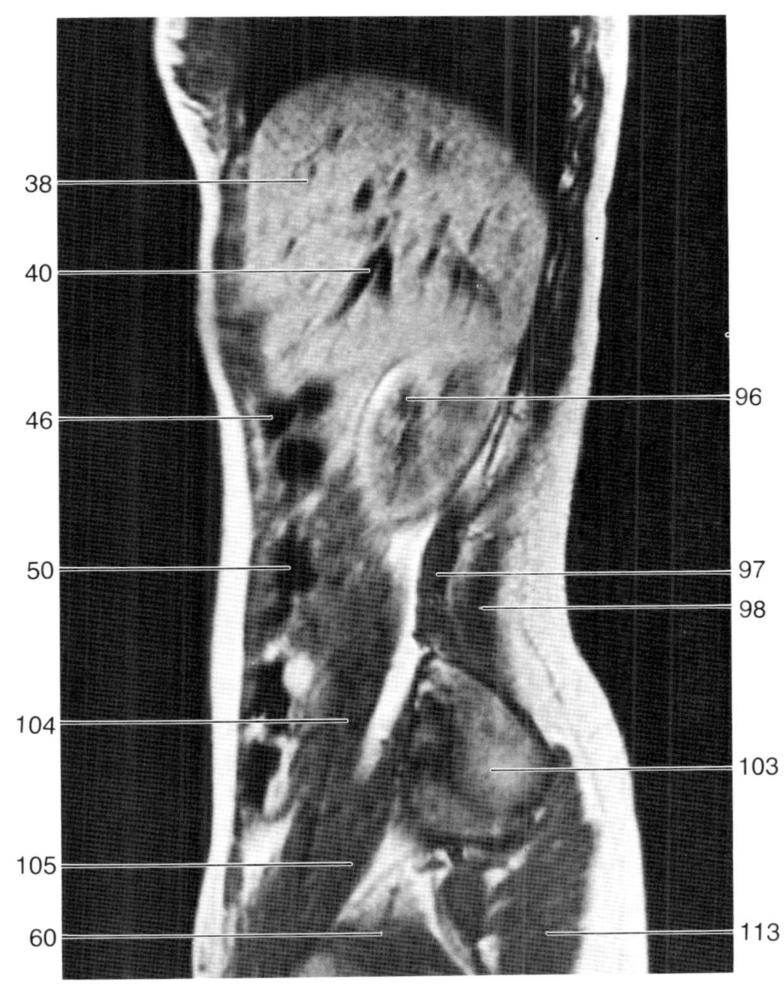

MRI, SE, ECG-triggered, $T_E = 30$

10.1 Temporal lobe
10.2 Cerebellum
31 Pectoralis major muscle
32 Upper lobe of the lung
38 Right lobe of the liver
40 Bronchi of the lung
46 Right colic flexure
50 Ascending colon
60 External obturator muscle
68 Occipital gyri
73 Splenius capitis muscle
75 Sternocleidomastoid muscle
77 Trapezius muscle
78 Levator scapulae muscle
84 Rhomboideus major muscle
96 Renal pyramid
97 Quadratus lumborum muscle
98 Iliocostalis lumborum muscle
103 Sacrum
105 Iliacus muscle
113 Gluteus maximus muscle

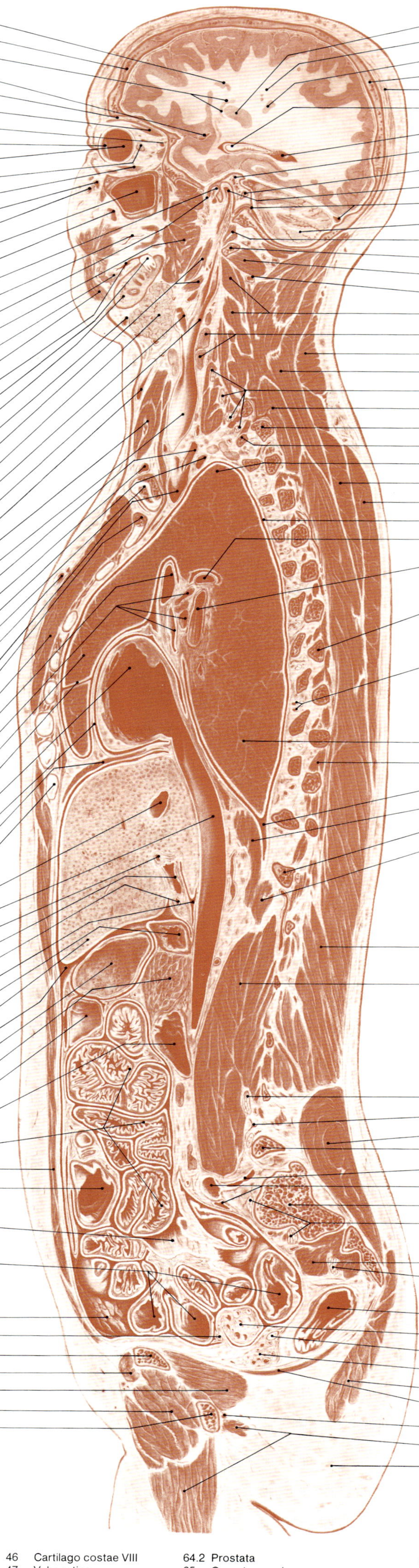

1 Corpus nuclei caudati
2 Os frontale
3 Claustrum
4 A. et V. cerebri media
5 M. levator palpebrae superioris
6 M. rectus superior
7 V. ophthalmica
8 Lens
9 Corpus vitreum
10 N. opticus
11 M. rectus inferior
12 V. angularis
13 V. labialis superior
14 Sinus maxillaris
15 V. facialis
16 A. meningea media
17 Cavum oris
18 N. mandibularis
19 Mm. pterygoideus lateralis et medialis
20 M. buccinator
21 M. depressor anguli oris
22 Dens molaris
23 Mandibula
24 V. submentalis
25 Mm. digastricus et stylohyoideus
26 Glandula submandibularis
27 V. jugularis interna
28 V. jugularis externa
29 M. sternocleidomastoideus
30 Bulbus inferior v. jugularis
31 V. vertebralis
32 Arcus venosus juguli
33 A. subclavia
34 Clavicula
35 Rr. cutanei anteriores a. et v. intercostalis
36 V. subclavia, V. brachiocephalica
37 Costa I
38 M. pectoralis major
39 A. pulmonalis dextra
39.1 Oesophagus
40 Vv. pulmonales dextrae
41 Lobus superior pulmonis
42 Fissura horizontalis
43 Atrium dextrum
44 Pericardium
45 Diaphragma, Pars costalis
46 Cartilago costae VIII
47 V. hepatica
47.1 Aorta descendens
47.2 A. coeliaca
47.3 A. mesenterica superior
48 V. cava inferior
49 A. hepatica communis
50 V. portae
51 Ductus choledochus
52 Foramen epiploicum
53 Pars superior duodeni
54 Lobus quadratus hepatis
55 Cavum peritonaei
56 Pars pylorica ventriculi
57 Caput pancreatis
58 Colon transversum
59 Flexura duodeni inferior
60 Jejunum
61 M. rectus abdominis
62 Caecum
63 Mesenterium
64 Ileum
64.1 Vesicula seminalis
64.2 Prostata
65 Omentum majus
65.1 Symphysis pubica
65.2 Urethra masculina
66 Lig. latum uteri
67 Os pubis
68 M. pectineus
69 M. obturatorius internus
70 M. obturatorius externus
71 Os ischii
72 Putamen
73 Radiatio corporis callosi
74 Cauda nuclei caudati
75 Os parietale
76 Galea aponeurotica
77 Pes hippocampi
78 Plexus choroideus ventriculi lateralis
79 Labyrinthum osseum
80 Cavum tympani
81 A. carotis interna
82 Sinus sigmoideus
83 Cerebellum
84 M. rectus capitis lateralis
85 Processus transversus atlantis
86 M. obliquus capitis inferior
87 A. vertebralis
88 M. levator scapulae
89 Nodi lymphatici cervicales profundi inferiores
90 M. trapezius
91 M. splenius capitis
92 Nn. cervicales V, VI, VII, VIII
93 M. levator scapulae
94 Processus transversus vertebrae thoracicae I
95 Apex pulmonis
96 M. rhomboideus major
97 Cavum pleurae
98 Bronchus lobaris superior dexter
99 Bronchus lobaris inferior dexter
100 Processus transversus vertebrae thoracicae VII
101 A. et V. intercostalis
102 Lobus inferior pulmonis dextri
103 M. intertransversarius
104 Recessus costodiaphragmaticus
105 Crus laterale diaphragmatis
106 Costa X
107 M. quadratus lumborum
108 M. longissimus thoracis
109 M. psoas major
110 N. femoralis
111 V. iliolumbalis dextra (R. dorsalis)
112 M. iliocostalis lumborum
113 Processus costarius vertebrae lumbalis V
114 V. iliolumbalis dextra
115 A. et V. iliaca communis dextra
116 Os sacrum
117 R. ventralis n. lumbalis V et n. sacralis I
118 M. piriformis
119 R. ventralis nervorum sacralium II et III
120 Rectum
120.1 Vesica urinaria
121 Ovarium
122 Ureter
123 Plexus uterovaginalis
124 M. glutaeus maximus
125 Diaphragma pelvis
126 V. pudenda interna
127 M. adductor magnus
128 Fossa ischiorectalis

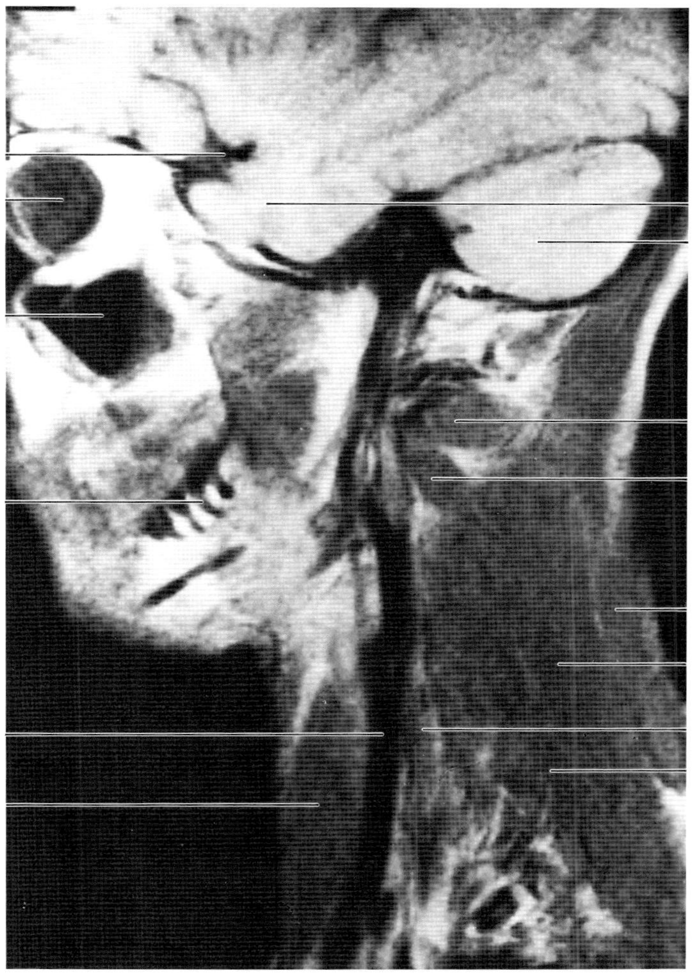

MRI, SE 600/30

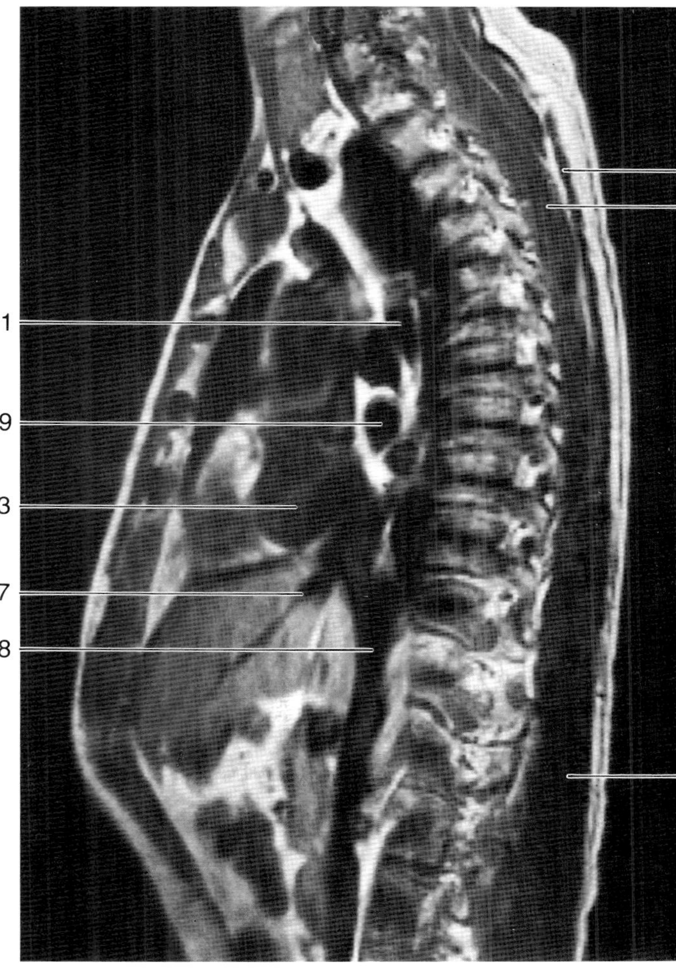

MRI, SE 970/22

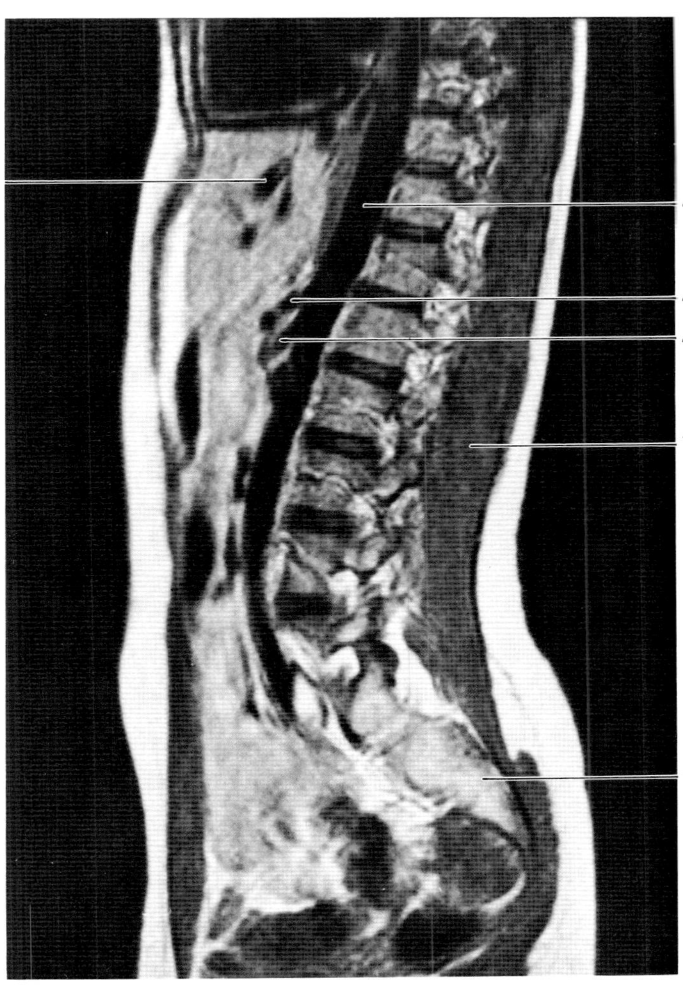

MRI, SE ECG-triggered, $T_E = 30$, ♀

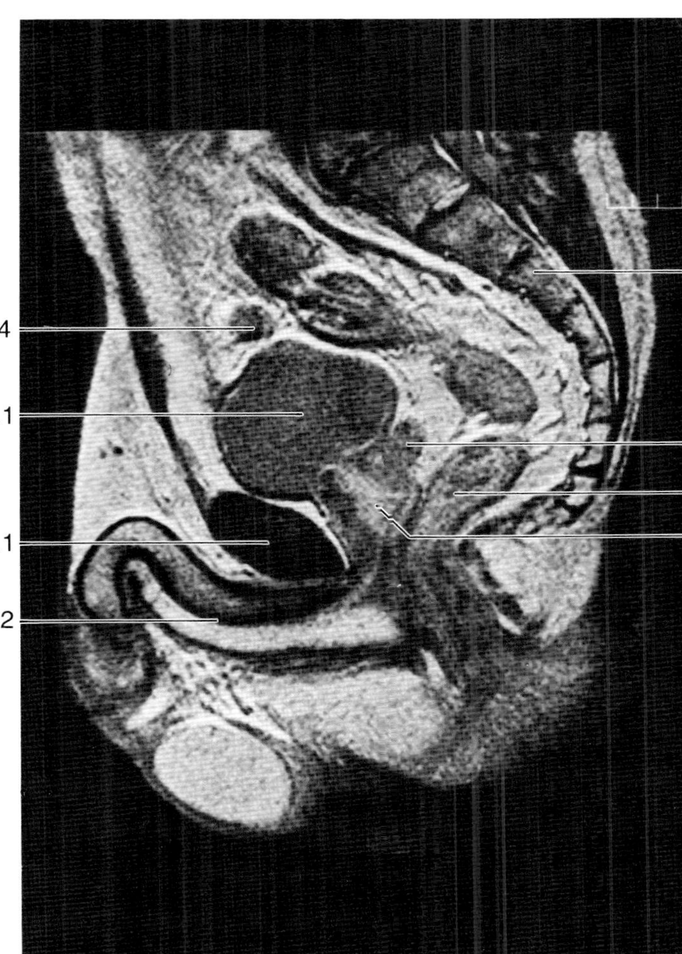

MRI, SE 1600/50, ♂

4 Middle cerebral artery and vein
9 Bulb of the right eye
14 Maxillary sinus
22 Molar tooth
27 Internal jugular vein
29 Sternocleidomastoid muscle
39 Right pulmonary artery
39.1 Esophagus
43 Right atrium
47 Hepatic vein
47.1 Descending aorta
47.2 Coeliac trunk
47.3 Superior mesenteric artery
48 Inferior vena cava
64 Ileum
64.1 Seminal vesicle
64.2 Prostate
65.1 Pubic symphysis
65.2 Male urethra
83 Cerebellum
83.1 Temporal lobe
86 Obliquus capitis inferior muscle
88 Levator scapulae muscle
90 Trapezius muscle
91 Splenius capitis muscle
91.1 Scalenus medius muscle
93 Levator scapulae muscle
96 Rhomboid major muscle
108 Longissimus thoracis muscle
116 Sacrum
120 Rectum
120.1 Urinary bladder

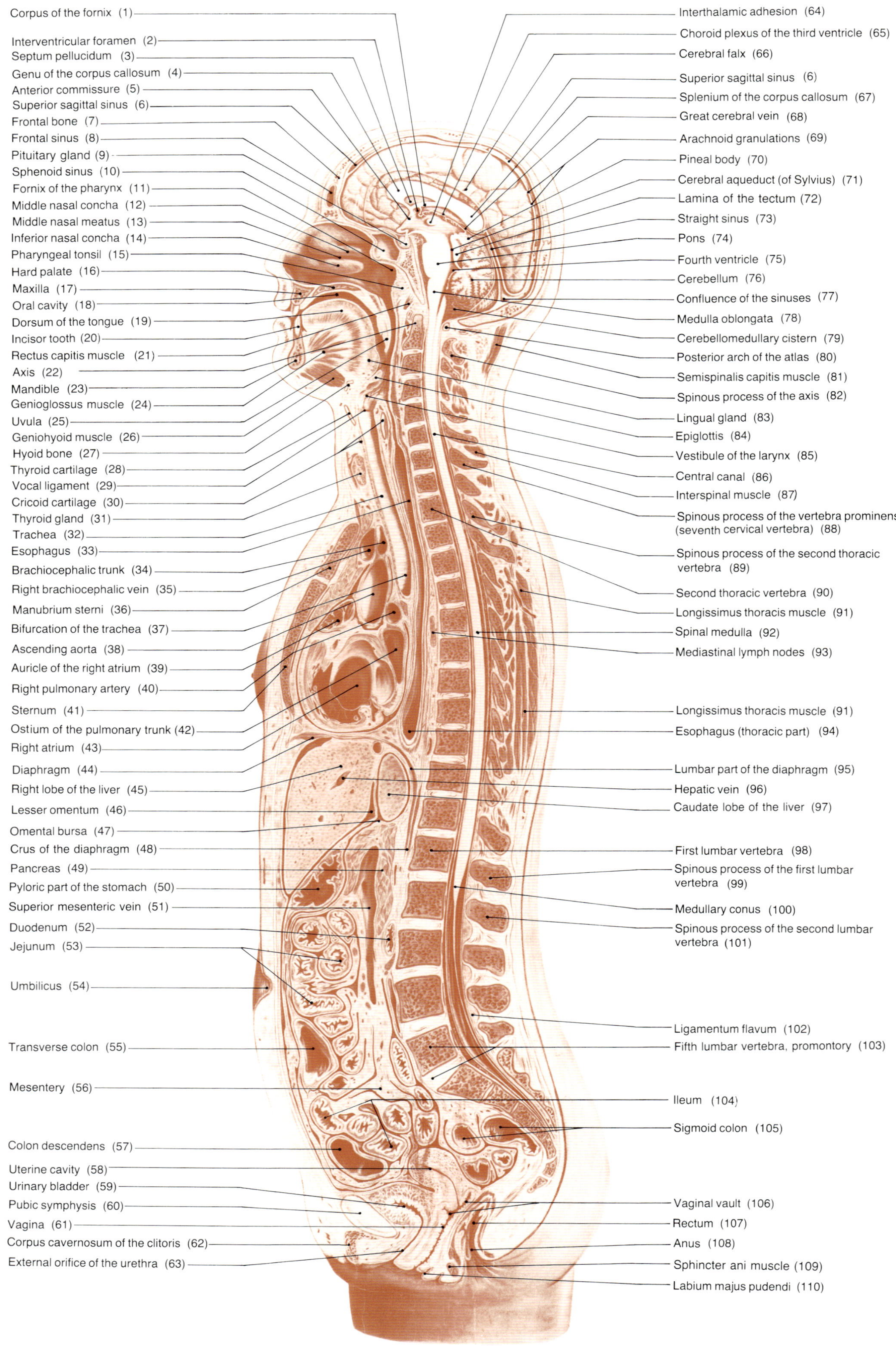

1 Corpus fornicis
2 Foramen interventriculare
3 Septum pellucidum
4 Genu corporis callosi
5 Commissura anterior
6 Sinus sagittalis superior
7 Os frontale
8 Sinus frontalis
9 Glandula pituitaria
10 Sinus sphenoidalis
11 Fornix pharyngis
12 Concha nasalis media
13 Meatus nasi medius
14 Concha nasalis inferior
15 Tonsilla pharyngea
16 Palatum durum
17 Maxilla
18 Cavitas oris
19 Dorsum linguae
20 Dens incisivus
21 M. rectus capitis
22 Axis
23 Mandibula
24 M. genioglossus
25 Uvula
26 M. geniohyoideus
27 Os hyoideum
28 Cartilago thyreoidea
29 Lig. vocale
30 Cartilago cricoidea
31 Glandula thyreoidea
32 Trachea
33 Oesophagus
34 Truncus brachiocephalicus
35 V. brachiocephalica dextra
36 Manubrium sterni
37 Bifurcatio tracheae
38 Aorta ascendens
39 Auricula atrii dextra
40 A. pulmonalis dextra
41 Sternum
42 Ostium trunci pulmonalis
43 Atrium dextrum
44 Diaphragma
45 Lobus hepatis dexter
46 Omentum minus
47 Bursa omentalis
48 Crus diaphragmatis
49 Pancreas
50 Pars pylorica ventriculi
51 V. mesenterica superior
52 Duodenum
53 Jejunum
54 Umbilicus
55 Colon transversum
56 Mesenterium
57 Colon descendens
58 Cavum uteri
59 Vesica urinaria
60 Symphysis pubica
61 Vagina
62 Corpus cavernosum clitoridis
63 Ostium urethrae externum
64 Adhaesio interthalamica
65 Plexus chorioideus ventriculi tertii
66 Falx cerebri
67 Splenium corporis callosi
68 V. cerebri magna
69 Granulationes arachnoideales
70 Corpus pineale
71 Aquaeductus cerebri (Sylvii)
72 Lamina tecti
73 Sinus rectus
74 Pons
75 Ventriculus IV
76 Cerebellum
77 Confluens sinuum
78 Medulla oblongata
79 Cisterna cerebellomedullaris
80 Arcus posterior atlantis
81 M. semispinalis capitis
82 Processus spinosus axis
83 Glandula lingualis
84 Epiglottis
85 Vestibulum laryngis
86 Canalis centralis
87 M. interspinalis
88 Processus spinosus vertebrae prominentis
89 Processus spinosus vertebrae thoracicae II
90 Vertebra thoracica II
91 M. longissimus thoracis
92 Medulla spinalis
93 Nodi lymphatici mediastinales
94 Oesophagus (Pars thoracica)
95 Diaphragma (Pars lumbalis)
96 V. hepatica
97 Lobus caudatus hepatis
98 Vertebra lumbalis I
99 Processus spinosus vertebrae lumbalis I
100 Conus medullaris
101 Processus spinosus vertebrae lumbalis II
102 Lig. flavum
103 Vertebra lumbalis V (Promontorium)
104 Ileum
105 Colon sigmoideum
106 Fornix vaginae
107 Rectum
108 Anus
109 M. sphincter ani
110 Labium majus pudendi

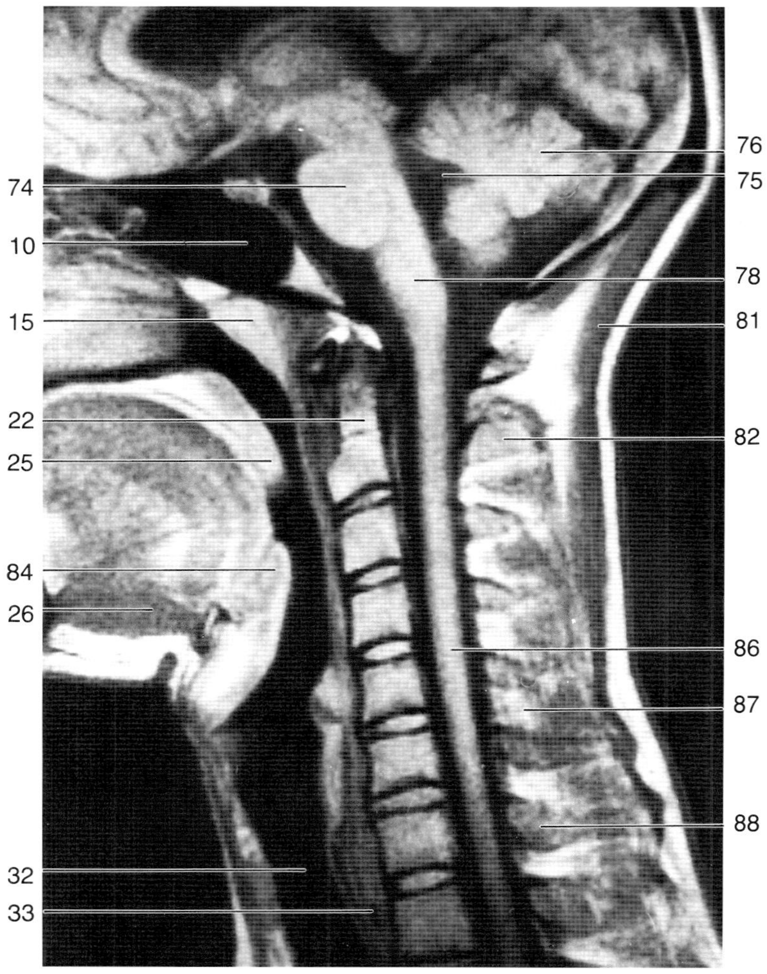

MRI, SE 600/30

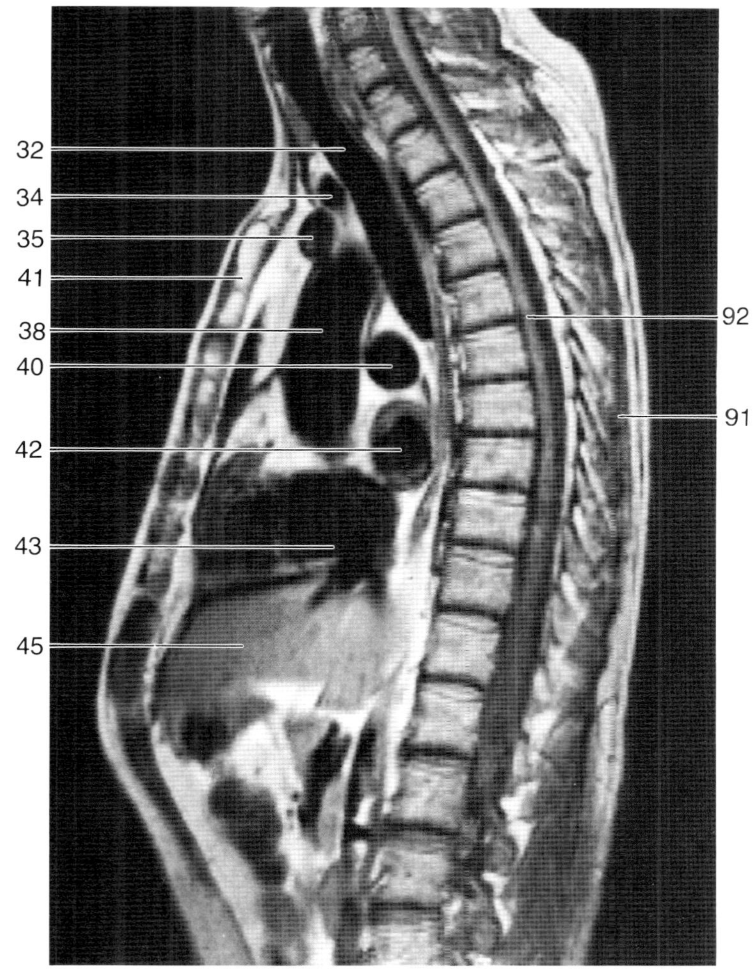

MRI, SE 970/22

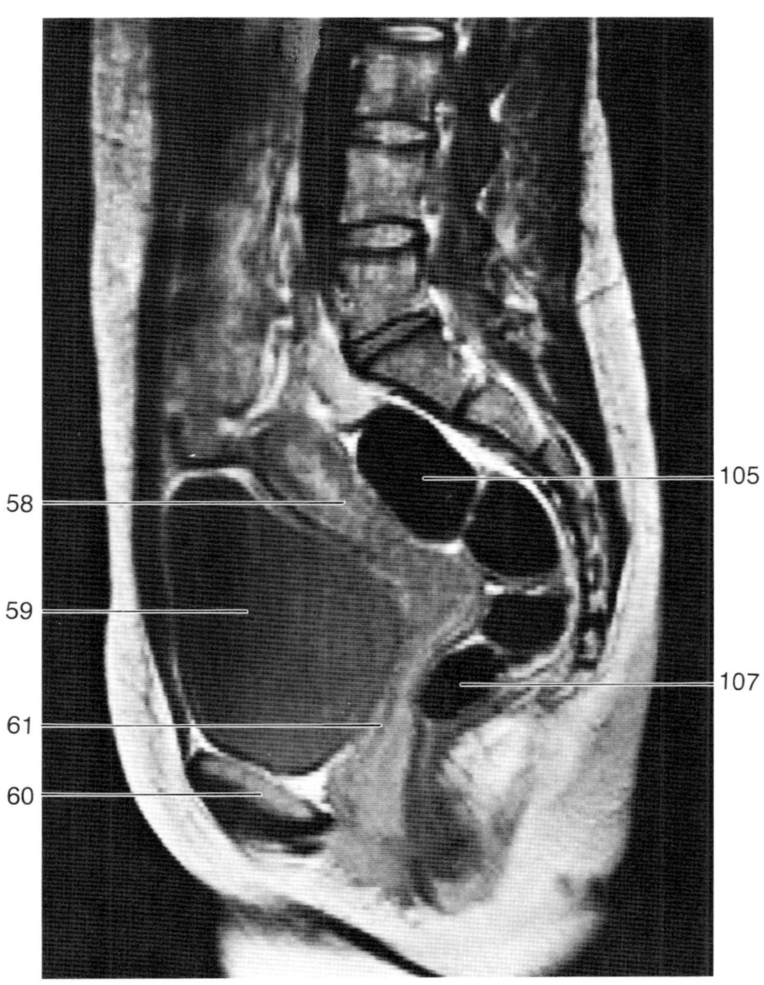

MRI, SE 1600/22, ♀

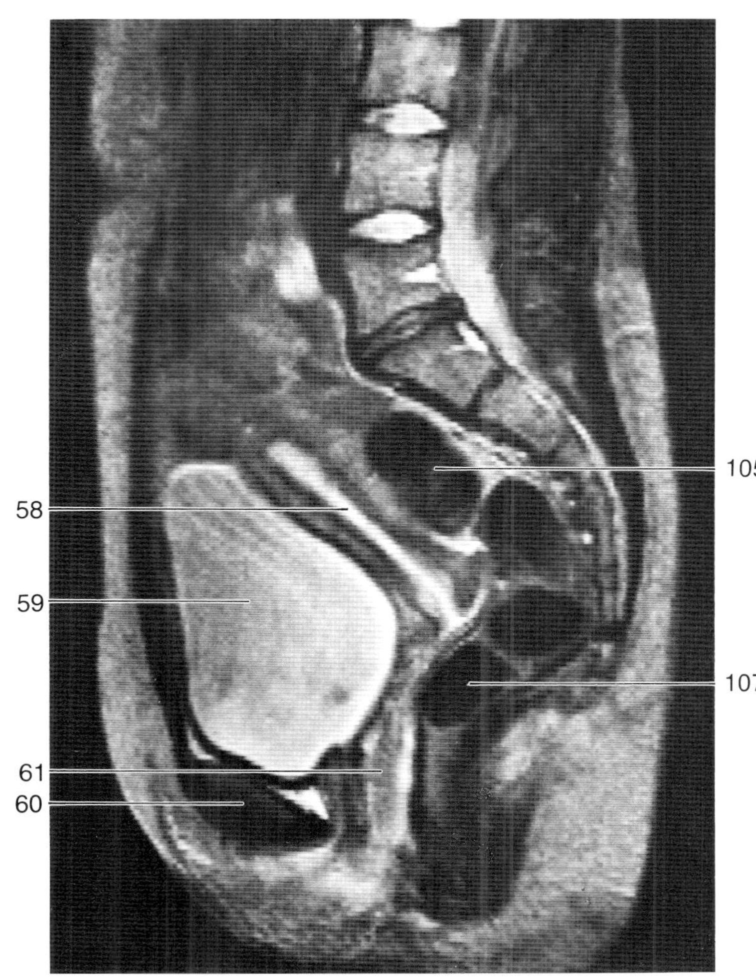

MRI, SE 1600/80, ♀

10 Sphenoid sinus
15 Pharyngeal tonsil
22 Axis
25 Uvula
26 Geniohyoid muscle
32 Trachea
33 Esophagus
34 Brachiocephalic trunk
35 Right brachiocephalic vein
38 Ascending aorta
40 Right pulmonary artery
41 Sternum
42 Ostium of the pulmonary trunk
43 Right atrium
45 Right lobe of the liver
58 Uterine cavity
59 Urinary bladder
60 Pubic symphysis
61 Vagina
74 Pons
75 Fourth ventricle
76 Cerebellum
78 Medulla oblongata
81 Semispinalis capitis muscle
82 Spinous process of the axis
84 Epiglottis
86 Central canal
87 Interspinal muscle
88 Spinous process of the vertebra prominens (seventh cervical vertebra)
91 Longissimus thoracis muscle
92 Spinal medulla
105 Sigmoid colon
107 Rectum

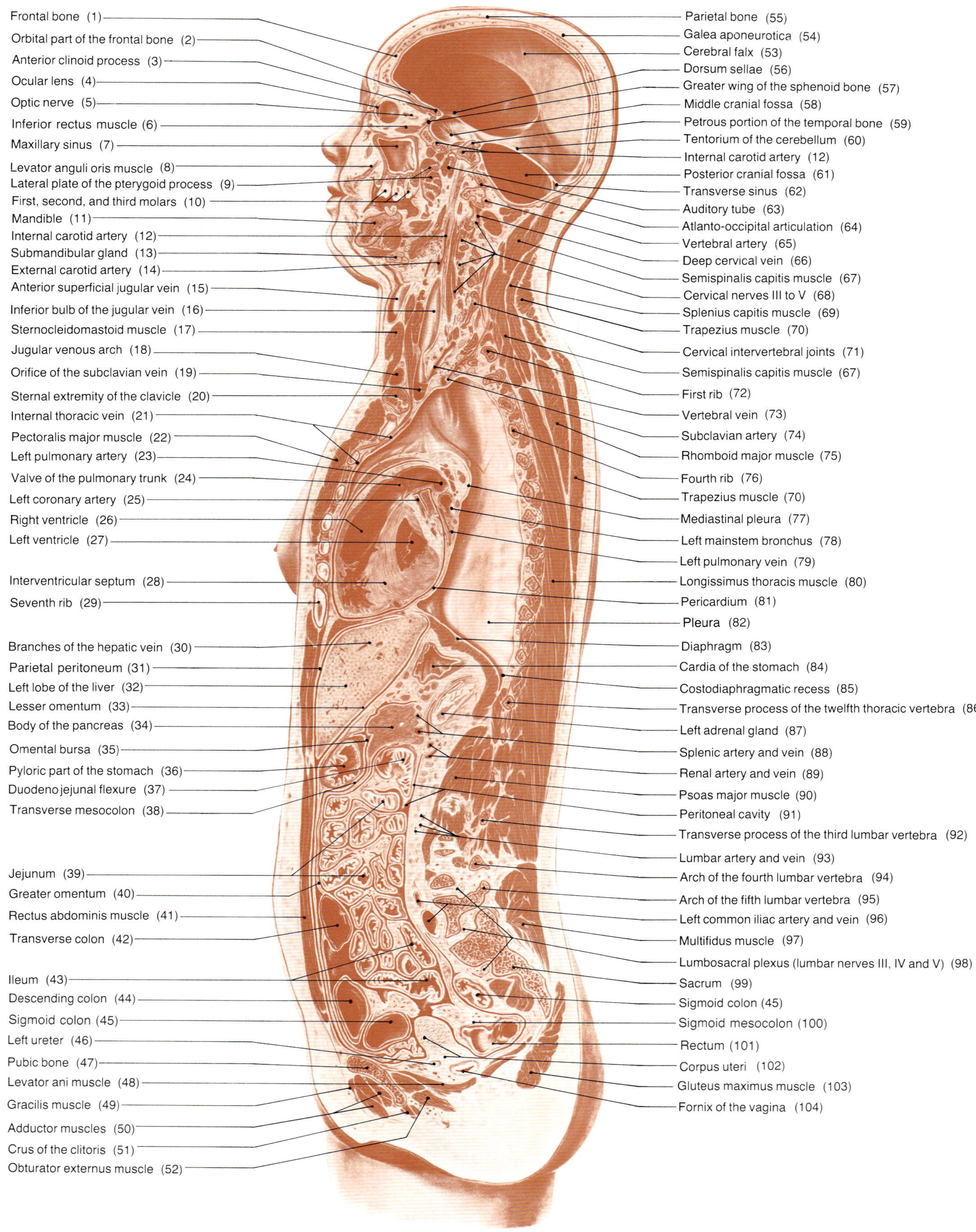

1 Os frontale
2 Pars orbitalis ossis frontalis
3 Processus clinoideus anterior
4 Lens oculi
5 N. opticus
6 M. rectus inferior
7 Sinus maxillaris
7.1 Capsula adiposa
7.2 Sinus sphenoidalis
7.3 Cerebellum
7.4 M. obliquus inferior
8 M. levator anguli oris
9 Lamina lateralis processus pterygoidei
10 Dentes molares I, II, III
11 Mandibula
12 A. carotis interna
13 Glandula submandibularis
14 A. carotis externa
15 V. jugularis superficialis anterior
16 Bulbus inferior v. jugularis
17 M. sternocleido-mastoideus
18 Arcus venosus juguli
19 Ostium v. subclaviae
20 Extremitas sternalis claviculae
21 V. thoracica interna
22 M. pectoralis major
23 A. pulmonalis sinistra
23.1 Atrium dexter
23.2 Aorta descendens
24 Valva trunci pulmonalis
25 A. coronaria sinistra
26 Ventriculus dexter
27 Ventriculus sinister
28 Septum interventriculare
29 Costa VII
30 Rr. v. hepaticae
31 Peritoneum
32 Lobus hepatis sinister
33 Omentum minus
34 Corpus pancreatis
35 Bursa omentalis
36 Pars pylorica ventriculi
37 Flexura duodenojejunalis
38 Mesocolon transversum
39 Jejunum
40 Omentum majus
41 M. rectus abdominis
42 Colon transversum
43 Ileum
44 Colon descendens
45 Colon sigmoideum
46 Ureter sinister
47 Os pubis
48 M. levator ani
49 M. gracialis
50 Mm. adductores
51 Crus clitoridis
52 M. obturatorius externus
53 Os parietale
54 Galea aponeurotica
55 Falx cerebri
56 Dorsum sellae
57 Ala major ossis sphenoidalis
58 Fossa cranii media
59 Pars petrosa ossis temporalis
60 Tentorium cerebelli
61 Fossa cranii posterior
62 Sinus transversus
63 Tuba auditiva
64 Articulatio atlantooccipitalis
65 A. vertebralis
65.1 A. carotis communis
66 V. cervicalis profunda
67 M. semispinalis capitis
68 Nn. cervicales III–V
69 M. splenius capitis
70 M. trapezius
71 Articulationes intervertebrales cervicales
72 Costa I
73 V. vertebralis
74 A. subclavia
75 M. rhomboideus major
76 Costa IV
77 Pleura mediastinalis
78 Bronchus principalis sinister
79 V. pulmonalis sinistra
80 M. longissimus thoracis
80.1 Aorta ascendens
80.2 V. brachiocephalica
81 Pericardium
82 Pleura
83 Diaphragma
84 Cardia ventriculi
85 Recessus costodiaphragmaticus
86 Processus transversus vertebrae thoracis XII
87 Glandula suprarenalis sinistra
88 A. et V. lienalis
89 A. et V. renalis
90 M. psoas major
91 Cavum peritoneale
92 Processus transversus vertebrae lumbalis III
93 A. et V. lumbalis
94 Arcus vertebrae lumbalis IV
95 Arcus vertebrae lumbalis V
96 A. et V. iliaca communis sinistra
97 M. multifidus
98 Plexus lumbosacralis (Nn. lumbales III, IV, V)
99 Os sacrum
100 Mesocolon sigmoideum
101 Rectum
102 Corpus uteri
102.1 Vesica urinaria
103 M. glutaeus maximus
104 Fornix vaginae

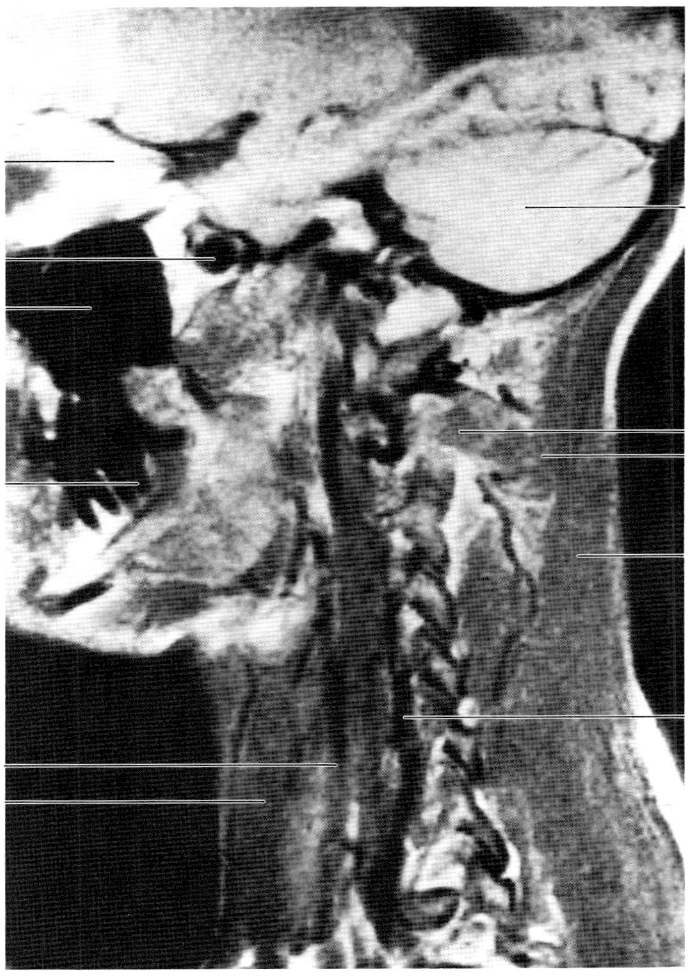

MRI, SE, $T_R/T_E = 0.6$ s/30 ms (M.S.)

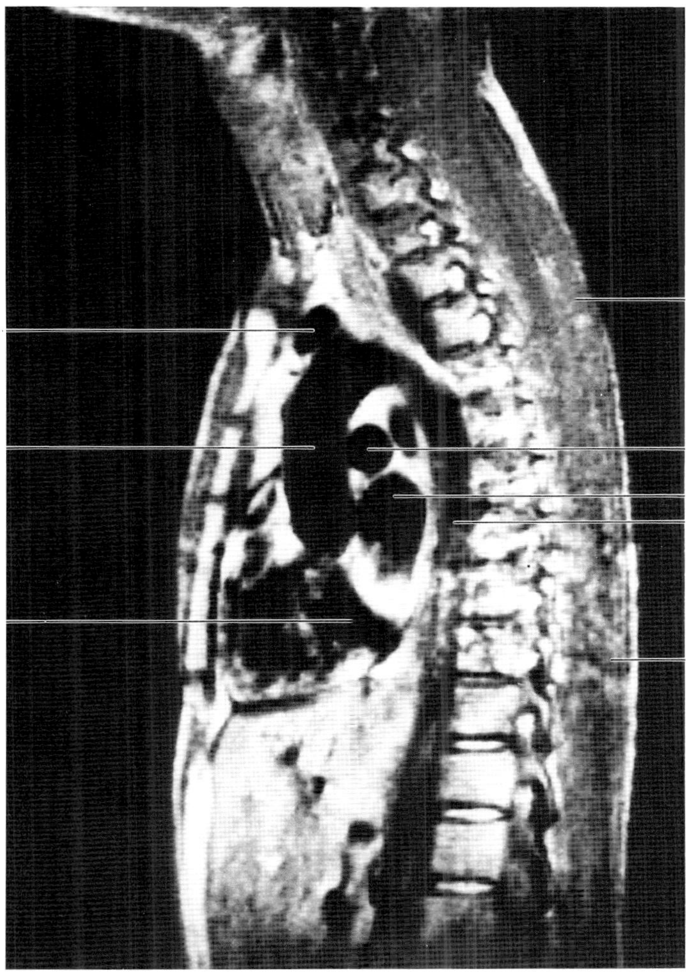

MRI, SE, ECG-triggered, $T_E = 30$ ms

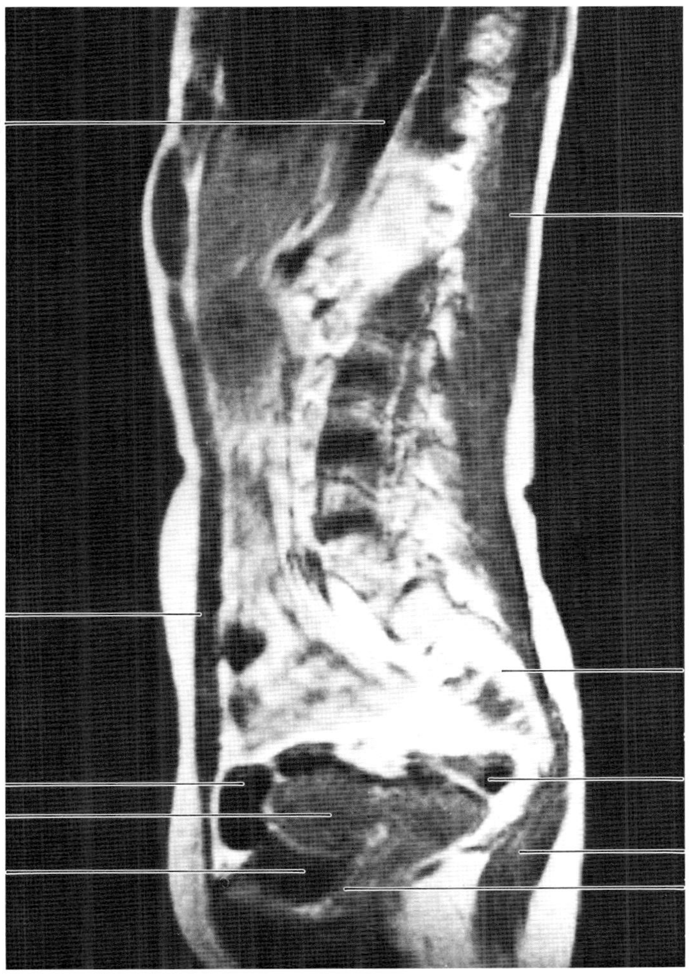

MRI, SE, $T_R/T_E = 0.6$ s/30 ms (M.S.)

7 Maxillary sinus
7.1 Orbital fat
7.2 Sphenoidal sinus
7.3 Cerebellum
7.4 Inferior oblique muscle
10 First, second and third molars
17 Sternocleidomastoid muscle
23 Left pulmonary artery
23.1 Left atrium
23.2 Descending aorta
27 Left ventricle
41 Rectus abdominis muscle
45 Sigmoid colon
65 Vertebral artery
65.1 Common carotid artery
67 Semispinalis capitis muscle
69 Splenius capitis muscle
70 Trapezius muscle
80 Longissimus thoracis muscle
80.1 Ascending aorta
80.2 Brachiocephalic vein
99 Sacrum
100 Sigmoid mesocolon
102 Corpus uteri
102.1 Urinary bladder
103 Gluteus maximus muscle
104 Fornix of the vagina

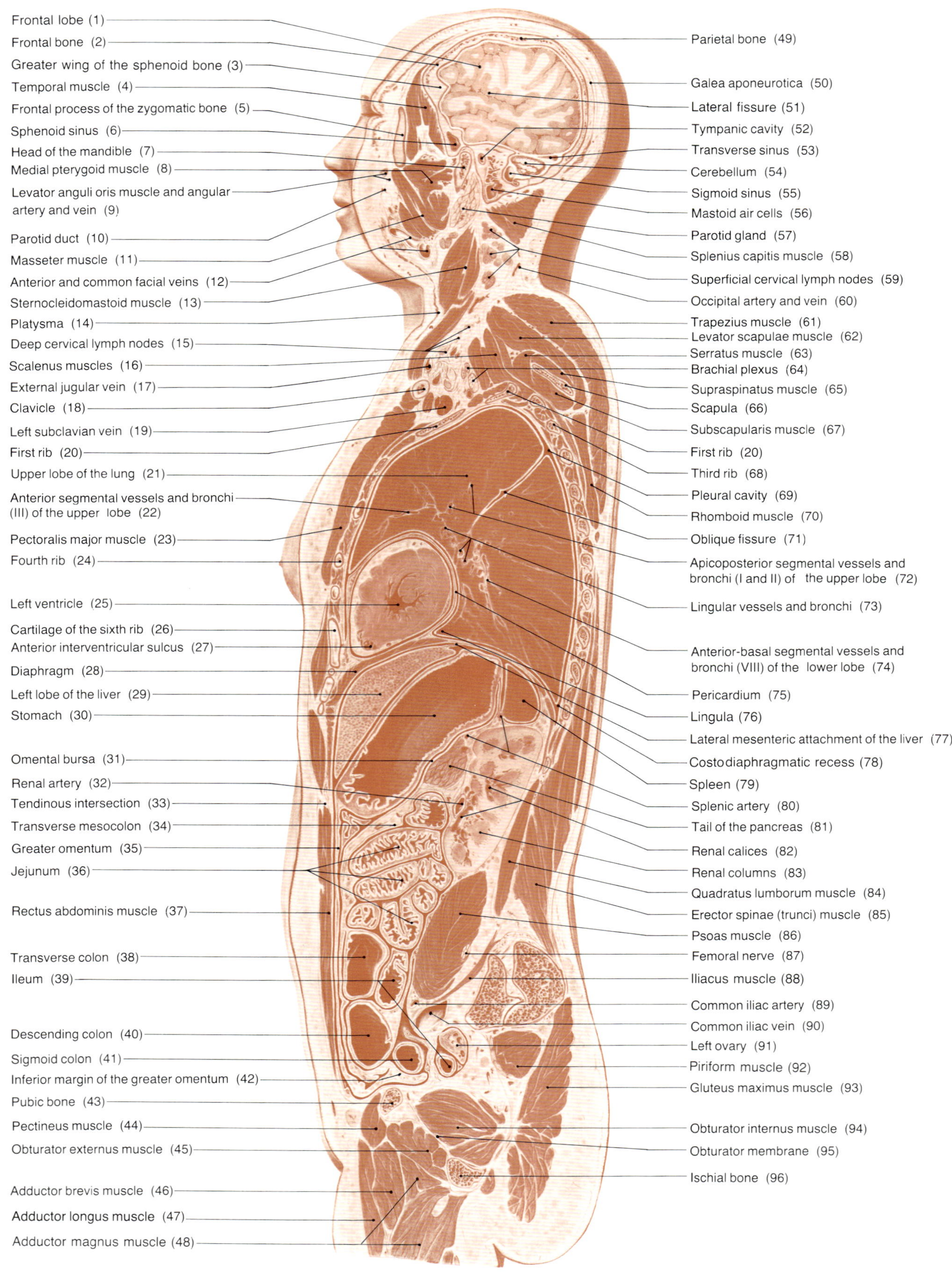

1 Lobus frontalis
2 Os frontale
3 Ala minor ossis sphenoidalis
4 M. temporalis
5 Processus frontalis (ossis zygomatici)
6 Sinus sphenoidalis
7 Caput mandibulae
8 M. pterygoideus medialis
9 M. levator anguli oris et A. et V. angularis
10 Ductus parotideus
11 M. masseter
12 Vv. facialis anterior et communis
13 M. sternocleidomastoideus
14 Platysma
15 Nodi lymphatici cervicales profundi
16 Mm. scaleni
17 V. jugularis externa
18 Clavicula
19 V. subclavia sinistra
20 Costa I
21 Lobus superior pulmonis
22 Vasa et Bronchi segmenti anterioris (III) lobi superioris
23 M. pectoralis major
24 Costa IV
25 Ventriculus sinister
26 Cartilago costa VI
27 Sulcus interventricularis anterior
28 Diaphragma
29 Lobus sinister hepatis
30 Ventriculus
31 Bursa omentalis
32 A. renalis
33 Intersectio tendinea
34 Mesocolon transversum
35 Omentum majus
36 Jejunum
37 M. rectus abdominis
38 Colon transversum
39 Ileum
40 Colon descendens
41 Colon sigmoideum
42 Margo inferior omenti majoris
43 Os pubis
44 M. pectineus
45 M. obturatorius externus
46 M. adductor brevis
47 M. adductor longus
48 M. adductor magnus
49 Os parietale
50 Galea aponeurotica
51 Fissura lateralis
52 Tympanum
53 Sinus transversus
54 Cerebellum
55 Sinus sigmoideus
56 Cellulae mastoideae
57 Glandula parotis
58 M. splenus capitis
59 Nodi lymphatici cervicales superficiales
60 A. et V. occipitalis
61 M. trapezius
62 M. levator scapulae
63 M. serratus
64 Plexus brachialis
65 M. supraspinatus
66 Scapula
67 M. subscapularis
68 Costa III
69 Cavum pleurae
70 M. rhomboideus
71 Fissura obliqua
72 Vasa et Bronchi segmenti apicoposterioris (I + II) lobi superioris
73 Vasa et Bronchi lingulares
74 Vasa et Bronchi segmenti anterobasalis (VIII) lobi inferioris
75 Pericardium
76 Lingula
77 Mesohepaticum laterale
78 Recessus costodiaphragmaticus
79 Lien
80 A. lienalis
81 Cauda pancreatis
82 Calices renales
83 Columnae renales
84 M. quadratus lumborum
85 M. erector spinae (trunci)
86 M. psoas
87 N. femoralis
88 M. iliacus
89 A. iliaca communis
90 V. iliaca communis
91 Ovarium sinistrum
92 M. piriformis
93 M. glutaeus maximus
94 M. obturatorius internus
95 Membrana obturatoria
96 Os ischii

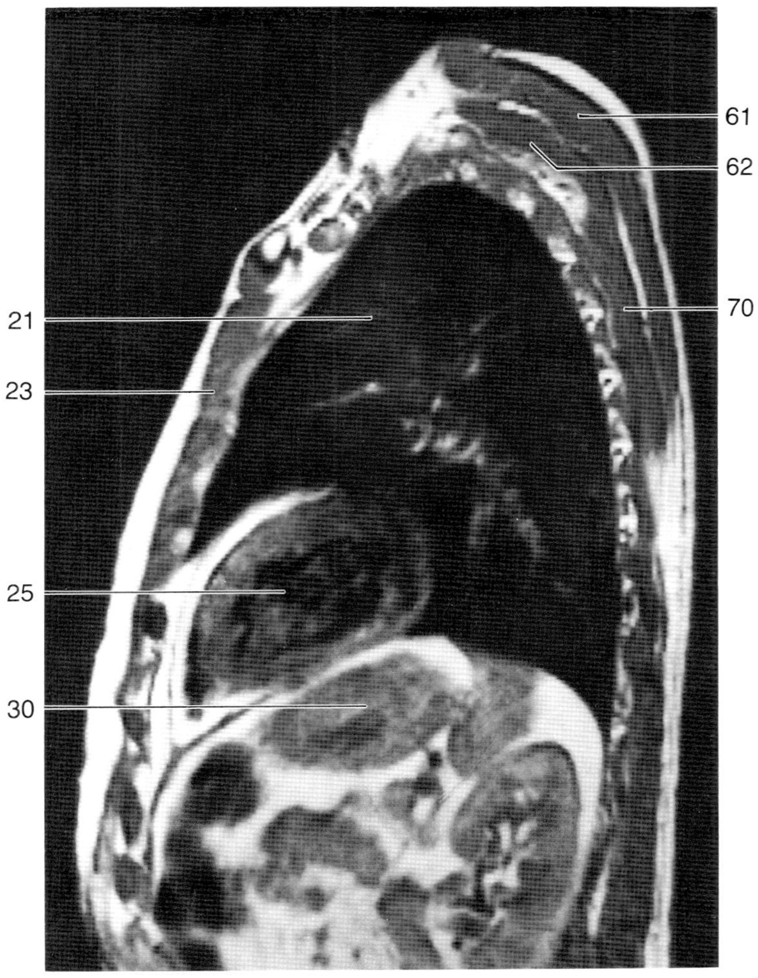

MRI, SE 970/22

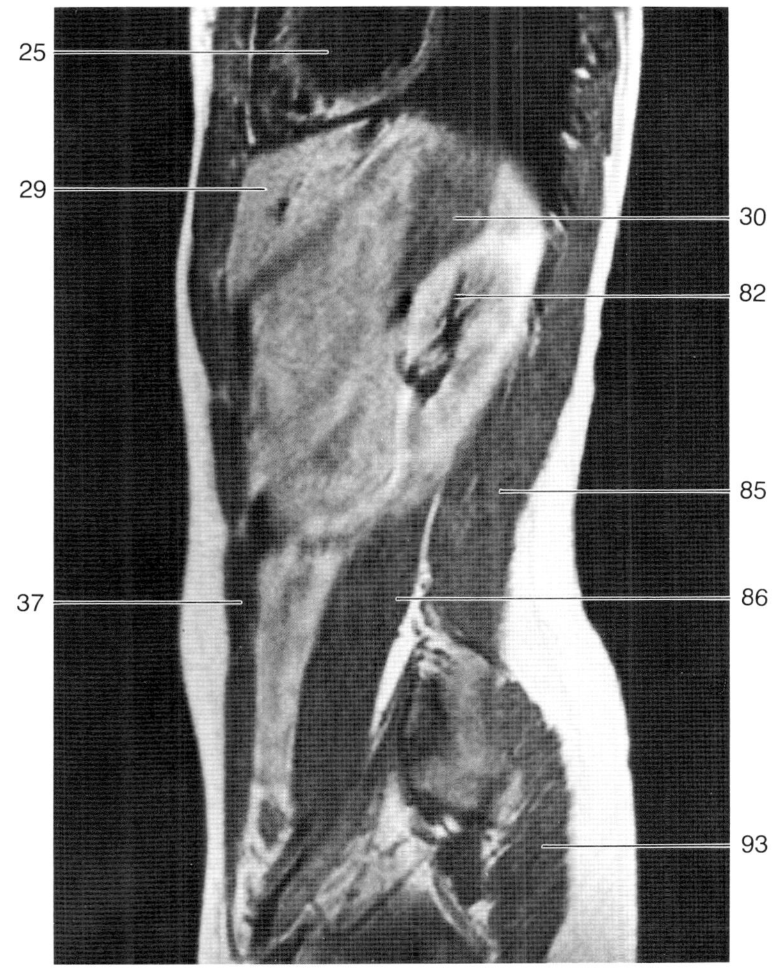

MRI, SE ECG-triggered, $T_E = 30$

21 Upper lobe of the lung
23 Pectoralis major muscle
25 Left ventricle
29 Left lobe of the liver
30 Stomach
37 Rectus abdominis muscle
61 Trapezius muscle
62 Levator scapulae muscle
70 Rhomboid muscle
82 Renal calices
85 Erector spinae (trunci) muscle
86 Psoas muscle
93 Gluteus maximus muscle

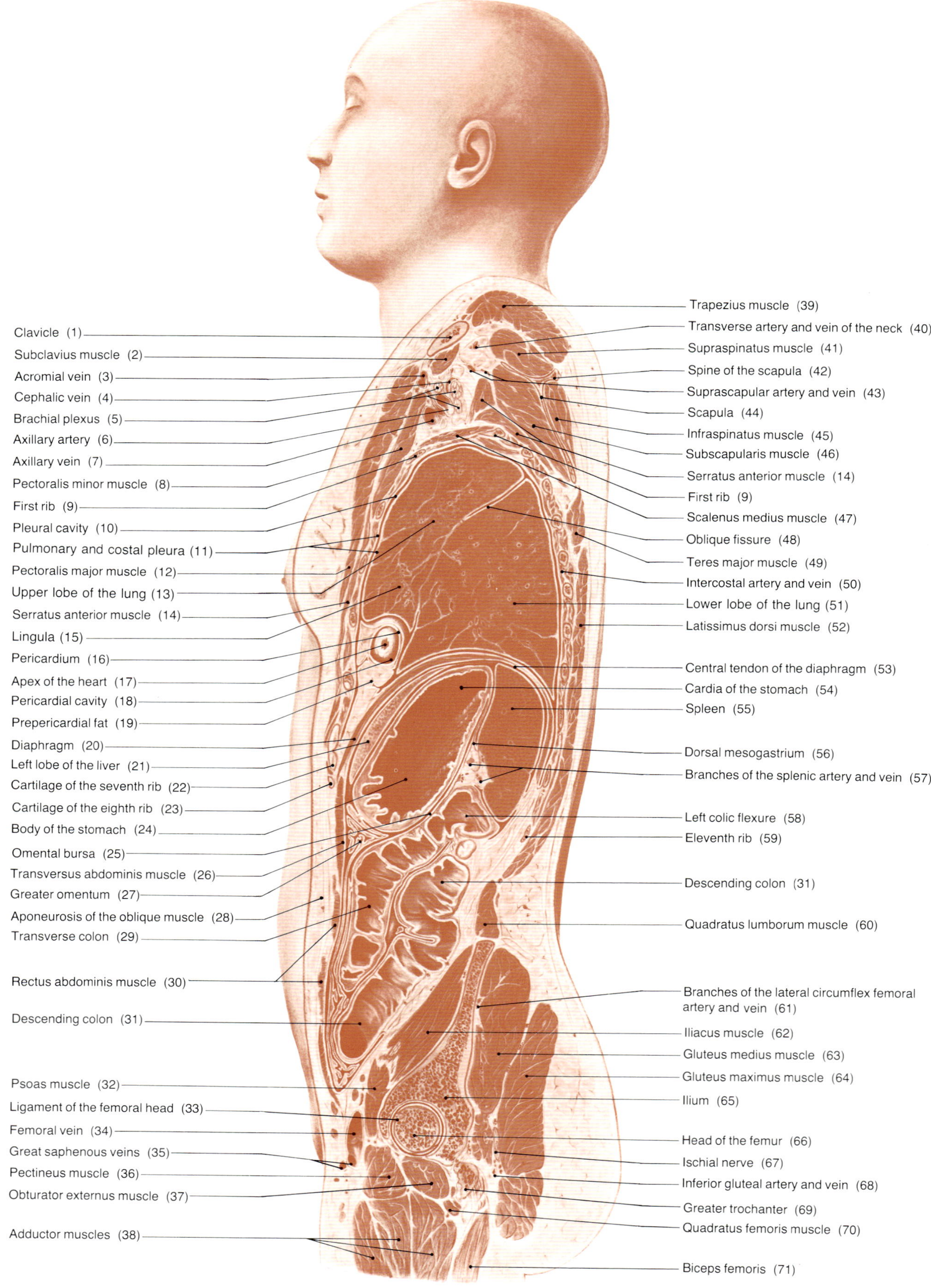

1 Clavicula
2 M. subclavius
3 V. acromialis
4 V. cephalica
5 Plexus brachialis
6 A. axillaris
7 V. axillaris
8 M. pectoralis minor
9 Costa I
10 Cavum pleurae
11 Pleura pulmonis et costalis
12 M. pectoralis major
13 Lobus superior pulmonis
14 M. serratus anterior
15 Lingula
16 Pericardium
17 Apex cordis
18 Cavum pericardii
19 Corpus adiposum praecardiale
20 Diaphragma
21 Lobus hepatis sinister
22 Cartilago costalis VII
23 Cartilago costalis VIII
24 Corpus ventriculi
25 Bursa omentalis
26 M. transversus abdominis
27 Omentum majus
28 Aponeurosis m. obliqui
29 Colon transversum
30 M. rectus abdominis
31 Colon descendens
32 M. psoas
33 Lig. capitis femoris
34 V. femoralis
35 Vv. saphenae magnae
36 M. pectineus
37 M. obturatorius externus
38 Mm. adductores
39 M. trapezius
40 A. et V. transversa colli
41 M. supraspinatus
42 Spina scapulae
43 V. et A. suprascapularis
44 Scapula
45 M. infraspinatus
46 M. subscapularis
47 M. scalenus medius
48 Fissura obliqua
49 M. teres major
50 A. et V. intercostalis
51 Lobus inferior pulmonis
52 M. latissimus dorsi
53 Centrum tendineum diaphragmatis
54 Cardia ventriculi
55 Lien
55.1 Ren sinister
56 Mesogastrium dorsale
57 Rr. a. et v. lienalis
58 Flexura coli sinistra
59 Costa XI
60 M. quadratus lumborum
61 Rr. a. et v. circumflexae femoris lateralis
62 M. iliacus
63 M. glutaeus medius
64 M. glutaeus maximus
65 Os ilium
66 Caput femoris
67 N. ischiadicus
68 A. et V. glutaea inferior
69 Trochanter major
70 M. quadratus femoris
71 M. biceps femoris

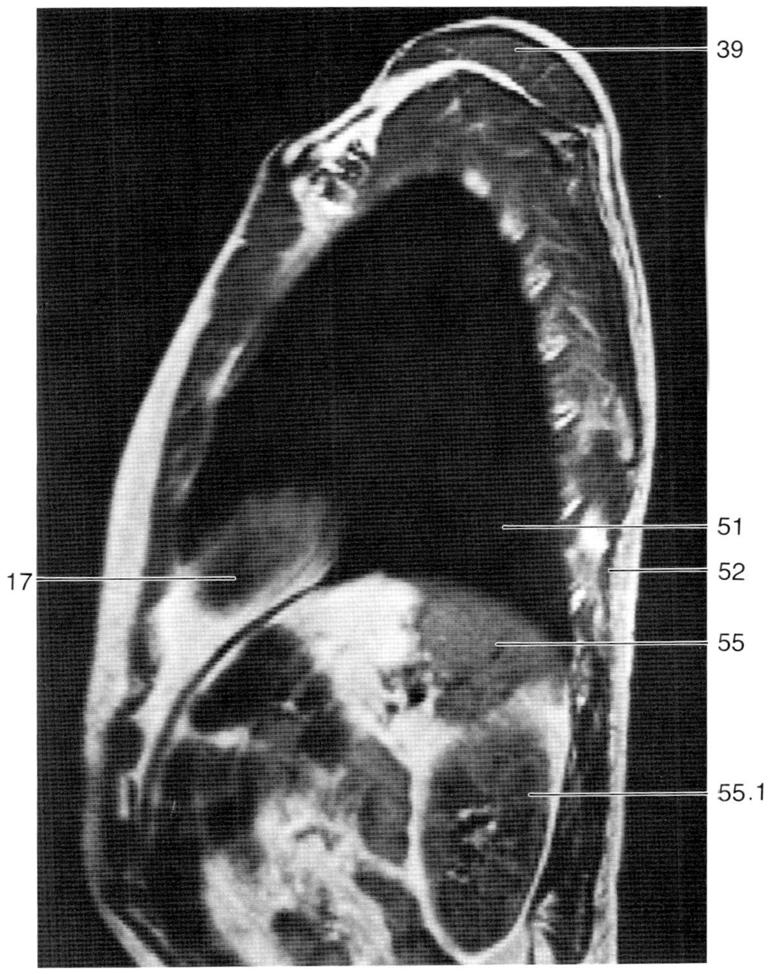

MRI, SE 1940/22

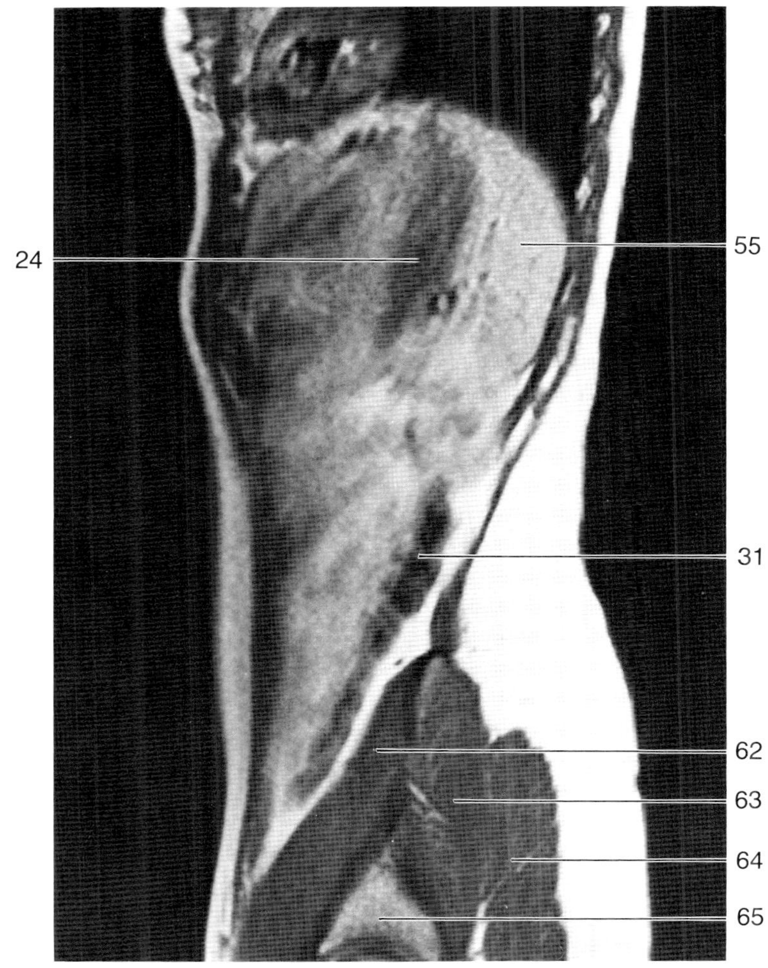

MRI, SE 1940/22

17 Apex of the heart
24 Body of the stomach
31 Descending colon
39 Trapezius muscle
51 Lower lobe of the lung
52 Latissimus dorsi muscle
55 Spleen
55.1 Left kidney
62 Iliacus muscle
63 Gluteus medius muscle
64 Gluteus maximus muscle
65 Ilium

Coronal Sections of the Head

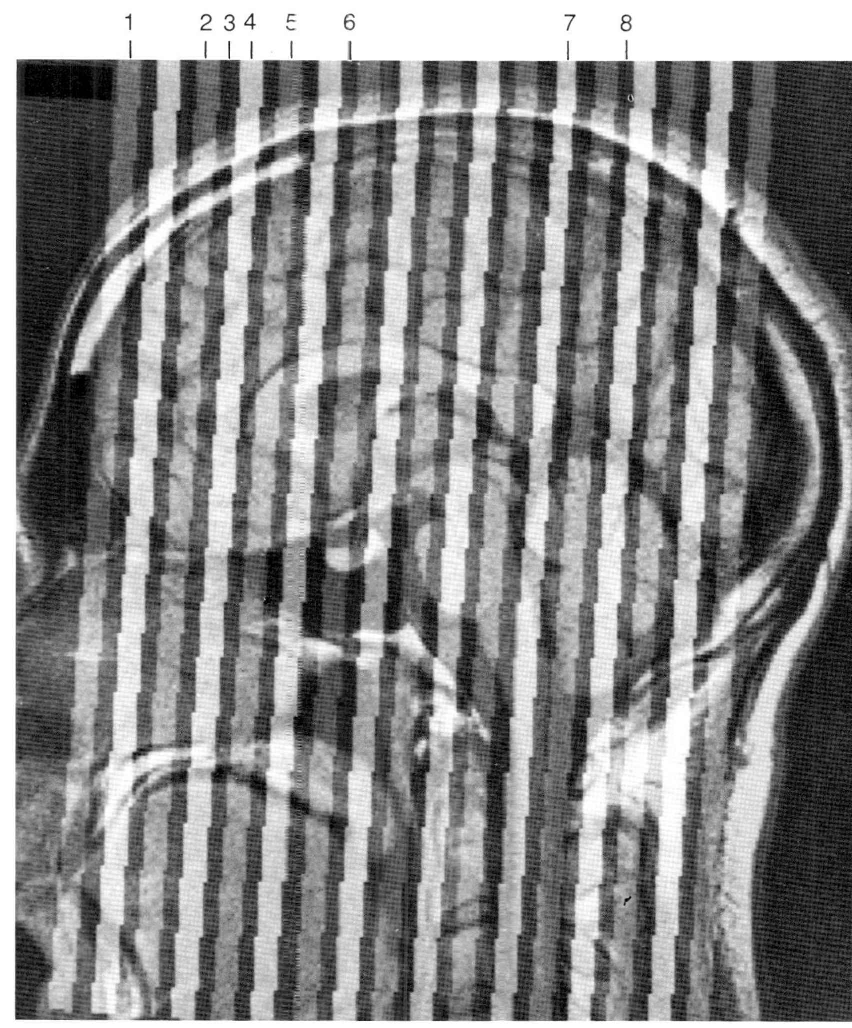

Sagittal MRI section. Coronal slices at levels no. 1–8. Slice thickness 5 mm.

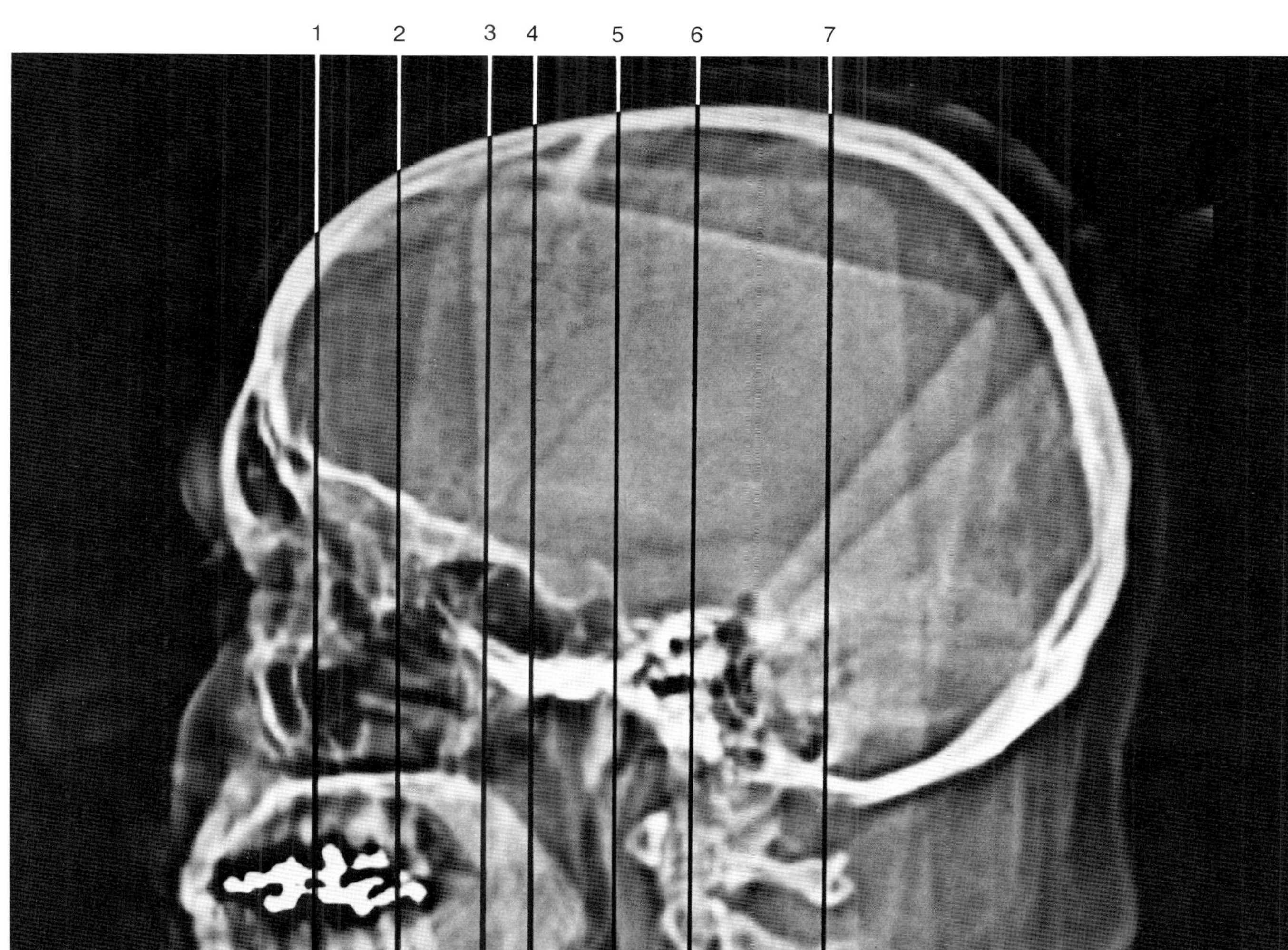

Lateral computed radiograph. Coronal rconstructions at levels no. 1–7. Slice thickness 3 mm.

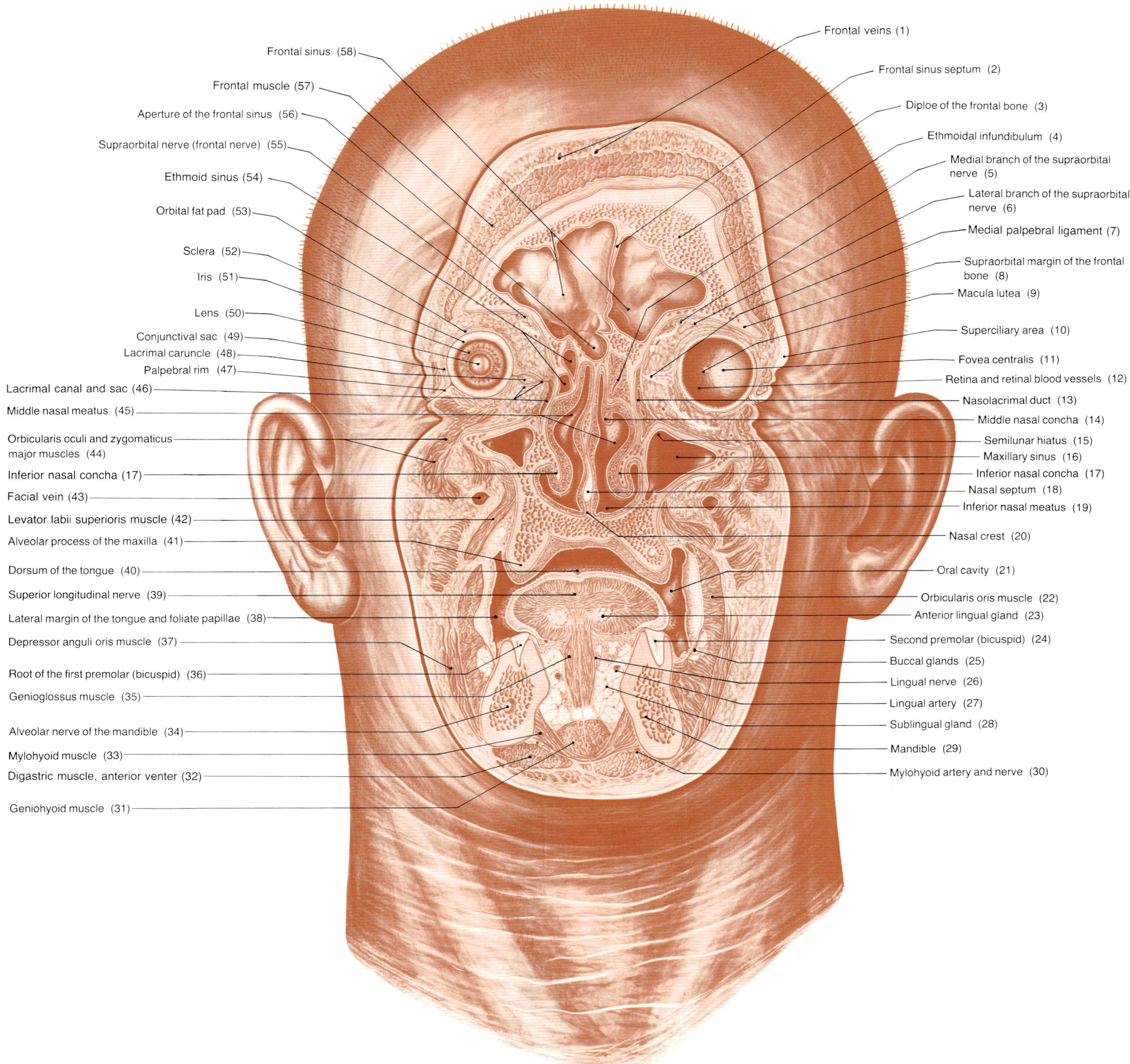

1 Vv. frontales
2 Septum sinuum frontalium
3 Diploe ossis frontalis
4 Infundibulum ethmoidale
5 R. medialis n. supraorbitalis
6 R. lateralis n. supraorbitalis
7 Lig. palpebrale mediale
7.1 Os frontale
8 Margo supraorbitalis (oss. front.)
9 Macula lutea
10 Supercilia
11 Fovea centralis
12 Retina et Vasa sanguinea retinae
13 Ductus nasolacrimalis
14 Concha nasalis media
15 Hiatus semilunaris
16 Sinus maxillaris
16.1 Corpus linguae
17 Concha nasalis inferior
17.1 Falx cerebri
17.2 Gyrus frontalis superior
17.3 Corpus vitreum
18 Septum nasi
19 Meatus nasi inferior
20 Crista nasalis
21 Cavum oris
21.1 Processus frontalis maxillae
22 M. orbicularis oris
23 Glandula lingualis anterior
24 Dens praemolaris II
25 Glandulae buccales
26 N. lingualis
27 A. lingualis
28 Glandula sublingualis
29 Mandibula
30 A. et N. mylohyoideus
31 M. geniohyoideus
32 M. digastricus, Venter anterior
33 M. mylohyoideus
34 N. alveolaris mandibulae
35 M. genioglossus
35.1 M. buccalis
36 Dens praemolaris I
37 M. depressor anguli oris
38 Margo lateralis linguae, Papillae foliatae
39 N. longitudinalis superior linguae
40 Dorsum linguae
41 Processus alveolaris maxillae
42 M. levator labii superioris
43 V. facialis
44 Mm. orbicularis oculi et zygomaticus major
44.1 M. rectus inferior
45 Meatus nasi medius
46 Canaliculus et Saccus lacrimalis
47 Rima palpebrarum
48 Caruncula lacrimalis
48.1 M. rectus bulbi lateralis
49 Conjunctiva
50 Lens
51 Iris
52 Sclera
53 Corpus adiposum orbitae
54 Sinus ethmoidalis
55 N. supraorbitalis (N. frontalis)
56 Apertura sinus frontalis
57 M. frontalis
58 Sinus frontalis
58.1 Paries superior orbitae
58.2 M. rectus bulbi superioris
58.3 M. levator palpebrae superioris
58.4 Crista galli
58.5 M. obliquus superior
58.6 M. rectus medialis
58.7 Glandula lacrimalis

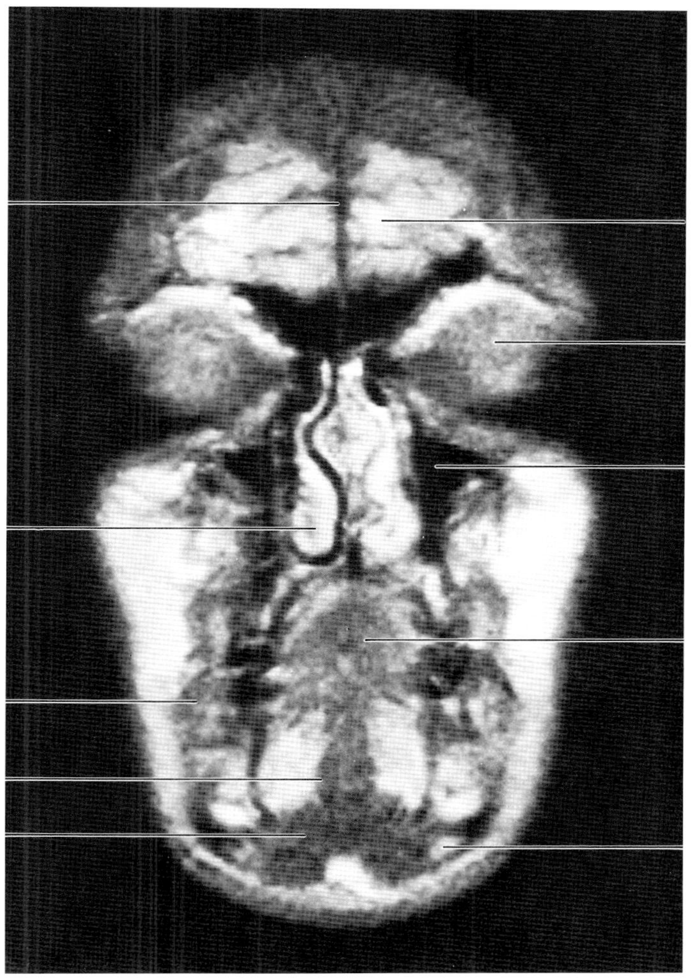

MRI, SE 1100/50

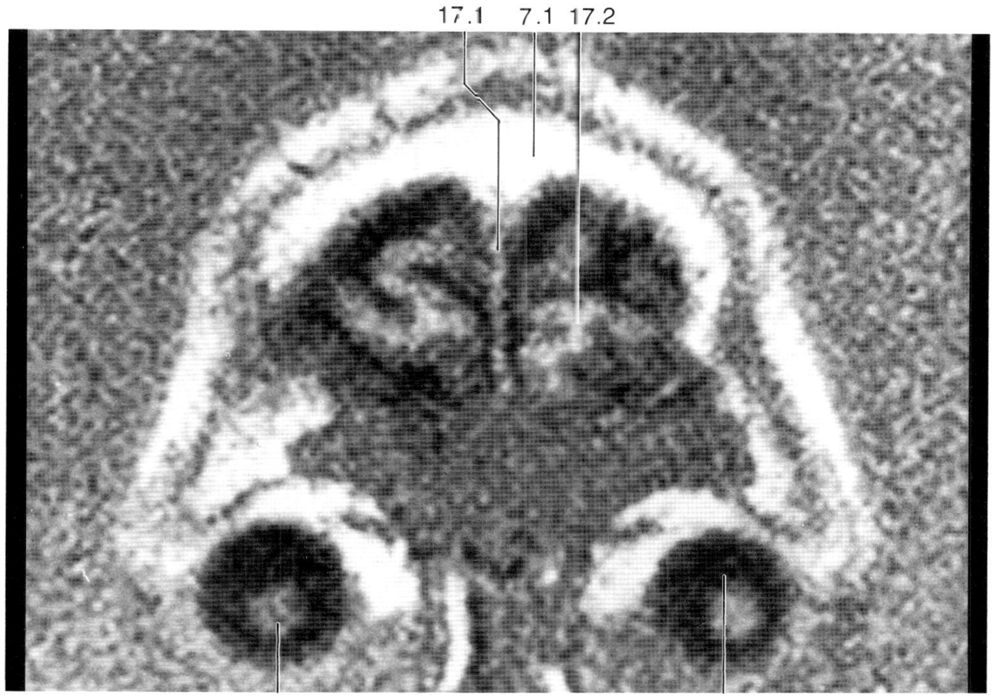

MRI, IR 1800/400/30, level 1

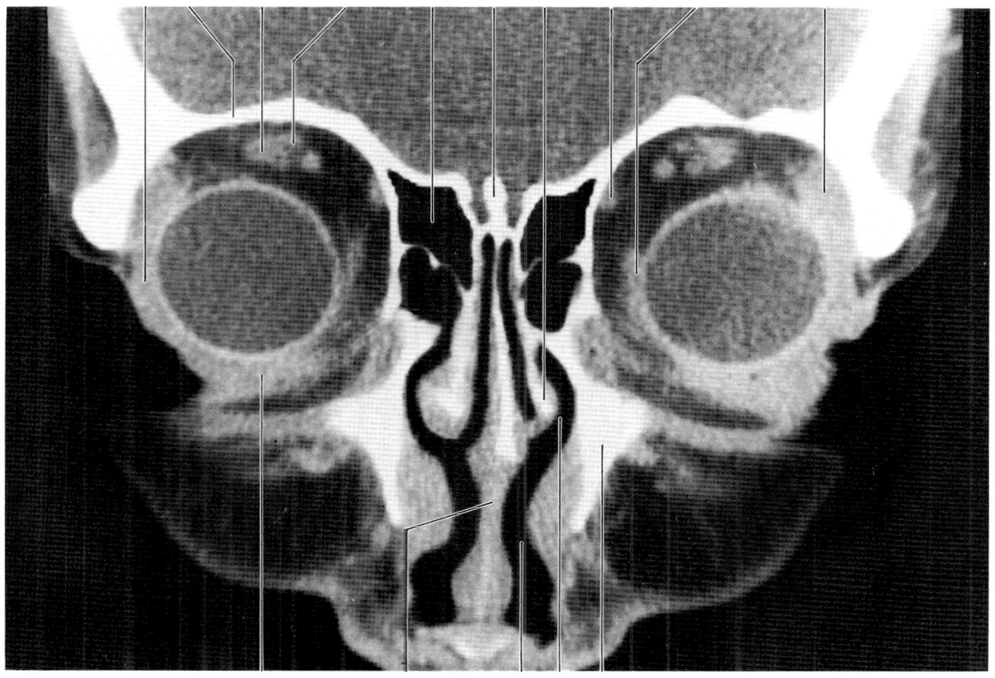

CT without contrast medium

7.1 Frontal bone
14 Middle nasal concha
16 Maxillary sinus
16.1 Corpus of the tongue
17 Inferior nasal concha
17.1 Falx cerebri
17.2 Superior frontal gyrus
17.3 Vitreous body
18 Nasal septum
19 Inferior nasal meatus
21.1 Frontal process of the maxilla
29 Mandible
31 Geniohyoid muscle
35 Genioglossus muscle
35.1 Buccinator muscle
44.1 Inferior rectus muscle
45 Middle nasal meatus
48.1 Lateral rectus muscle
50 Lens
54 Ethmoid sinus
58.1 Superior orbital wall
58.2 Superior rectus muscle
58.3 Levator palpebrae superioris muscle
58.4 Crista galli
58.5 Obliquus superior muscle
58.6 Medial rectus muscle
58.7 Lacrimal gland

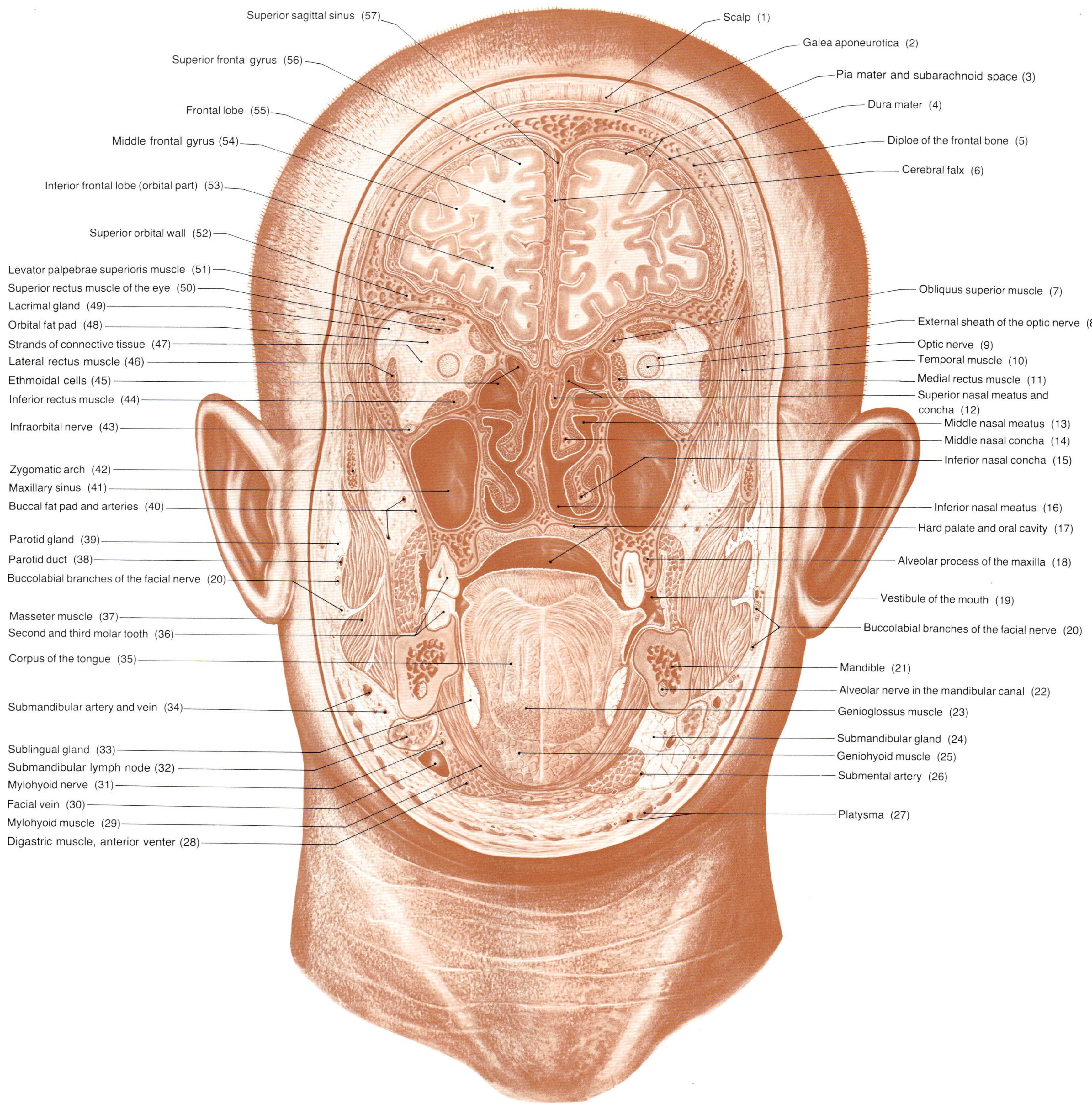

1 Epicranium
2 Galea aponeurotica
3 Pia mater et Spatium subarachnoideale
4 Dura mater
4.1 Os frontale
5 Diploe ossis frontalis
6 Falx cerebri
7 M. obliquus superior
7.1 Crista galli
8 Vagina externa n. optici
9 N. opticus
10 M. temporalis
11 M. rectus medialis
12 Meatus nasi superior et Concha nasalis superior
13 Meatus nasi medius
13.1 Septum nasi
14 Concha nasalis media
15 Concha nasalis inferior
15.1 Palatum durum
16 Meatus nasi inferior
17 Palatum durum et Cavum oris
18 Processus alveolaris maxillae
19 Vestibulum oris
20 Rr. buccolabiales n. facialis
21 Mandibula
22 N. alveolaris canalis mandibulae
23 M. genioglossus
24 Glandula submandibularis
25 M. geniohyoideus
26 A. submentalis
27 Platysma
28 M. digastricus (venter anterior)
29 M. mylohyoideus
30 V. facialis
31 N. mylohyoideus
32 Nodi lymphatici submandibulares
33 Glandula sublingualis
34 A. et V. submandibularis
35 Corpus linguae
36 Dentes molares II et III
37 M. masseter
37.1 M. zygomaticus
38 Ductus parotideus
39 Glandula parotis
40 Corpus adiposum buccae et Aa. buccales
41 Sinus maxillaris
41.1 Sclera
42 Arcus zygomaticus
43 N. infraorbitalis
43.1 Gyrus rectus
44 M. rectus inferior
45 Cellulae ethmoidales
46 M. rectus bulbi lateralis
47 Fasciculi textus connectivi
48 Corpus adiposum orbitae
49 Glandula lacrimalis
50 M. rectus bulbi superior
51 M. levator palpebrae superioris
52 Paries superior orbitae
53 Lobus frontalis inferior (Pars orbitalis)
54 Gyrus frontalis medius
55 Lobus frontalis
56 Gyrus frontalis superior
57 Sinus sagittalis superior

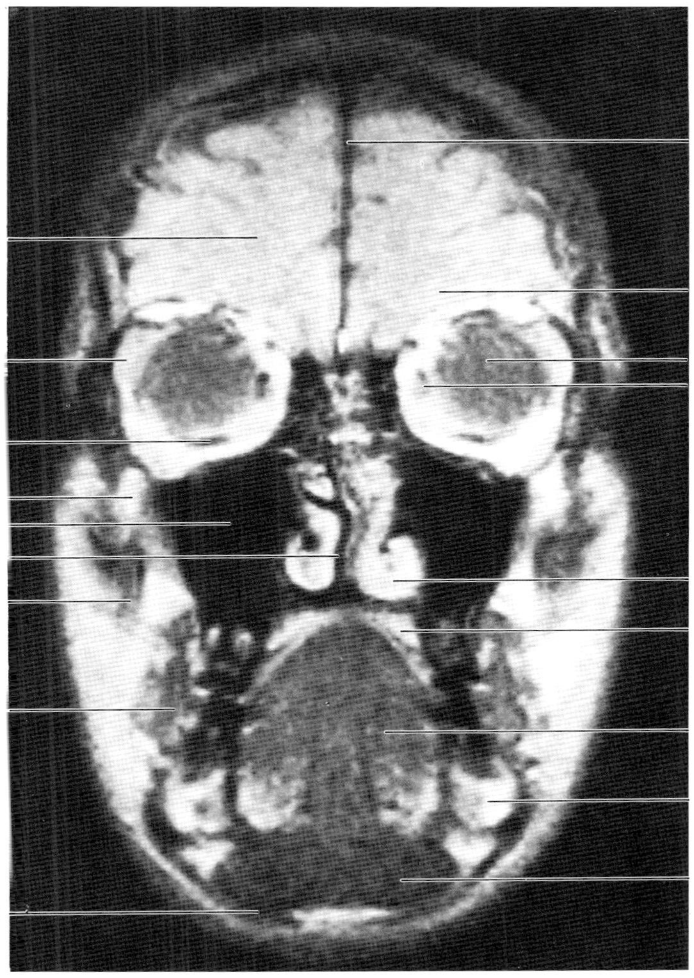

MRI, SE 1100/50

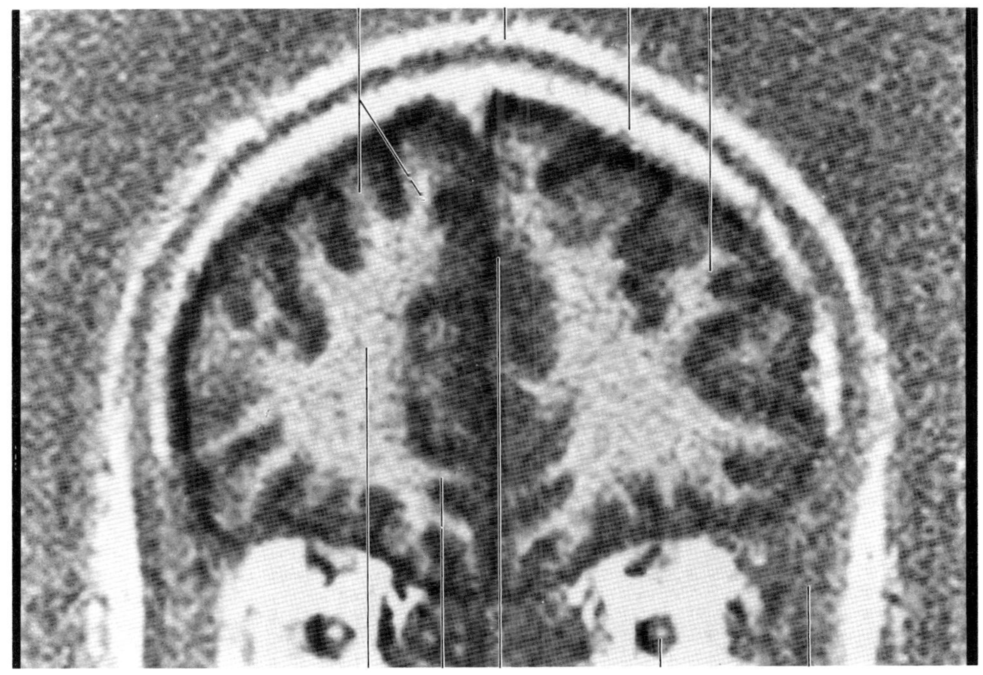

MRI, IR 1800/400/30, level 2

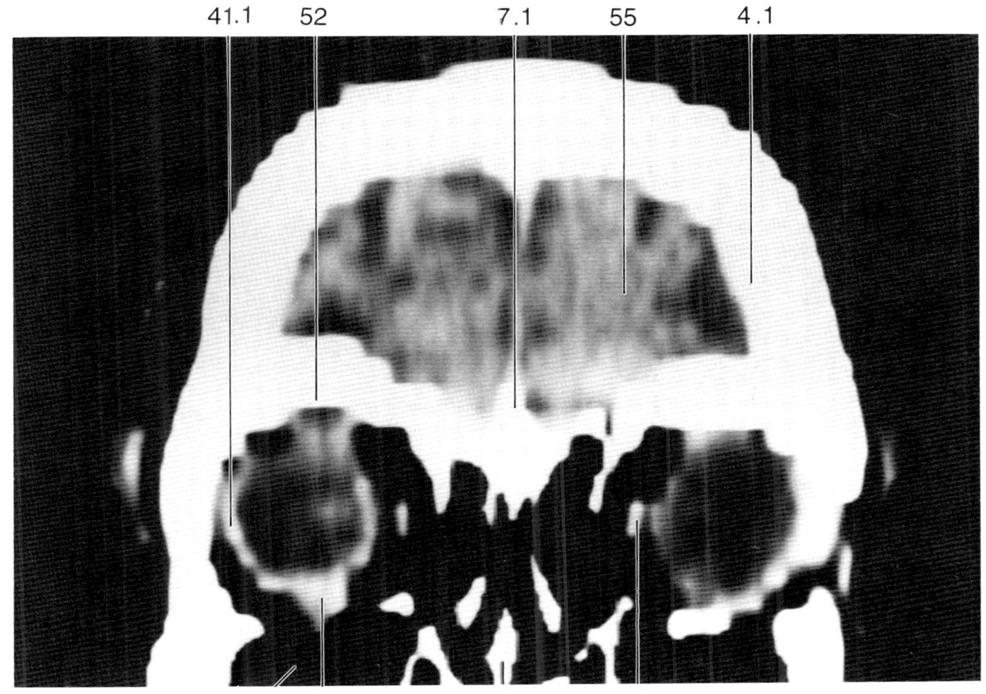

CT, coronal reconstruction, level 1

1 Scalp
4.1 Frontal bone
6 Cerebral falx
7.1 Crista galli
9 Optic nerve
10 Temporal muscle
11 Medial rectus muscle
11.1 Vitreous body
13.1 Nasal septum
15 Inferior nasal concha
15.1 Hard palate
16 Inferior nasal meatus
21 Mandible
25 Geniohyoid muscle
28 Digastric muscle, anterior venter
35 Corpus of the tongue
37 Masseter muscle
37.1 Zygomatic muscle
41 Maxillary sinus
41.1 Sclera
42 Zygomatic arch
43.1 Rectal gyrus
44 Inferior rectus muscle
48 Orbital fat pad
52 Superior orbital wall
53 Inferior frontal lobe (orbital part)
54 Middle frontal gyrus
55 Frontal lobe
56 Superior frontal gyrus
57 Superior sagittal sinus

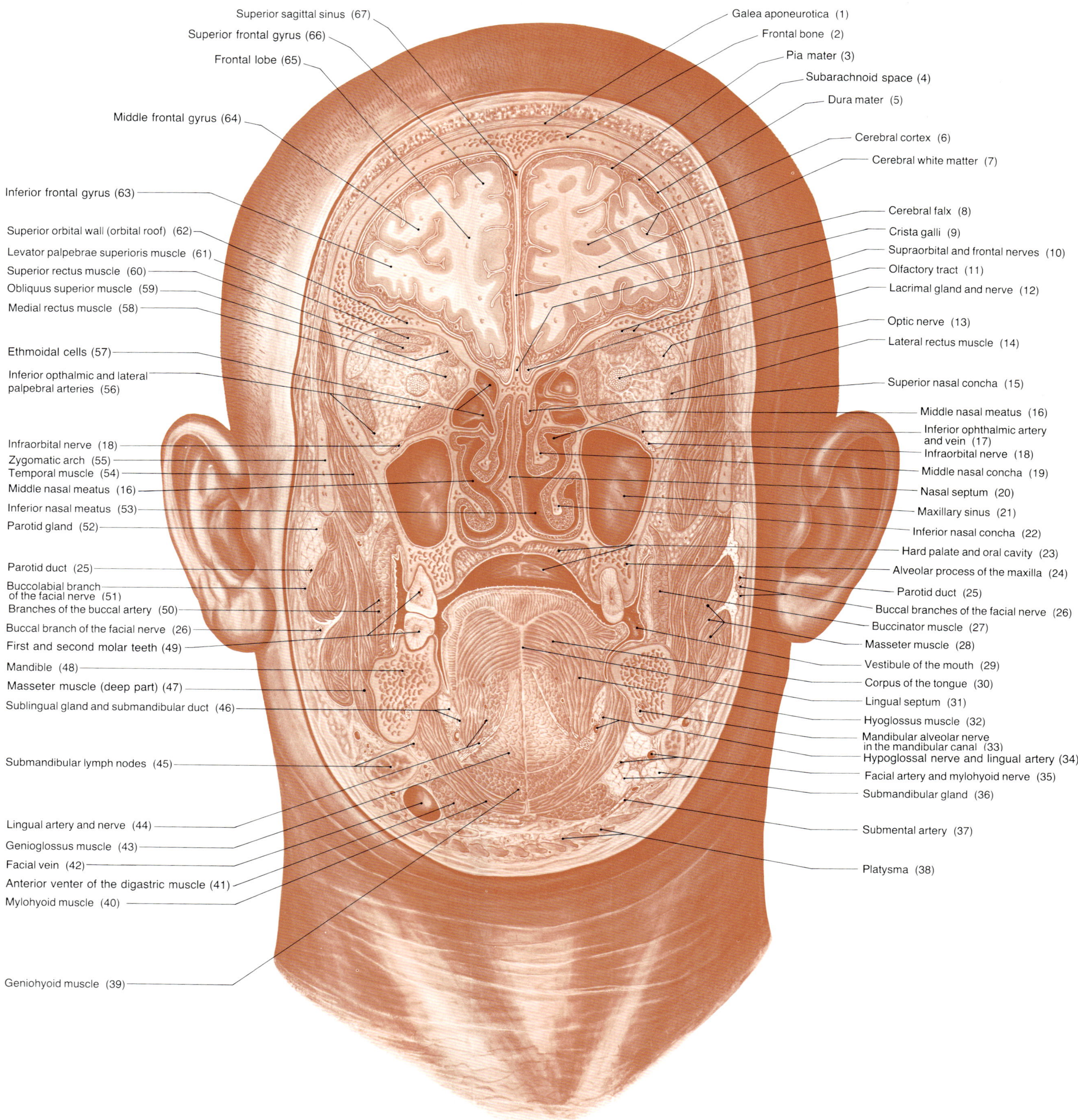

1 Galea aponeurotica
2 Os frontale
3 Pia mater
4 Spatium subarachnoideale
5 Dura mater
6 Cortex cerebri
7 Substantia alba cerebri
8 Falx cerebri
9 Crista galli
10 Nn. supraorbitalis et frontalis
11 Tractus olfactorius
12 Glandula et N. lacrimalis
13 N. opticus
13.1 M. rectus inferior
14 M. rectus lateralis
15 Concha nasalis superior
16 Meatus nasi medius
17 A. et V. ophthalmica inferior
18 N. infraorbitalis
19 Concha nasalis media
20 Septum nasi
21 Sinus maxillaris
22 Concha nasalis inferior Palatum
23 Palatum durum et Cavum oris
24 Processus alveolaris maxillae
25 Ductus parotideus
26 Rr. buccales n. facialis
27 M. buccalis
28 M. masseter
29 Vestibulum oris
30 Corpus linguae
31 Septum linguae
32 M. hypoglossus
33 N. alveolaris mandibulae (Canalis mandibulae)
34 Nn. hypoglossus et lingualis
35 A. facialis et N. mylohyoideus
36 Glandula submandibularis
37 A. submentalis
38 Platysma
39 M. geniohyoideus
40 M. mylohyoideus
41 M. digastricus (Venter anterior)
42 V. facialis
43 M. genioglossus
44 A. et N. lingualis
45 Nodi lymphatici submandibulares
46 Glandula sublingualis et Ductus submandibularis
47 M. masseter (pars profunda)
48 Mandibula
49 Dentes molares I et II
50 Rr. a. buccalis
51 R. buccolabialis n. facialis
52 Glandula parotis
53 Meatus nasi inferior
54 M. temporalis
55 Arcus zygomaticus
56 Aa. ophthalmica inferior et palpebralis lateralis
57 Cellulae ethmoidales
58 M. rectus medius
59 M. obliquus superior
60 M. rectus superior
61 M. levator palpebrae superioris
62 Paries superior orbitae
63 Gyrus frontalis inferior
64 Gyrus frontalis medius
65 Lobus frontalis
66 Gyrus frontalis superior
67 Sinus sagittalis superior
68 Gyrus rectus
69 Gyri orbitales
70 Gyrus cinguli
71 Sulcus frontalis superior
72 Genu corporis callosi
73 A. pericallosa

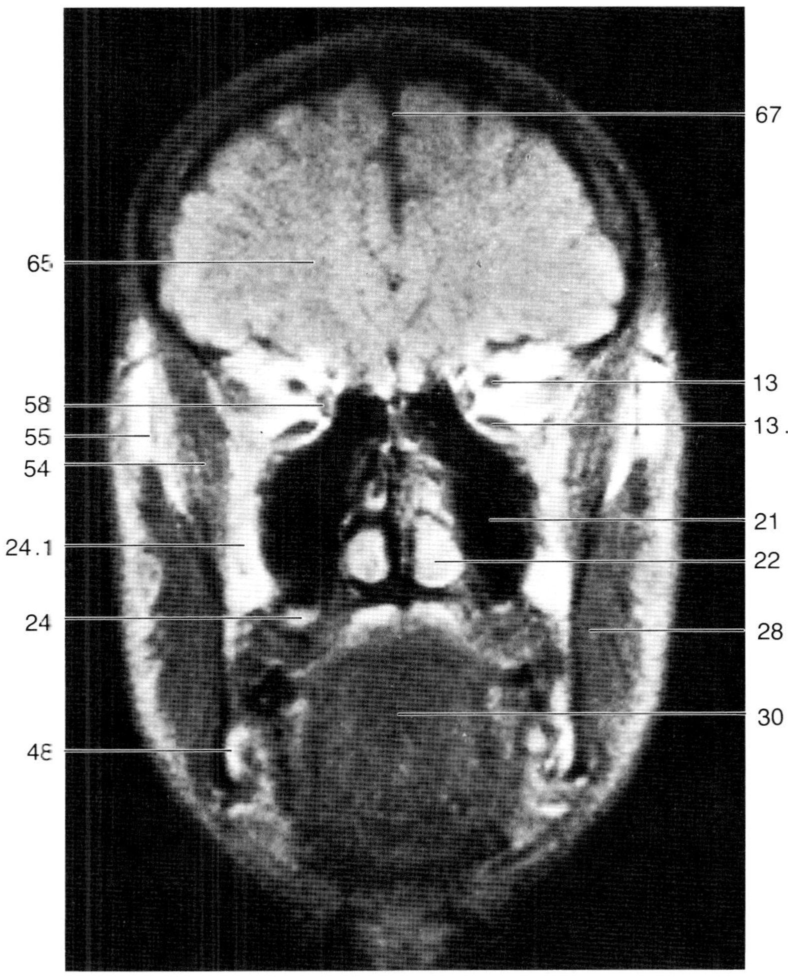

MRI, SE 1100/50

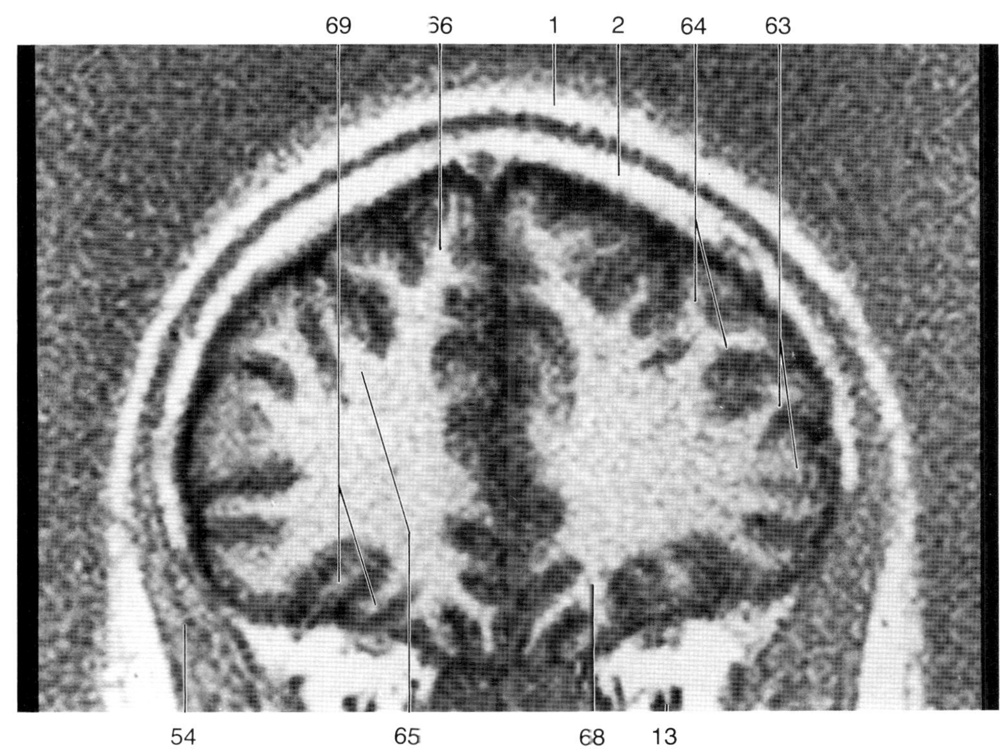

MRI, IR 1800/400/30, level 3

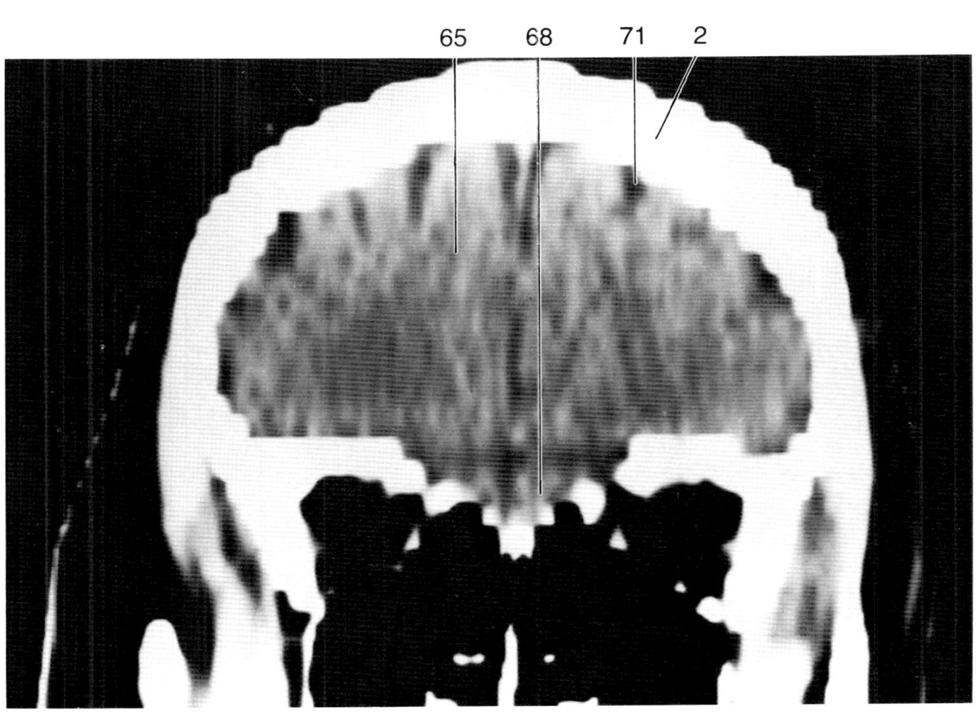

CT, coronal reconstruction, level 2

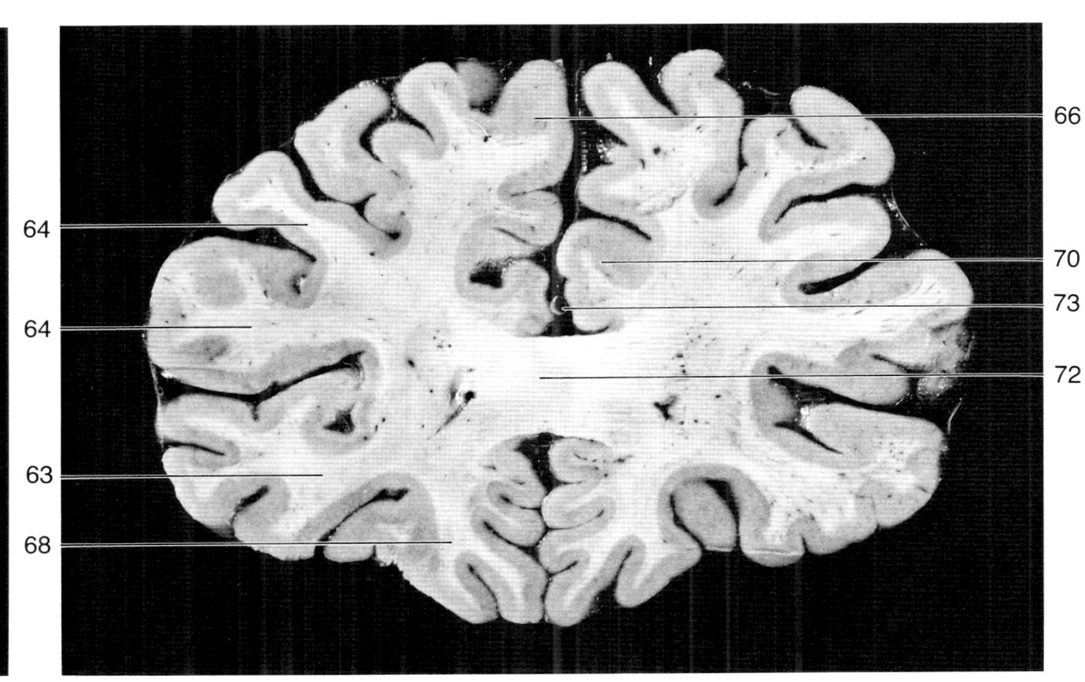

Anatomical section

1 Scalp
2 Frontal bone
13 Optic nerve
13.1 Inferior rectus muscle
21 Maxillary sinus
22 Inferior nasal concha
24 Alveolar process of the maxilla
24.1 Temporal process of the zygomatic bone
28 Masseter muscle
30 Corpus of the tongue
48 Mandible
54 Temporal muscle
55 Zygomatic arch
58 Medial rectus muscle
63 Inferior frontal gyrus
64 Middle frontal gyrus
65 Frontal lobe
66 Superior frontal gyrus
67 Superior sagittal sinus
68 Rectal gyrus
69 Orbital gyri
70 Cingulate gyrus
71 Superior frontal sulcus
72 Genu of the corpus callosum
73 Pericallosal artery

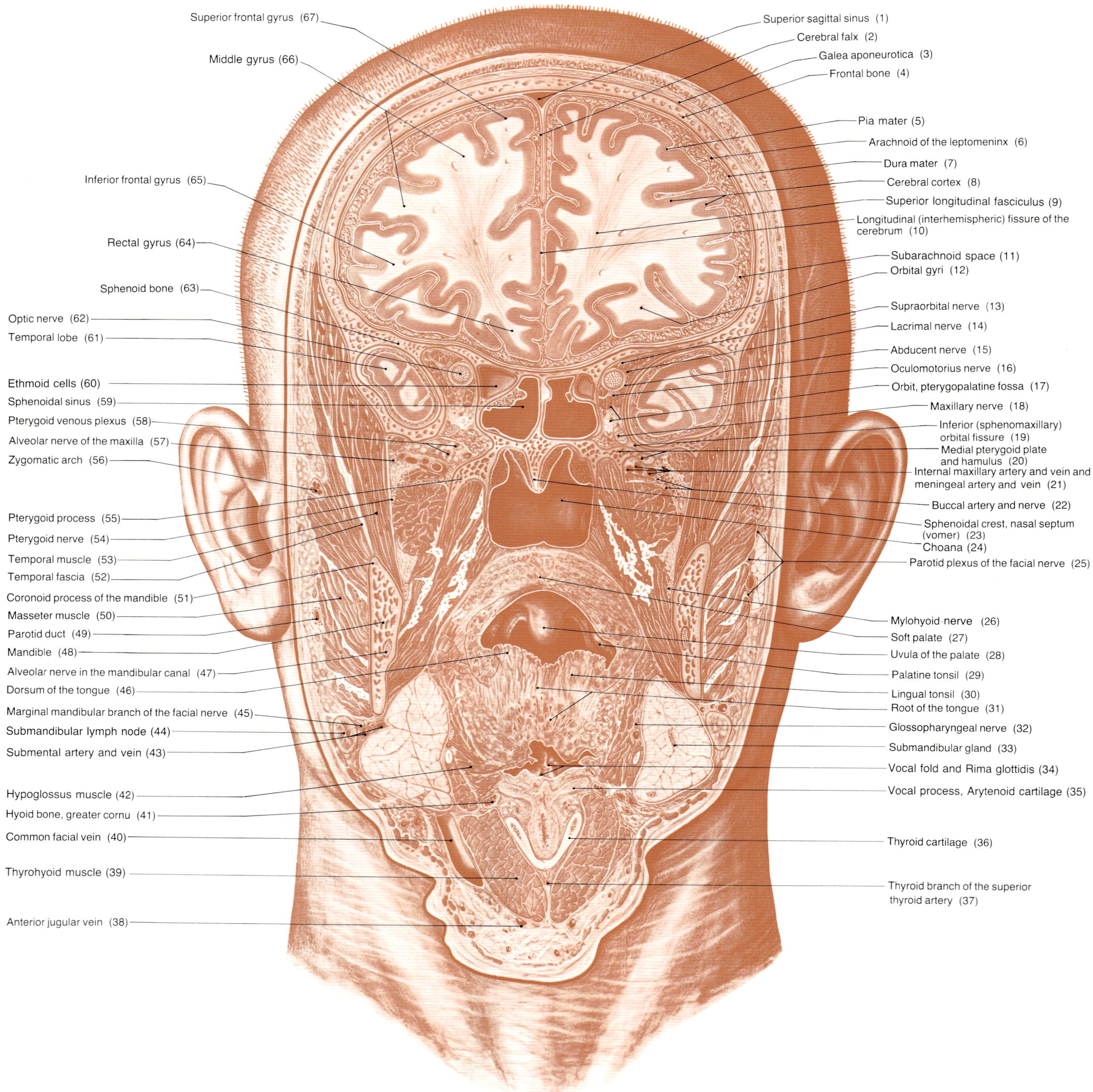

1 Sinus sagittalis superior
2 Falx cerebri
3 Galea aponeurotica
4 Os frontale
5 Pia mater leptomeninx
6 Arachnoidea leptomeninx
7 Dura mater
8 Cortex cerebri
9 Fasciculus longitudinalis superior
10 Fissura longitudinalis cerebri
11 Cavum subarachnoideale
12 Gyri orbitales
13 N. supraorbitalis
14 N. lacrimalis
15 N. abducens
16 N. oculomotorius
17 Orbita, Fossa pterygopalatina
18 N. maxillaris
19 Fissura orbitalis sphenomaxillaris inferior
20 Lamina perpendicularis et Hamulus pterygoideus
21 A. et V. maxillaris interna et A. et V. meningea
22 A. et N. buccalis
23 Crista sphenoidalis, Septum nasi (vomer)
24 Choana
25 Plexus parotideus n. facialis
26 N. mylohyoideus
27 Palatium molle
28 Uvula palatina
29 Tonsilla palatina
30 Tonsilla lingualis
31 Radix linguae
32 N. glossopharyngeus
33 Glandula submandibularis
34 Plica vocalis et Rima glottidis
35 Processus vocalis, Cartilago arytaenoidea
36 Cartilago thyroidea
37 R. thyroideus a. thyroidea superior
38 V. jugularis anterior
39 M. thyrohyoideus
40 V. facialis communis
41 Cornu majus ossis hyoidei
42 M. hypoglossus
43 A. et V. submentalis
44 Nodus lymphaticus submandibularis
45 R. marginalis mandibulae n. facialis
46 Dorsum linguae
47 N. alveolaris (canalis mandibulae)
48 Mandibula
49 Ductus parotideus
50 M. masseter
51 Processus coronoideus mandibulae
52 Fascia temporalis
53 M. temporalis
54 N. pterygoideus
55 Processus pterygoideus
56 Arcus zygomaticus
57 Nn. alveolaris et maxillaris
58 Plexus venosus pterygoideus
59 Sinus sphenoidalis
60 Cellulae ethmoidales
61 Lobus temporalis
62 N. opticus
63 Os sphenoidale
64 Gyrus rectus
65 Gyrus frontalis inferior
66 Gyrus frontalis medialis
67 Gyrus frontalis superior
67.1 M. pterygoideus lateralis
67.2 Nasopharynx
67.3 M. pterygoideus medialis
68 Gyrus praecentralis
69 Gyrus temporalis superior
70 Corpus callosum
71 Insula
72 Nucleus caudatus
73 Cornu anterius ventriculi lateralis
74 Gyrus cinguli

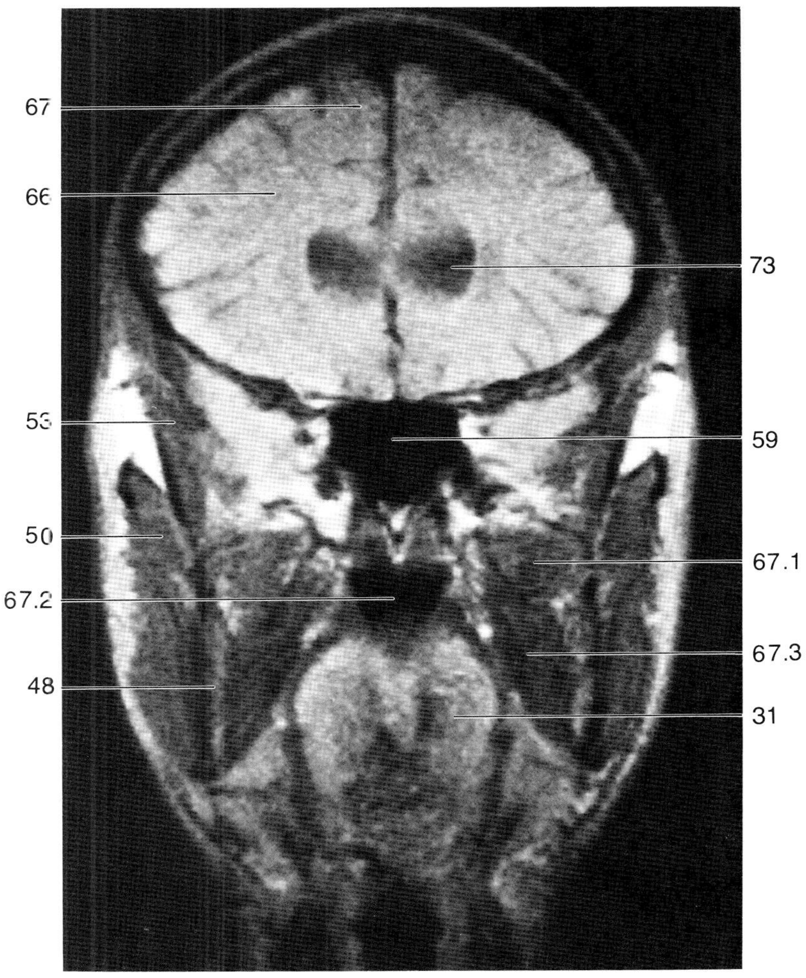

MRI, SE 1100/50

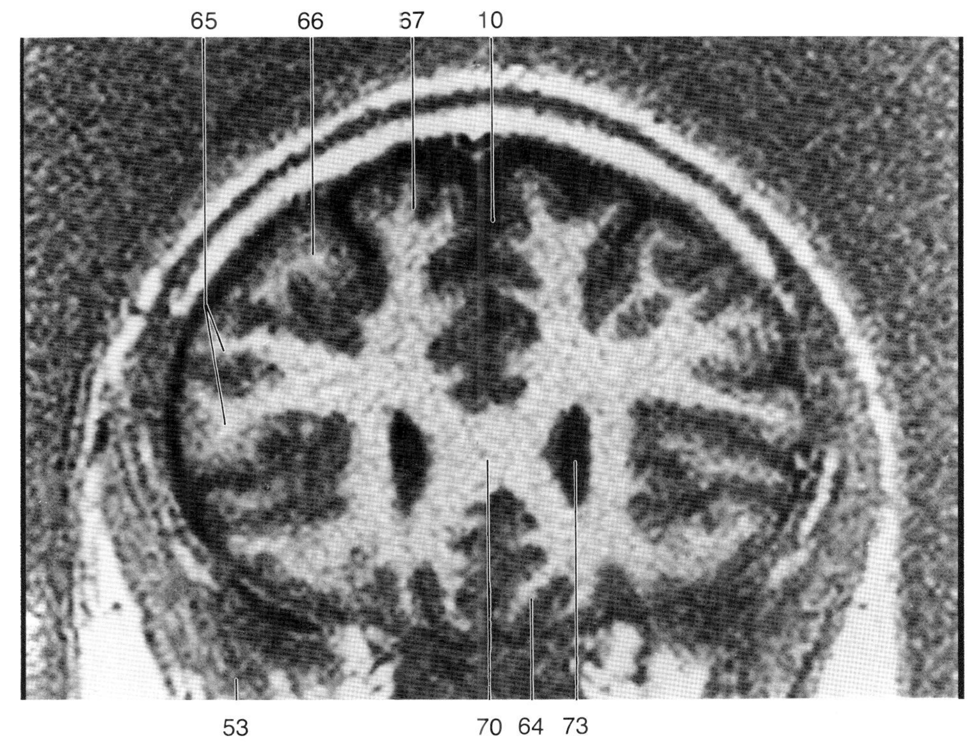

MRI, IR 1800/400/30, level 4

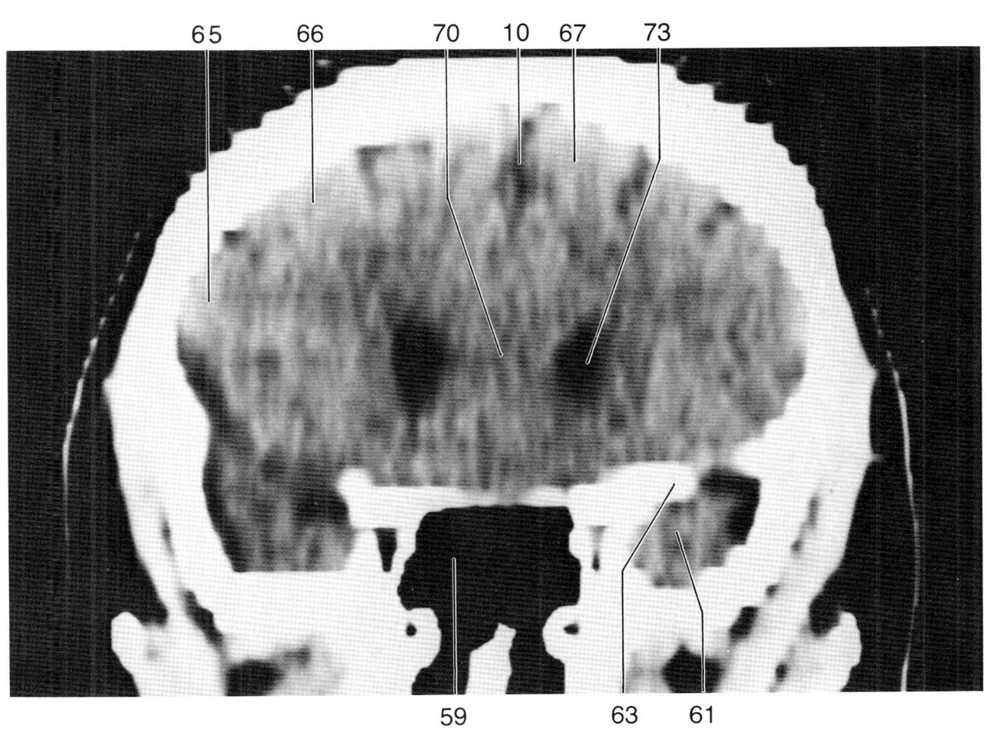

CT, coronal reconstruction, level 3

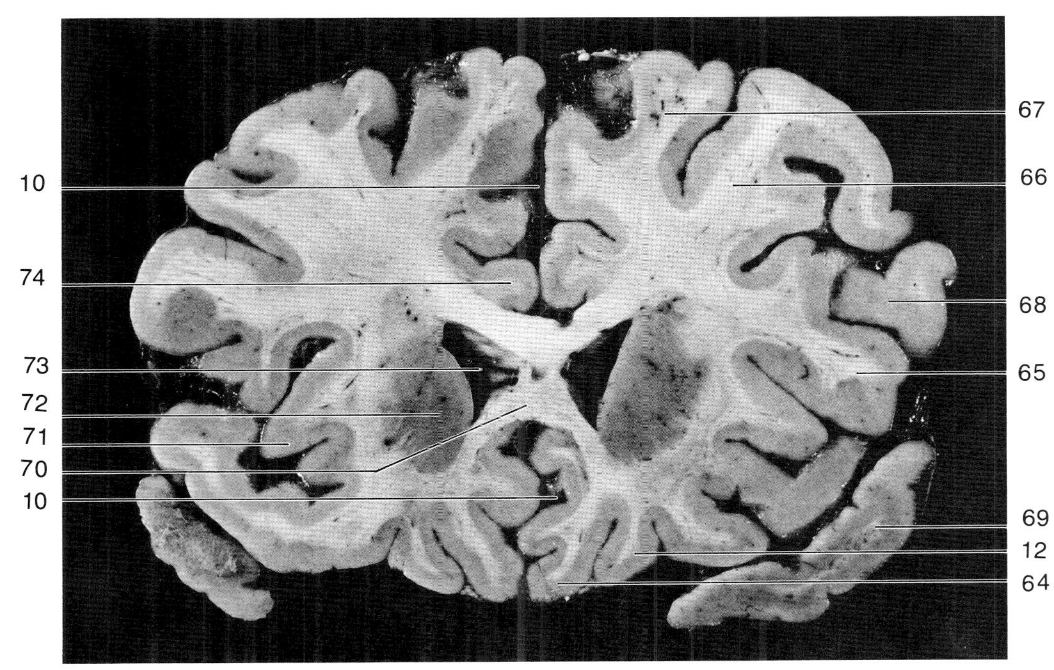

Anatomical section at level 3–4

10 Longitudinal fissure
12 Orbital gyrus
31 Root of the tongue
48 Mandible
50 Masseter muscle
53 Temporal muscle
59 Sphenoidal sinus
61 Temporal lobe
63 Sphenoid bone
64 Rectal gyrus
65 Inferior frontal gyrus
66 Middle frontal gyrus
67 Superior frontal gyrus
67.1 Lateral pterygoid muscle
67.2 Nasopharynx
67.3 Medial pterygoid muscle
68 Precentral gyrus
69 Superior temporal gyrus
70 Corpus callosum
71 Insula
72 Caudate nucleus
73 Anterior horn of the lateral ventricle
74 Cingulate gyrus

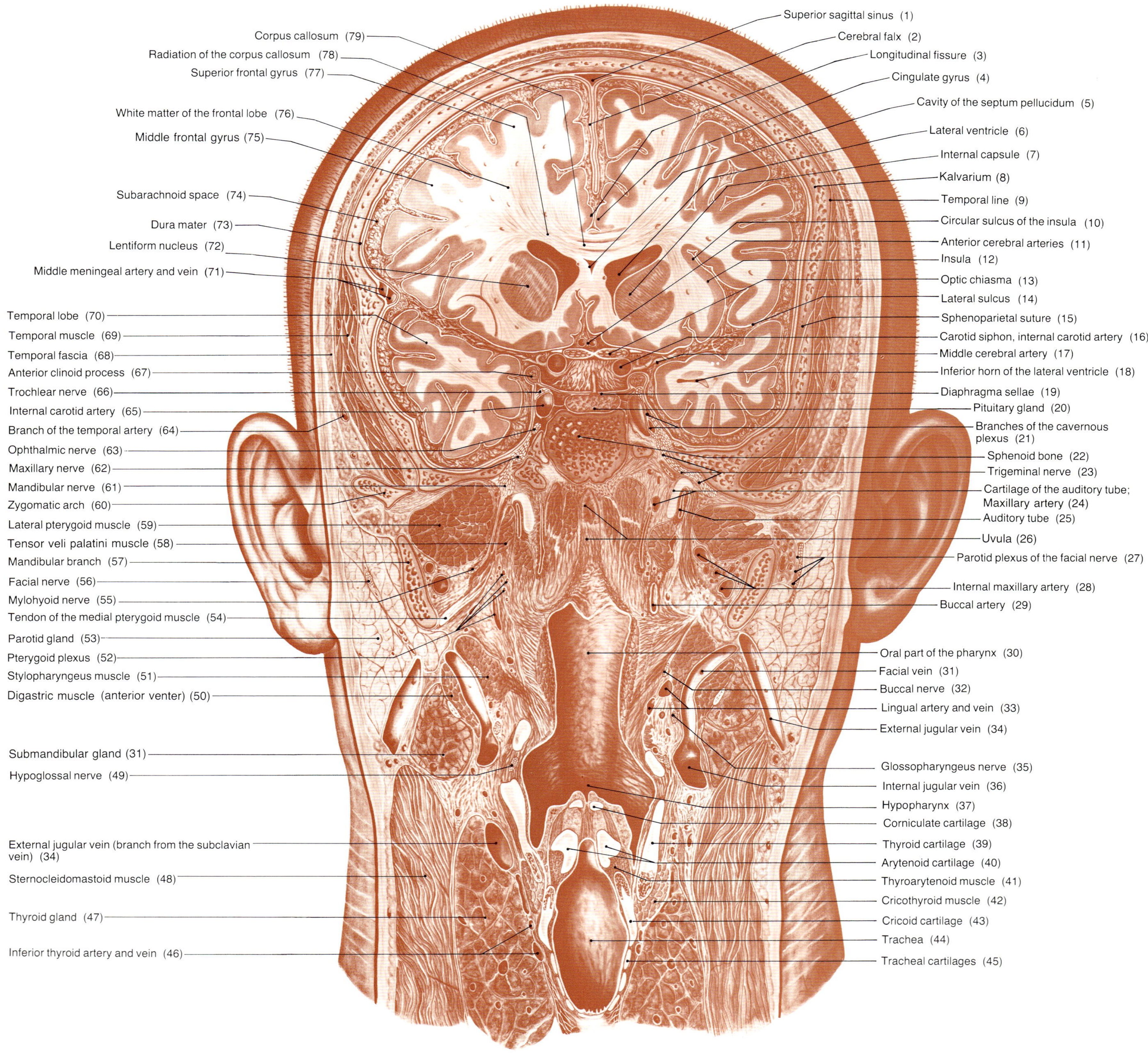

1 Sinus sagittalis superior
2 Falx cerebri
3 Fissura longitudinalis
4 Gyrus cinguli
5 Cavum septi pellucidi
6 Ventriculus lateralis
7 Capsula interna
8 Calvarium
9 Linea temporalis
10 Sulcus circularis insulae
11 Aa. cerebri anteriores
12 Insula
13 Chiasma opticum
13.1 Nasopharynx
14 Fissura lateralis
15 Sutura sphenoparietalis
16 A. carotis interna
17 A. cerebri media
18 Cornu inferius ventriculi lateralis
19 Diaphragma sellae
20 Glandula pituitaria
21 Rr. plexus cavernosus
22 Os sphenoidale
23 N. trigeminus
24 Cartilago tubae auditivae
25 Tuba auditiva
26 Uvula
27 Plexus parotideus n. facialis
28 A. maxillaris
29 A. buccalis
30 Pars oralis pharyngis
31 Glandula submandibularis
32 N. buccalis
33 A. et V. lingualis
34 V. jugularis externa
35 N. glossopharyngeus
36 V. jugularis interna
37 Hypopharynx
38 Cartilago corniculata
39 Cartilago thyroidea
40 Cartilago arytaenoidea
41 M. thyroarytaenoideus
42 M. cricothyroideus
43 Cartilago cricoidea
44 Trachea
45 Cartilagines tracheales
46 A. et V. thyroidea inferior
47 Glandula thyroidea
48 M. sternocleidomastoideus
49 M. hypoglossus
50 M. digastricus (Venter anterior)
51 M. stylopharyngeus
52 Plexus pterygoideus
52.1 M. masseter
52.2 M. pterygoideus medialis
53 Glandula parotis
54 Tendo m. pterygoidei medialis
55 N. mylohyoideus
56 N. facialis
57 R. mandibularis
58 M. tensor veli palatini
59 M. pterygoideus lateralis
60 Arcus zygomaticus
61 N. mandibularis
62 N. maxillaris
63 N. ophthalmicus
64 R. a. temporalis
65 A. carotis interna
66 N. trochlearis
67 Processus clinoideus anterior
68 Fascia temporalis
69 M. temporalis
70 Lobus temporalis
71 A. et V. meningea media
72 Nucleus lentiformis
73 Dura mater
74 Cavum subarachnoidea
75 Gyrus frontalis medius
76 Substantia alba lobi frontalis
77 Gyrus frontalis superior
78 Radiatio corporis callosi
79 Corpus callosum
80 Operculum frontale
81 Capsula externa
82 Gyrus frontalis inferior
83 Gyrus temporalis superior
84 Gyrus orbitalis
85 Gyrus temporalis medius
86 Gyrus rectus
87 Nucleus caudatus
88 Putamen
89 Cornu anterius ventriculi lateralis
90 Septum pellucidum
91 Cisterna laminae terminalis

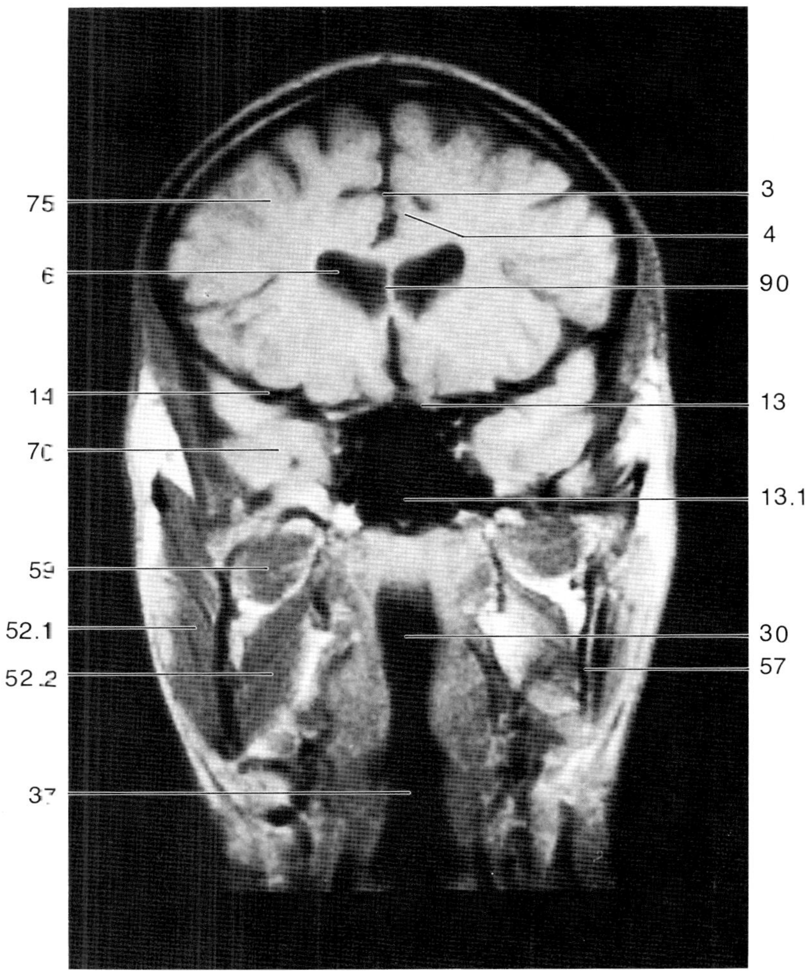

MRI, SE 600/30

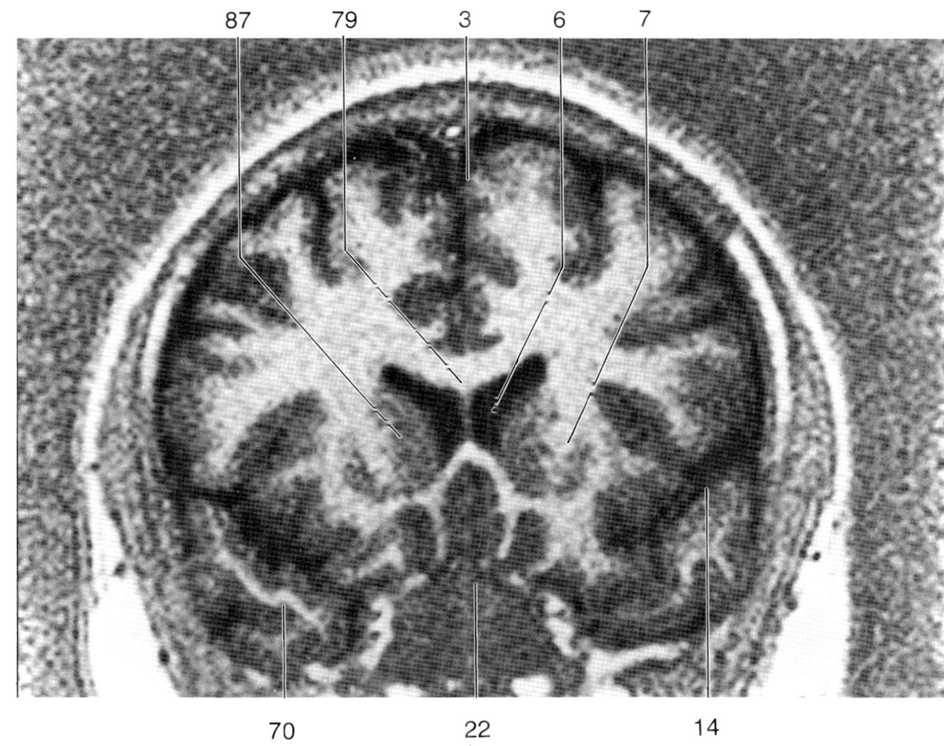

MRI, IR 1800/400/30, level 5

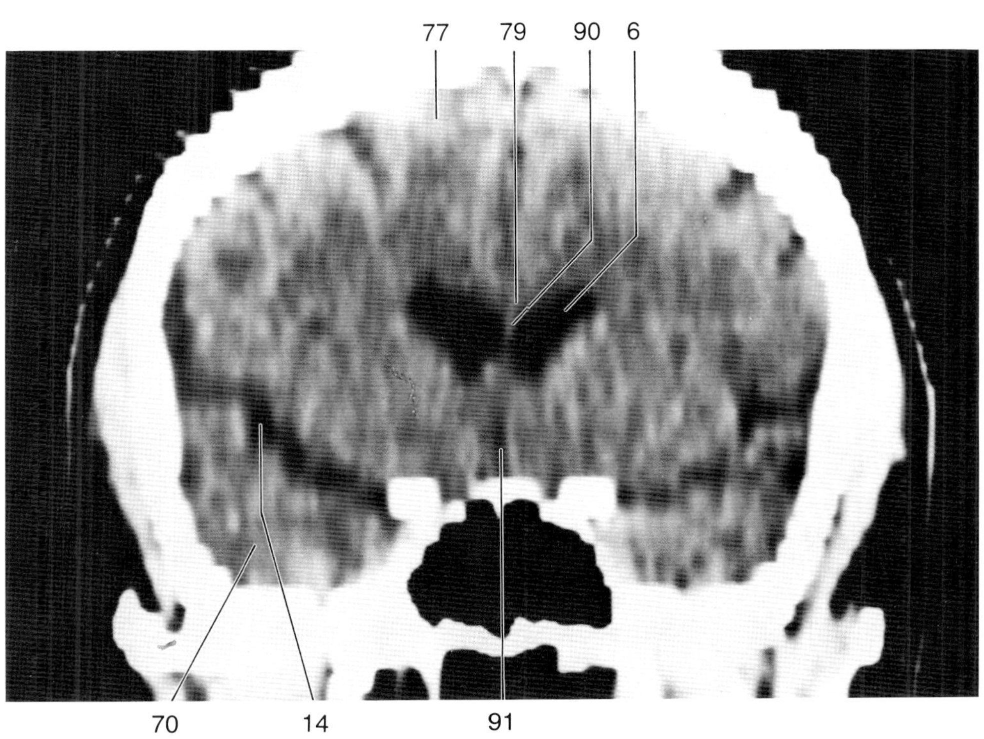

CT, coronal reconstruction, level 4

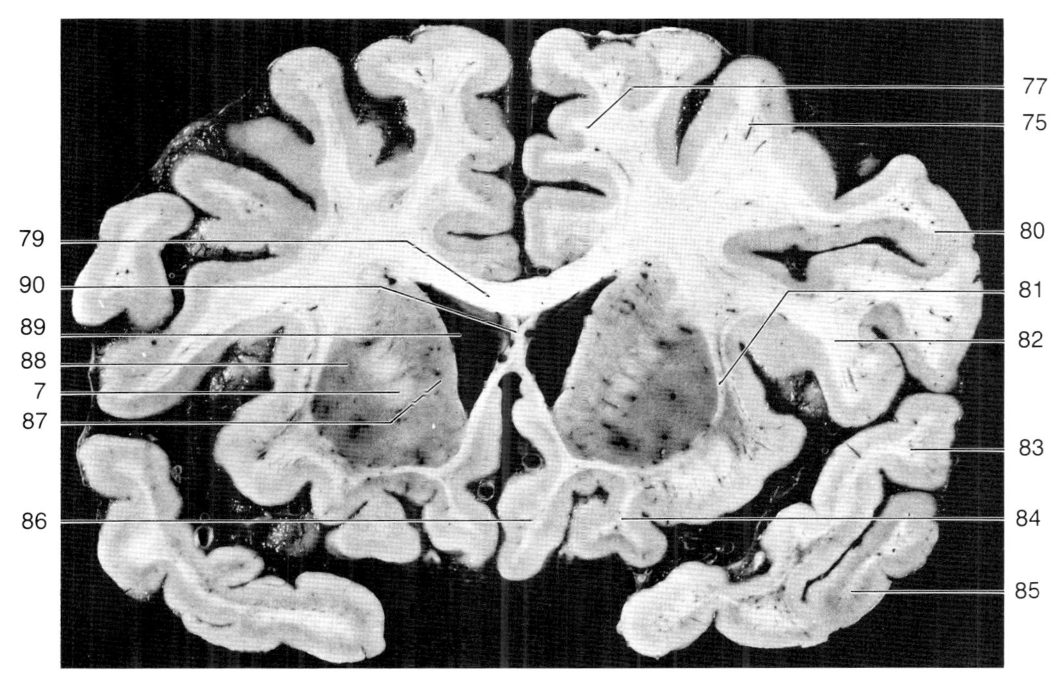

Anatomical section at level 4–5

- 3 Longitudinal fissure
- 4 Cingulate gyrus
- 6 Lateral ventricle
- 7 Internal capsule
- 13 Optic chiasma
- 13.1 Nasopharynx
- 14 Lateral fissure
- 22 Sphenoid bone
- 30 Oral part of the pharynx
- 37 Hypopharynx
- 52.1 Masseter muscle
- 52.2 Medial pterygoid muscle
- 57 Mandibular branch
- 59 Lateral pterygoid muscle
- 70 Temporal lobe
- 75 Medial frontal gyrus
- 77 Superior frontal gyrus
- 79 Corpus callosum
- 80 Frontal operculum
- 81 External capsule
- 82 Inferior frontal gyrus
- 83 Superior temporal gyrus
- 84 Orbital gyrus
- 85 Middle temporal gyrus
- 86 Rectal gyrus
- 87 Caudate nucleus
- 88 Putamen
- 89 Anterior horn of the lateral ventricle
- 90 Septum pellucidum
- 91 Cistern of the lamina terminalis

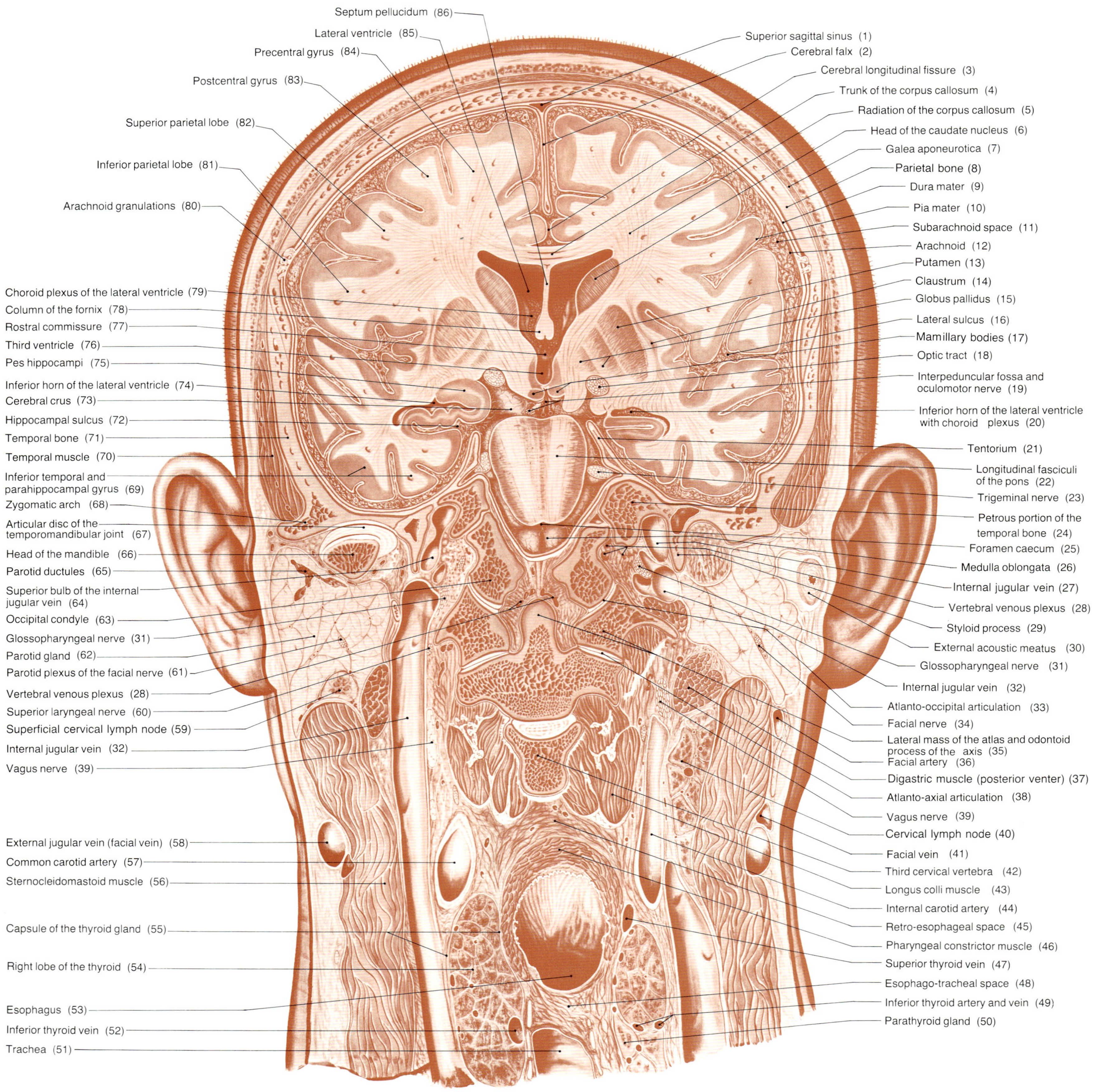

1 Sinus sagittalis superior
2 Falx cerebri
3 Fissura longitudinalis cerebri
4 Truncus corporis callosi
5 Radiatio corporis callosi
6 Caput nuclei caudati
7 Galea aponeurotica
8 Os frontale
9 Dura mater
10 Pia mater
11 Cavum subarachnoideale
12 Arachnoidea
13 Putamen
14 Claustrum
15 Globus pallidus
16 Sulcus lateralis
17 Corpora maxillaria
18 Chiasma opticum
19 Fossa interpeduncularis et N. oculomotorius
20 Cornu inferius (ventr. lat.), Plexus choroideus
21 Tentorium
22 Fasciculi longitudinales pontis
23 N. trigeminus
24 Pars petrosa ossis temporalis
25 Foramen caecum
26 Medulla oblongata
27 V. jugularis interna
28 Plexus venosus vertebralis
29 Processus styloideus
30 Meatus acusticus externus
31 N. glossopharyngeus
32 V. jugularis interna
33 Articulatio atlantooccipitalis
34 N. facialis
35 Massa lateralis atlantis, Dens axis
36 A. facialis
37 M. digastricus (Venter posterior)
38 Articulatio atlantoaxialis
39 N. vagus
40 Nodi lymphatici colli
41 V. facialis
42 Vertebra cervicalis III
43 M. longus colli
44 A. carotis interna
45 Spatium retrooesophageale
46 M. constrictor pharyngis
47 V. thyroidea superior
48 Spatium oesophagotracheale
49 A. et V. thyroidea inferior
50 Glandula parathyroidea
51 Trachea
52 V. thyroidea inferior
53 Oesophagus
54 Glandula thyroidea, Lobus dexter
55 Glandula thyroidea, Capsula propria
56 M. sternocleidomastoideus
57 A. carotis communis
58 V. jugularis externa (V. facialis)
59 Nodi lymphatici cervicales superficiales
60 N. laryngeus superior
61 Plexus parotideus facialis
62 Glandula parotis
63 Condylus occipitalis
64 Bulbus superior v. jugularis internae
65 Ductuli glandulae parotidis
66 Caput mandibulae
67 Discus articularis articulationis temporomandibularis
68 Arcus zygomaticus
69 Gyri temporalis inferior et parahippocampalis
70 M. temporalis
71 Os temporale
72 Sulcus hippocampi
73 Crus cerebri
74 Cornu inferius ventriculi lateralis
75 Pes hippocampi
76 Ventriculus III
77 Commissura rostralis
78 Columna fornicis
79 Plexus choroideus ventriculi lateralis
80 Granulationes arachnoideales
81 Lobus parietalis inferior
82 Lobus parietalis superior
83 Gyrus postcentralis
84 Gyrus praecentralis
85 Ventriculus lateralis
86 Septum pellucidum
87 Gyrus frontalis superior
88 Gyrus frontalis medius
89 Gyrus temporalis superior
90 Gyrus hippocampi
91 Gyrus temporalis medius
92 Massa intermedia
93 Capsula interna
94 Fornix
95 Nucleus caudatus
96 Gyrus cinguli
97 Gyrus temporalis inferior
98 Cisterna chiasmatis

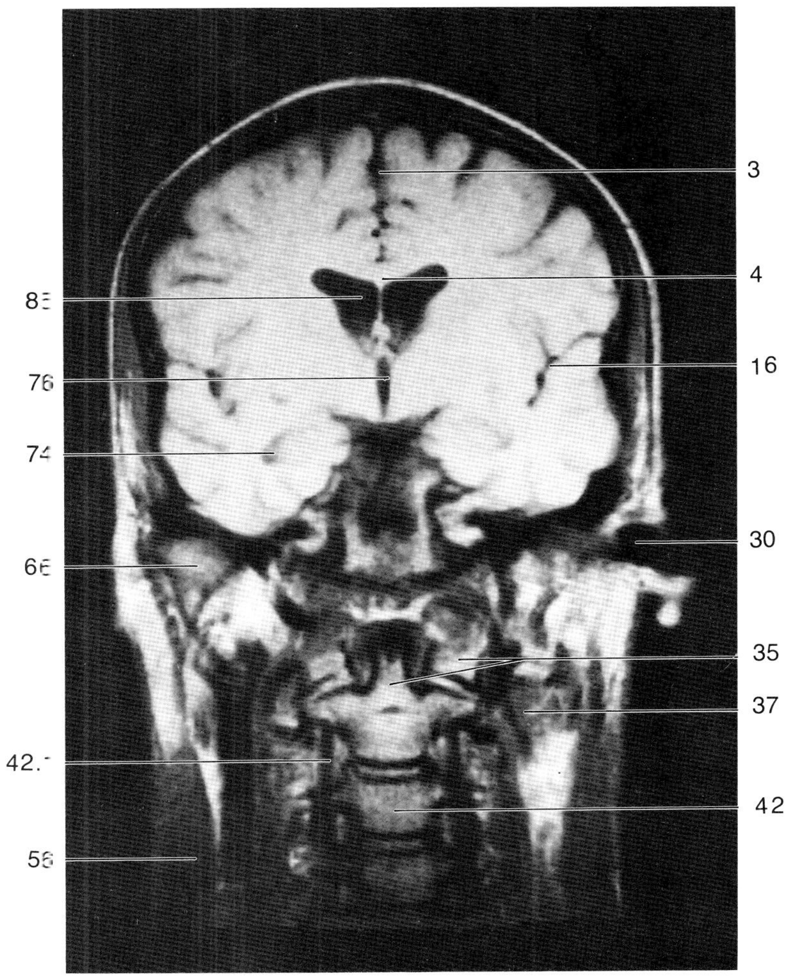

MRI, SE 600/30

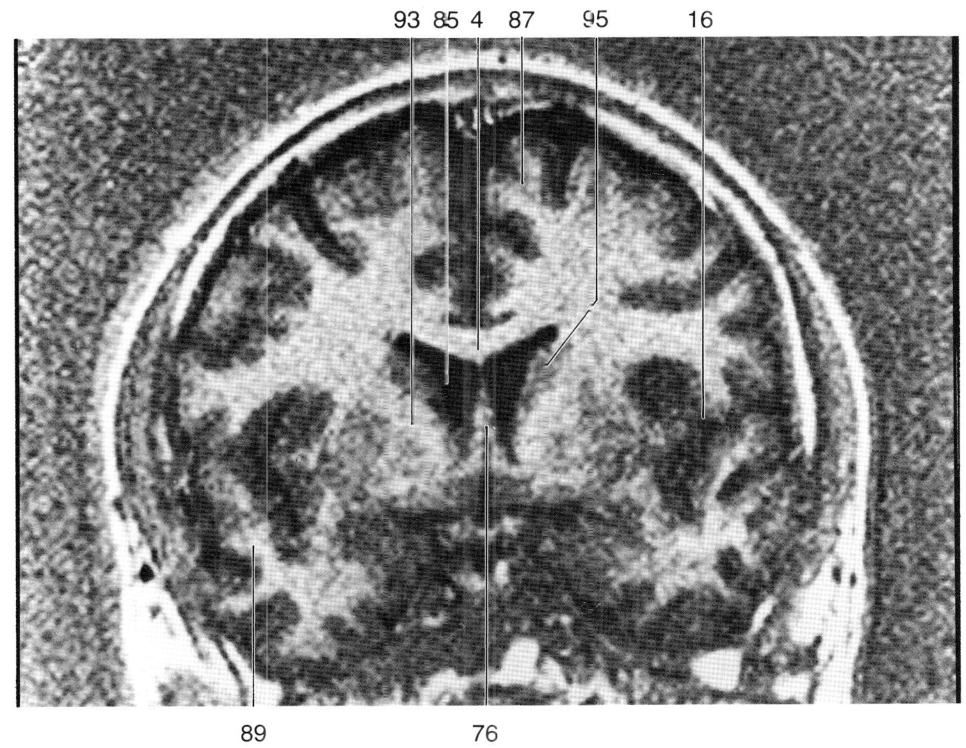

MRI, IR 1800/400/30, level 6

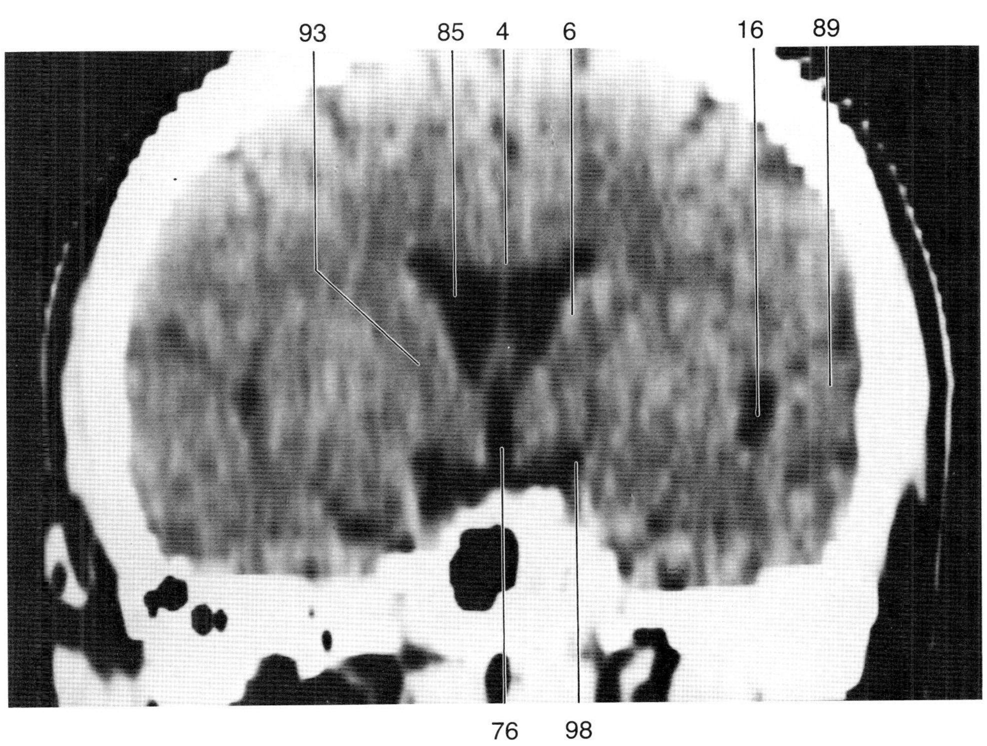

CT, coronal reconstruction, level 5

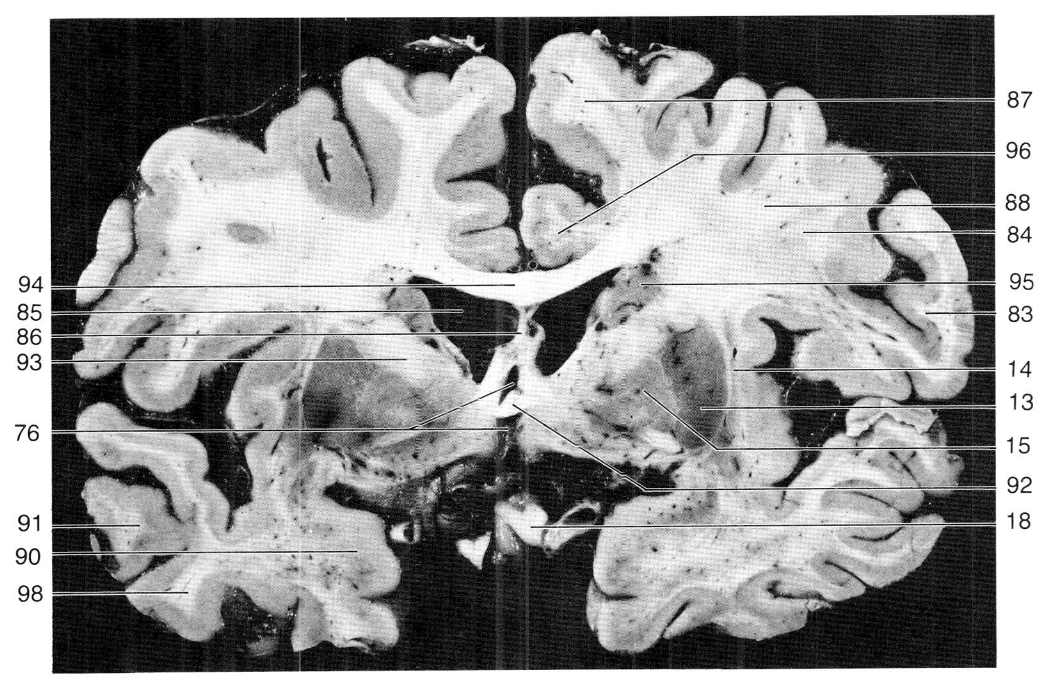

Anatomical section at level 5–6

3 Cerebral longitudinal fissure
4 Corpus callosum
6 Head of the caudate nucleus
13 Putamen
14 Claustrum
15 Globus pallidus
16 Lateral fissure
18 Optic chiasm
30 External acoustic meatus
35 Lateral mass of the atlas and odontoid process of the axis
37 Digastric muscle (posterior venter)
42 Third cervical vertebra
42.1 Vertebral artery
56 Sternocleidomastoid muscle
66 Head of the mandible
74 Inferior horn of the lateral ventricle
76 Third ventricle
83 Postcentral gyrus
84 Precentral gyrus
85 Lateral ventricle
86 Septum pellucidum
87 Superior frontal gyrus
88 Middle frontal gyrus
89 Superior temporal gyrus
90 Hippocampal gyrus
91 Middle temporal gyrus
92 Massa intermedia
93 Internal capsule
94 Fornix
95 Caudate nucleus
96 Cingulate gyrus
98 Chiasmatic cistern

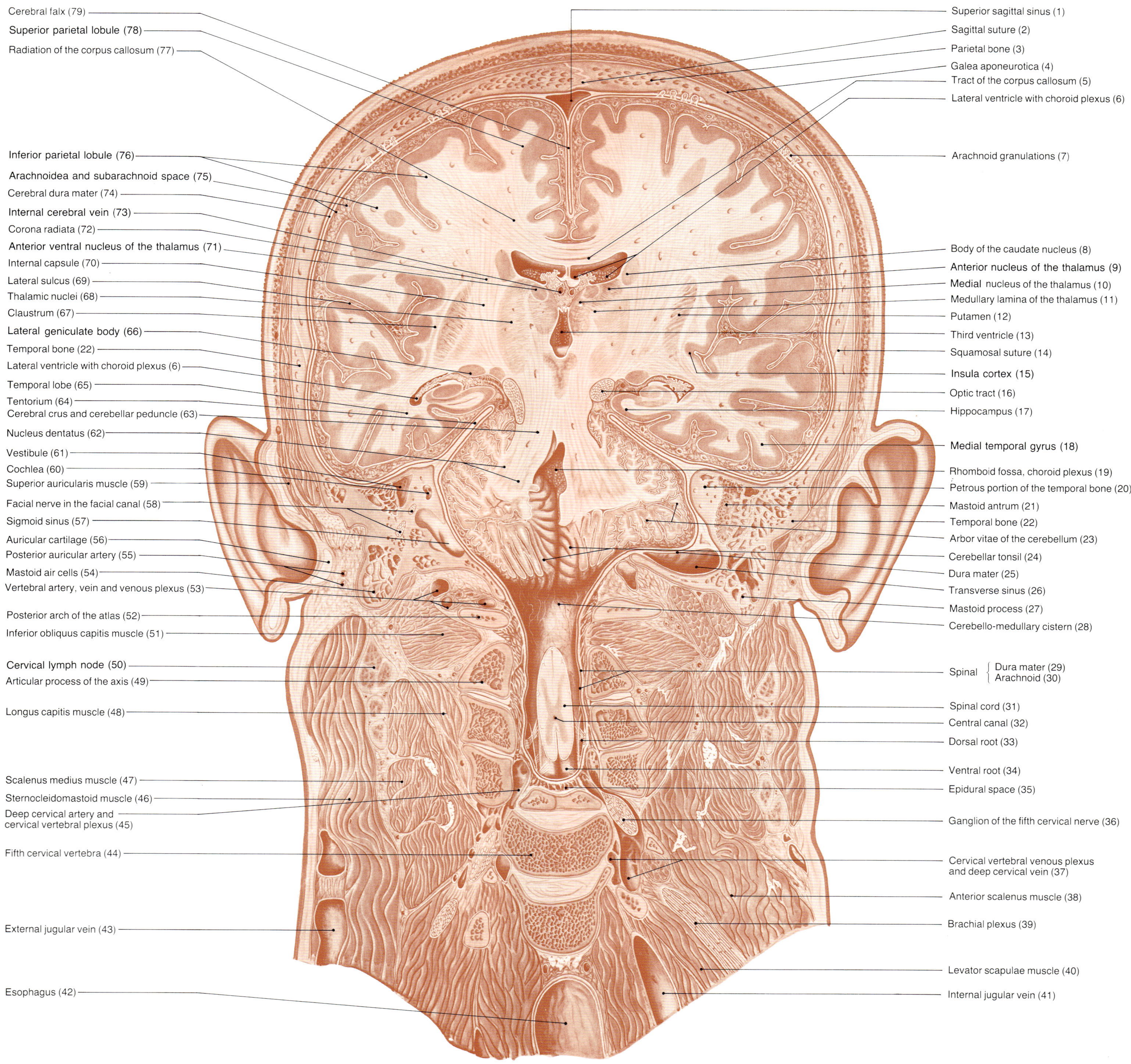

1 Sinus sagittalis superior
2 Sutura sagittalis
3 Os parietale
4 Galea aponeurotica
5 Tractus corporis callosi
6 Plexus choroideus ventriculi lateralis
7 Granulationes arachnoideales
8 Corpus nuclei caudati
9 Nucleus anterior thalami
10 Nucleus medialis thalami
11 Lamina medullaris thalami
12 Putamen
13 Ventriculus III
14 Sutura squamosa
15 Cortex insulae
16 Tractus opticus
17 Hippocampus
17.1 Pons
18 Gyrus temporalis medius
19 Fossa rhomboidea, Plexus choroideus
19.1 Ventriculus IV
20 Pars petrosa ossis temporalis
21 Antrum mastoideum
22 Os temporale
23 Arbor vitae cerebelli
24 Tonsilla cerebelli
24.1 Medulla oblongata
25 Dura mater
26 Sinus transversus
27 Processus mastoideus
28 Cisterna cerebellomedullaris
29 Dura mater spinalis
30 Arachnoidea spinalis
31 Medulla spinalis
32 Canalis centralis
33 Radix dorsalis
34 Radix ventralis
35 Spatium epidurale
36 Ganglion n. cervicalis V
37 Plexus venosus vertebralis cervicalis et V. cervicalis profunda
38 M. scalenus anterior
39 Plexus brachialis
40 M. levator scapulae
41 V. jugularis interna
42 Oesophagus
43 V. jugularis externa
44 Vertebra cervicalis V
45 A. cervicalis profunda et Plexus venosus vertebralis cervicalis
46 M. sternocleidomastoideus
47 M. scalenus medius
48 M. longus capitis
49 Processus articularis axis
50 N. lymphaticus
51 M. obliquus capitis inferior
51.1 Cerebellum
51.2 Pedunculus cerebellaris
52 Arcus posterior atlantis
53 A. et V. vertebralis et Plexus venosus
54 Cellulae mastoideae
55 A. auricularis posterior
56 Cartilago auriculae
57 Sinus sigmoideus
58 N. facialis
59 M. auriculus superior
60 Cochlea
61 Vestibulum
62 Nucleus dentatus
63 Crus cerebri, Pedunculus cerebellaris
64 Tentorium
65 Lobus temporalis
66 Corpus geniculatum laterale
67 Claustrum
68 Nucleus lateralis thalami
69 Sulcus lateralis
70 Capsula interna
71 Nucleus anteroventralis thalami
72 Corona radiata
73 V. cerebri interna
74 Dura mater cerebri
75 Arachnoidea et Cavum subarachnoideale
76 Lobulus parietalis inferior
76.1 Sulcus cinguli
77 Radiatio corporis callosi
78 Lobulus parietalis superior
79 Falx cerebri
80 Lobulus paracentralis
80.1 Splenium corporis callosi
81 Gyrus cinguli
82 Gyrus praecentralis
83 Gyrus postcentralis
84 Nucleus caudatus
85 Gyrus postcentralis
86 Globus pallidus
87 Commissura anterior
88 Gyrus temporalis superior
89 Gyrus temporalis inferior
90 Corpora mamillaria
91 Gyrus temporalis medius
92 Fornix
93 Massa intermedia

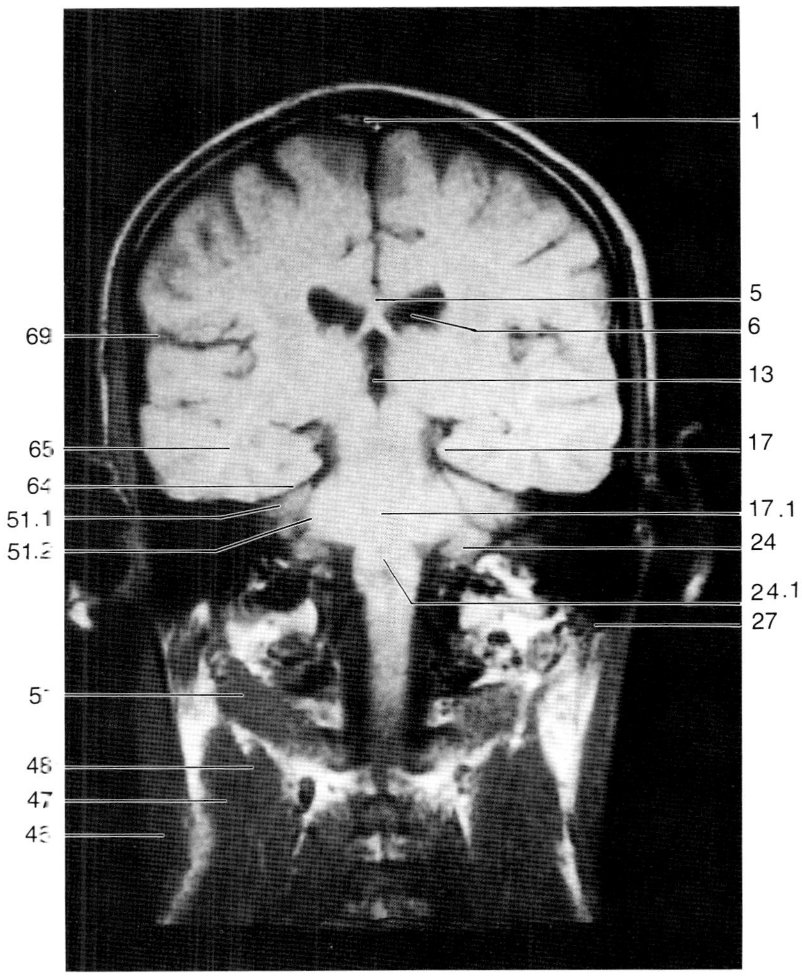

MRI, SE 600/30

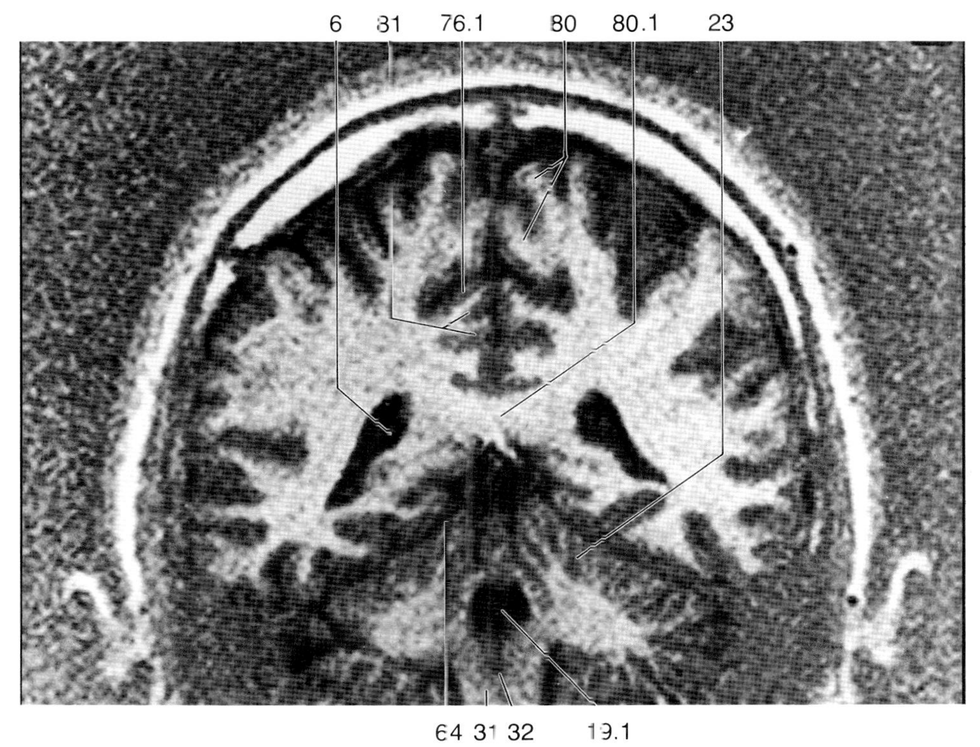

MRI, IR 1800/400/30, level 7

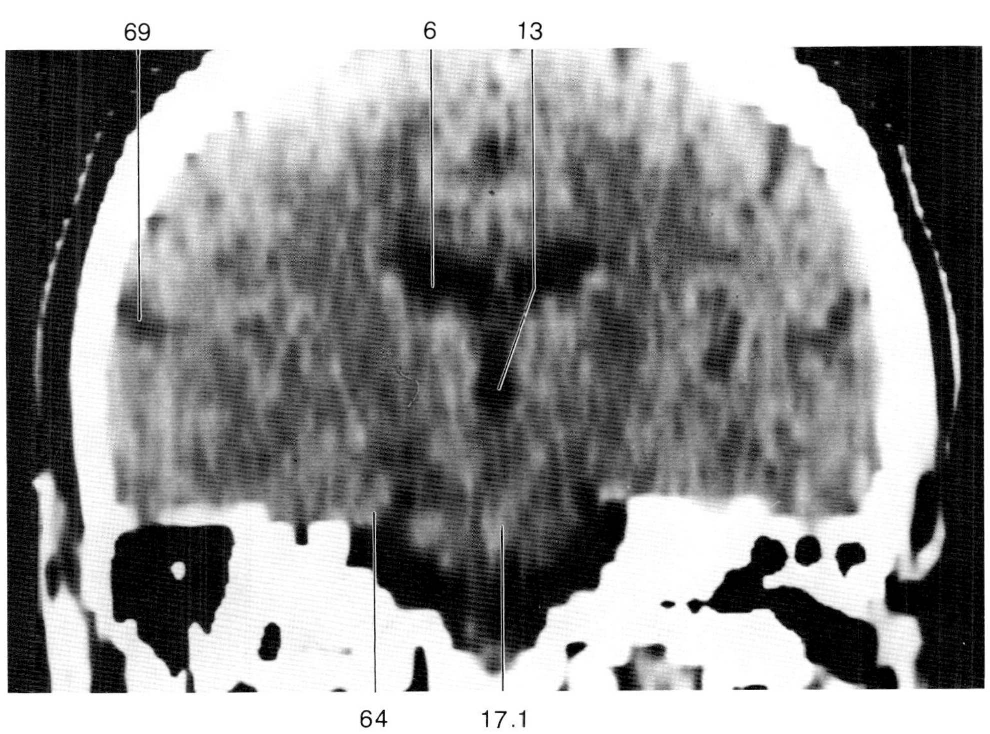

CT, coronal reconstruction, level 6

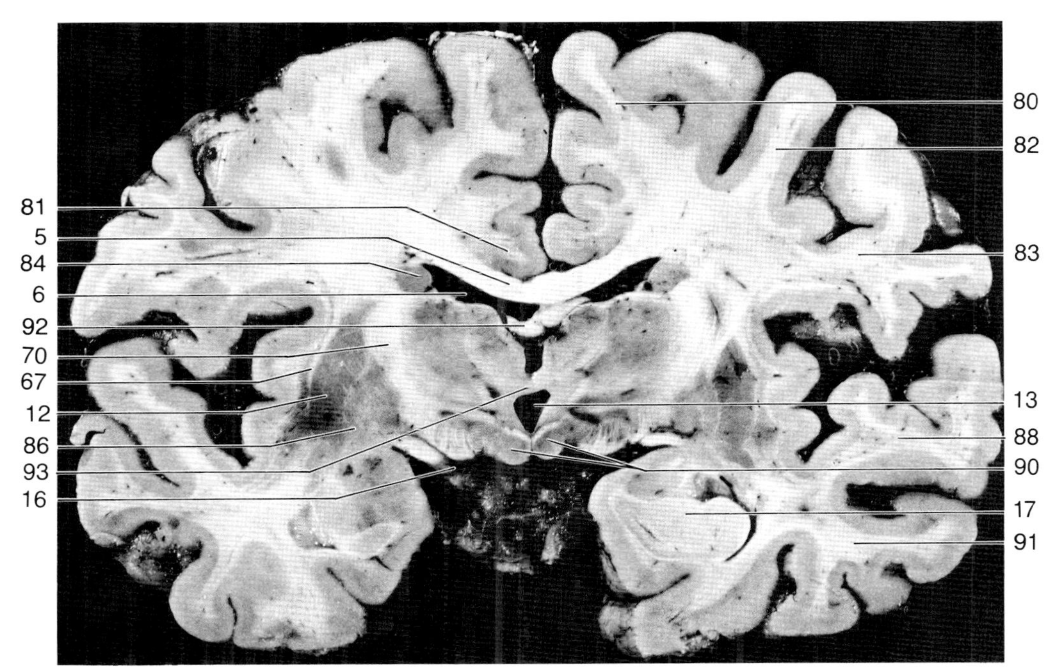

Anatomical section at level 6

1 Superior sagittal sinus
5 Trunk of the corpus callosum
6 Lateral ventricle with choroid plexus
12 Putamen
13 Third ventricle
16 Optic tract
17 Hippocampus
17.1 Pons
19.1 Fourth ventricle
23 Arbor vitae of the cerebellum
24 Cerebellar tonsil
24.1 Medulla oblongata
27 Mastoid process
31 Spinal cord
32 Central canal
46 Sternocleidomastoid muscle
47 Scalenus medius muscle
48 Longus capitis muscle
51 Inferior obliquus capitis muscle
51.1 Cerebellum
51.2 Cerebellar peduncle
64 Tentorium
65 Temporal lobe
67 Claustrum
69 Lateral sulcus
70 Internal capsule
76.1 Cingulate sulcus
80 Paracentral lobule
80.1 Splenium of the corporis callosum
81 Cingulate gyrus
82 Precentral gyrus
83 Postcentral gyrus
84 Caudate nucleus
86 Globus pallidus
88 Superior temporal gyrus
90 Mamillary bodies
91 Middle temporal gyrus
92 Fornix
93 Massa intermedia

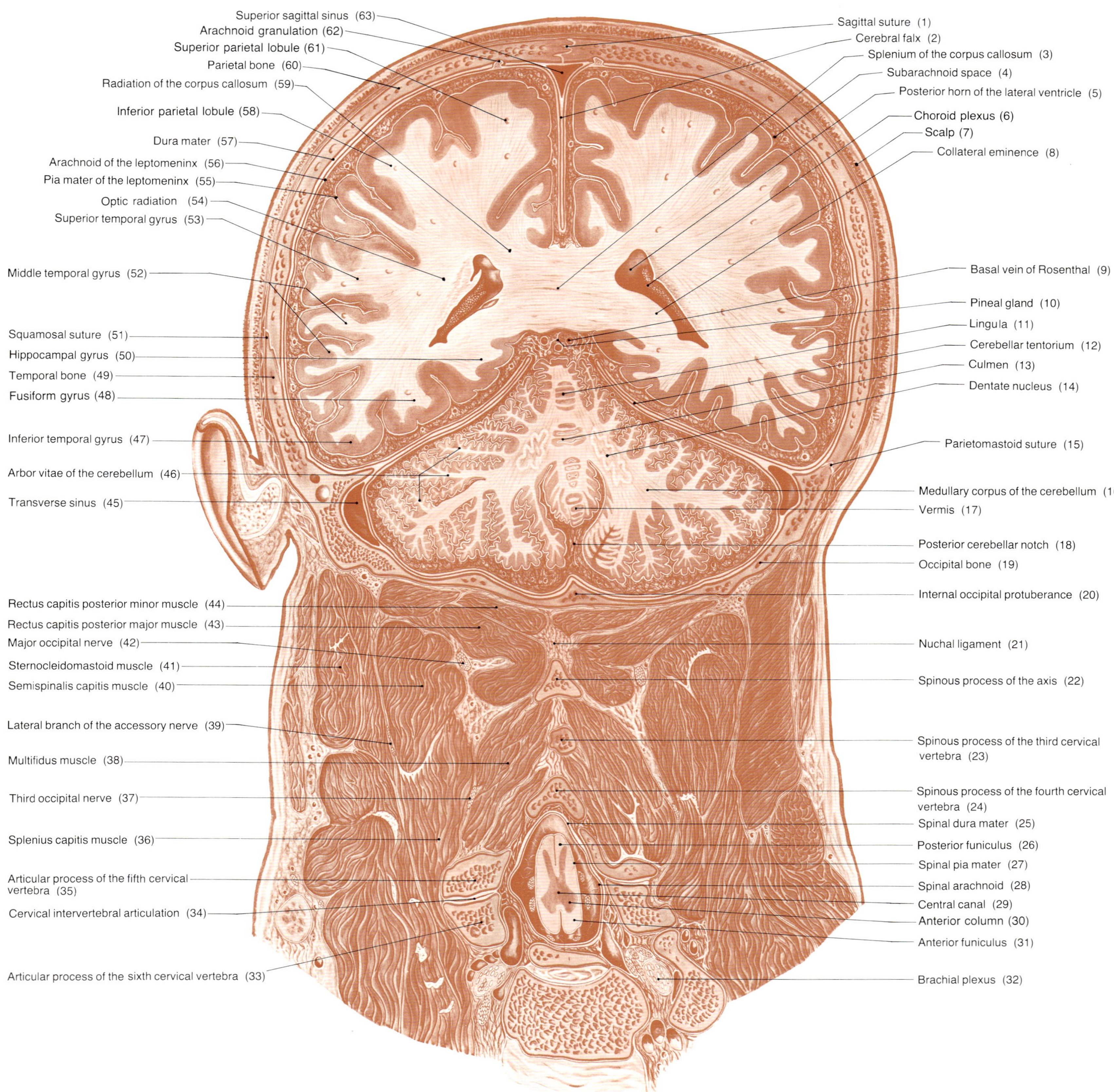

1 Sutura sagittalis
2 Falx cerebri
3 Splenium corporis callosi
4 Cavum subarachnoideale
5 Cornu posterius ventriculi lateralis
6 Plexus choroideus
7 Epicranium
8 Eminentia collateralis
9 V. basalis (Rosenthali)
10 Corpus pineale
11 Lingula
12 Tentorium cerebelli
12.1 Ventriculus IV
13 Culmen
14 Nucleus dentatus
15 Sutura parietomastoidea
16 Corpus medullare cerebelli
17 Vermis
18 Incisura cerebelli posterior
19 Os occipitale
20 Protuberantia occipitalis interna
21 Lig. nuchae
22 Processus spinosus axis
23 Processus spinosus vertebrae cervicalis III
24 Processus spinosus vertebrae cervicalis IV
25 Dura mater spinalis
26 Funiculus dorsalis
27 Pia mater spinalis
28 Arachnoidea spinalis
29 Canalis centralis
30 Columna anterior
31 Funiculus anterior
32 Plexus brachialis
33 Processus articularis vertebrae cervicalis VI
34 Articulatio intervertebralis cervicis
35 Processus articularis vertebrae cervicalis V
36 M. splenius capitis
37 N. occipitalis tertius
38 M. multifidus
39 R. lateralis n. accessorii
40 M. semispinalis capitis
40.1 M. obliquus inferior
41 M. sternocleidomastoideus
41.1 M. levator scapulae
42 N. occipitalis major
43 M. rectus capitis posterior major
43.1 Cisterna cerebellaris superior
43.2 Fissurae cerebellares
44 M. rectus capitis posterior minor
45 Sinus transversus
46 Arbor vitae cerebelli
47 Gyrus temporalis inferior
48 Gyrus occipitotemporalis
49 Os temporale
50 Gyrus hippocampi
51 Sutura squamosa
52 Gyrus temporalis medius
53 Gyrus temporalis superior
54 Radiatio optica
55 Leptomeninx (Pia mater)
56 Leptomeninx (Arachnoidea)
57 Dura mater
58 Lobulus parietalis inferior
59 Radiatio corporis callosi
60 Os parietale
61 Lobulus parietalis superior
62 Granulatio arachnoidealis
63 Sinus sagittalis superior
64 Lobulus paracentralis
64.1 Sulcus centralis
65 Gyrus postcentralis
65.1 Sulcus postcentralis
66 Gyrus cinguli
67 Corpus callosum
68 Gyrus fusiformis
69 Pons
70 Substantia nigra
71 Pedunculus cerebralis
72 Nucleus ruber
73 Ventriculus III
74 Putamen
75 Capsula interna
76 Thalamus
77 Ventriculus lateralis

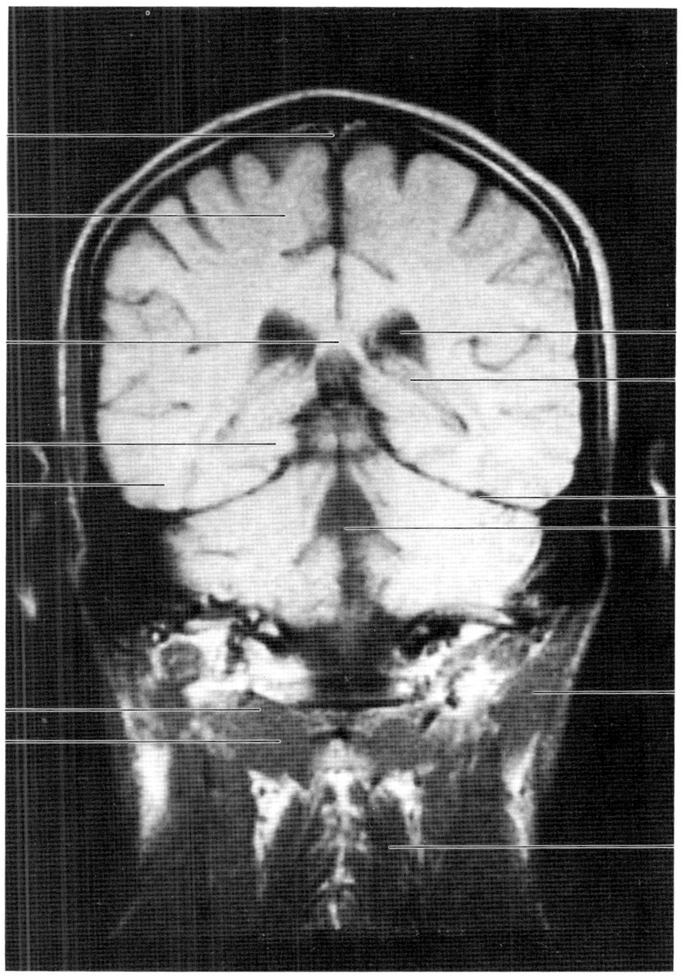

MRI, SE 600/30

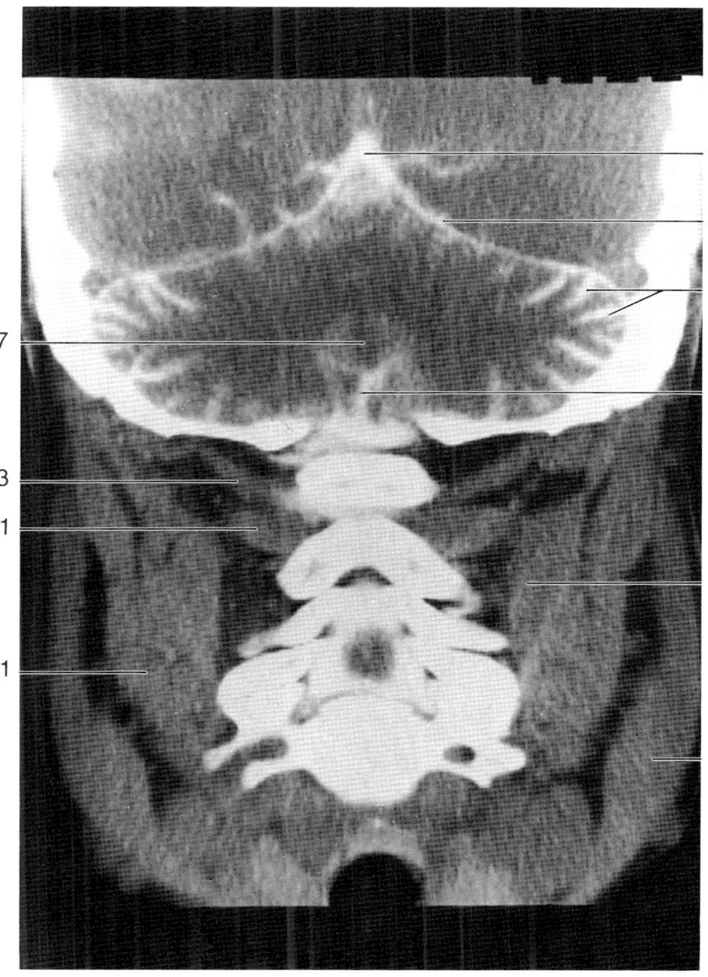

CT with contrast enhancement of the subarachnoid space

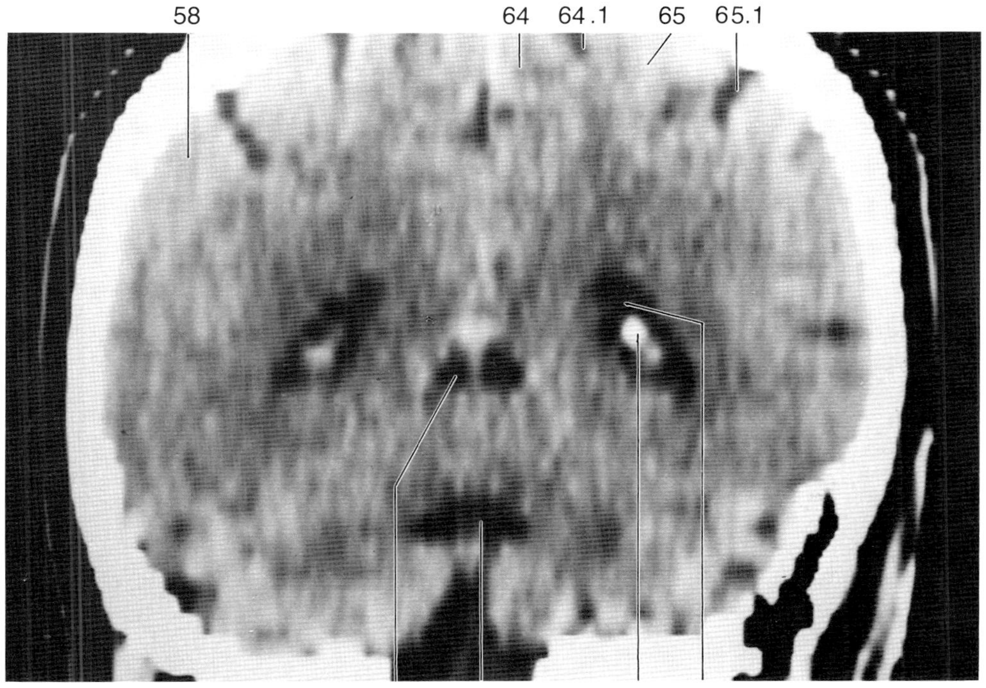

CT, coronal reconstruction, level 7

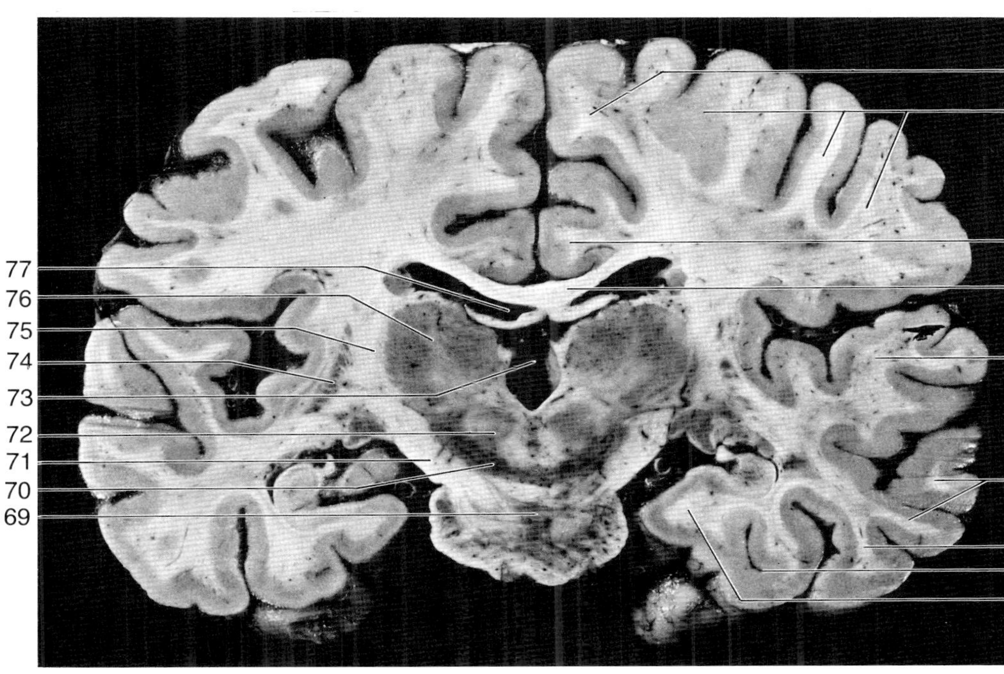

Anatomical section at the level of the third ventricle

3 Splenium of the corpus callosum
5 Posterior horn of the lateral ventricle
6 Choroid Plexus
12 Cerebellar tentorium
12.1 Fourth ventricle
17 Vermis
18 Posterior cerebellar notch
38 Multifidus muscle
40 Semispinalis capitis muscle
40.1 Inferior oblique muscle
41 Sternocleidomastoid muscle
41.1 Levator scapulae muscle
43 Rectus capitis posterior major muscle
43.1 Superior cerebellar cistern
43.2 Cerebellar fissures
44 Rectus capitis posterior minor muscle
47 Inferior temporal gyrus
50 Hippocampal gyrus
52 Middle temporal gyrus
53 Superior temporal gyrus
58 Inferior parietal lobule
61 Superior parietal lobule
63 Superior sagittal sinus
64 Paracentral lobule
64.1 Central sulcus
65 Postcentral gyrus
65.1 Postcentral sulcus
66 Cingulate gyrus
67 Corpus callosum
68 Fusiform gyrus
69 Pons
70 Substantia nigra
71 Cerebral peduncle
72 Red nucleus
73 Third ventricle
74 Putamen
75 Internal capsule
76 Thalamus
77 Lateral ventricle

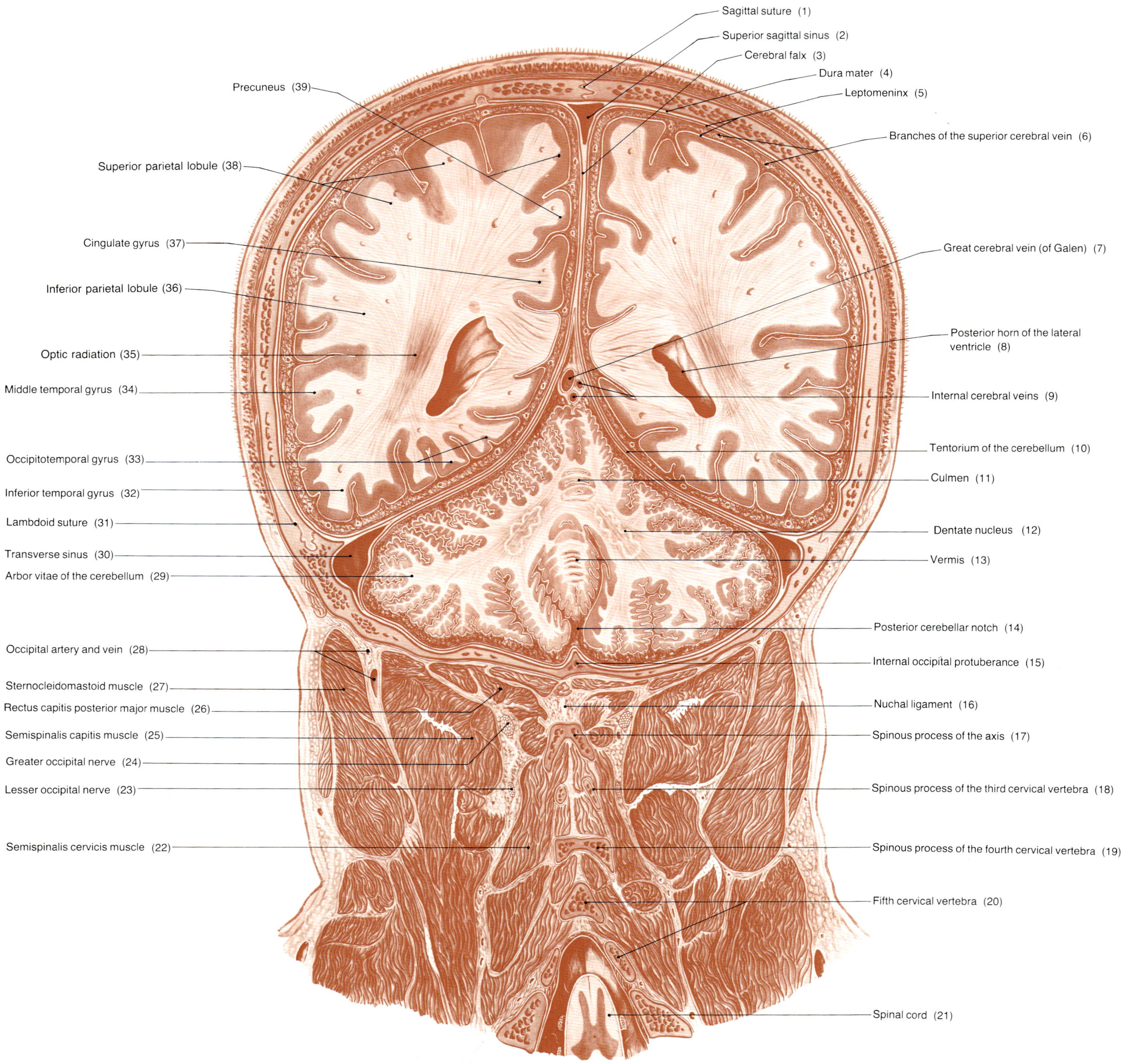

1 Sutura sagittalis
2 Sinus sagittalis superior
3 Falx cerebri
4 Dura mater
5 Leptomeninx
6 Rr. venae cerebri superioris
7 V. cerebri magna (Galeni)
8 Cornu posterius ventriculi lateralis
9 Vv. cerebri internae
10 Tentorium cerebelli
11 Culmen
12 Nucleus dentatus
13 Vermis
13.1 Cisterna cerebellaris superior
14 Incisura cerebelli posterior
15 Protuberantia occipitalis interna
16 Lig. nuchae
17 Processus spinosus axis
18 Processus spinosus vertebrae cervicalis III
19 Processus spinosus vertebrae cervicalis IV
20 Vertebra cervicalis V
21 Medulla spinalis
22 M. semispinalis cervicis
23 N. occipitalis minor
24 N. occipitalis major
25 M. semispinalis capitis
26 M. rectus capitis posterior major
27 M. sternocleidomastoideus
27.1 Sulcus calcarinus
27.2 Fissurae cerebellaris
28 A. et V. occipitalis
29 Arbor vitae cerebelli
30 Sinus transversus
31 Sutura lambdoidea
32 Gyrus temporalis inferior
33 Gyrus occipitotemporalis
34 Gyrus temporalis medius
35 Radiatio optica
36 Lobulus parietalis inferior
37 Gyrus cinguli
38 Lobulus parietalis superior
39 Praecuneus
40 Lobulus paracentralis
41 Gyrus postcentralis
42 Gyrus temporalis superior
43 Corpus pineale
44 Aquaeductus cerebri
45 Gyrus hippocampi
46 Gyrus fusiformis
47 Pedunculus cerebellaris medius
48 Pons
49 Pes hippocampi (Cornu ammonis)
50 Colliculus inferior
51 Colliculus superior
52 Pulvinar
53 Fornix
54 Ventriculus lateralis
55 Corpus callosum

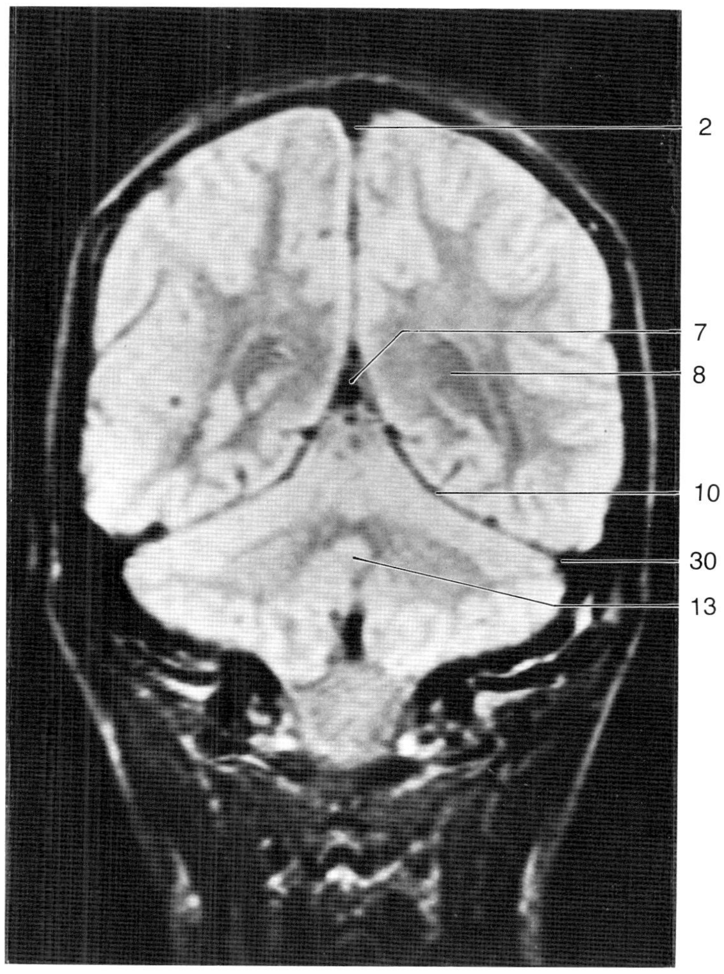

MRI, SE 2000/50

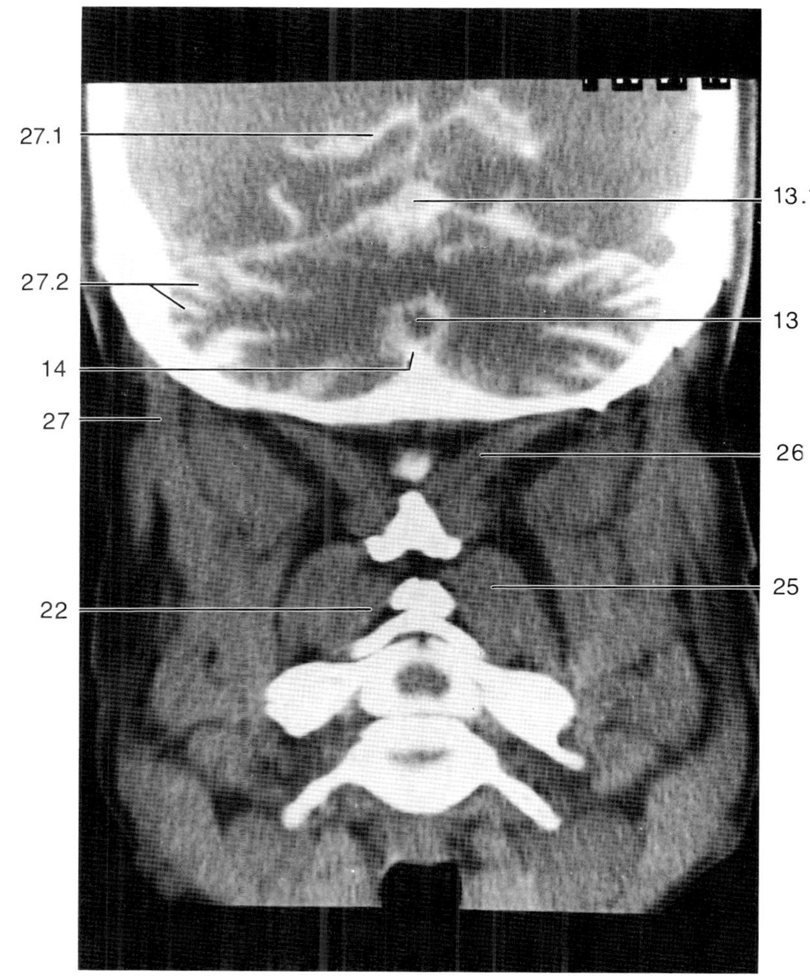

CT with contrast enhancement of the subarachnoid space

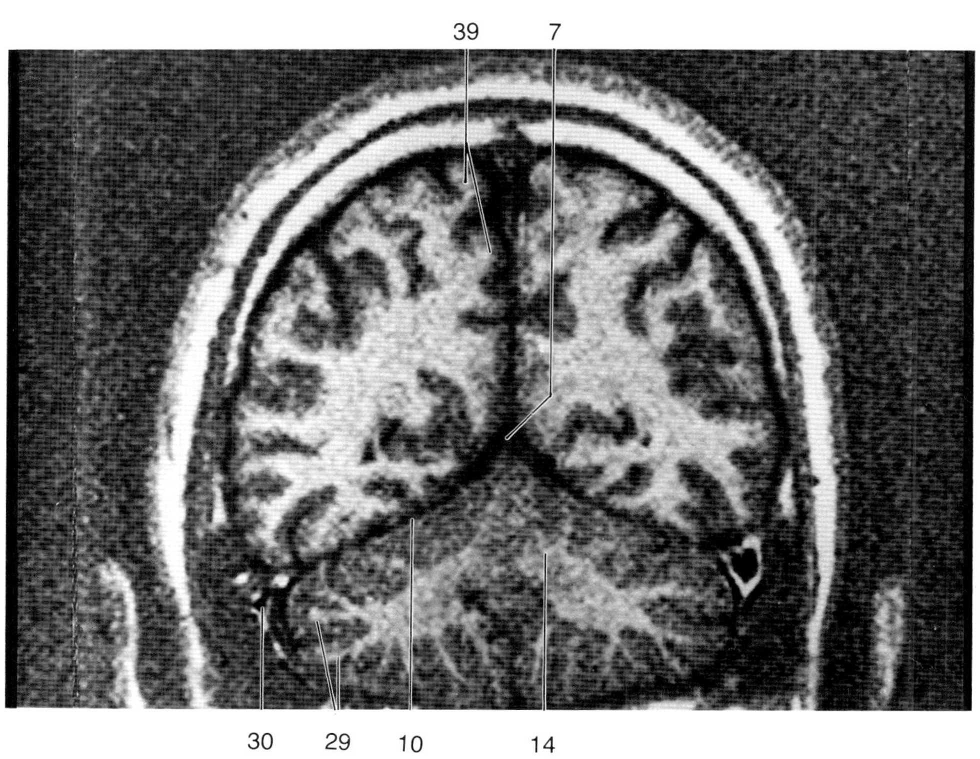

MRI, IR 1800/400/30, level 8

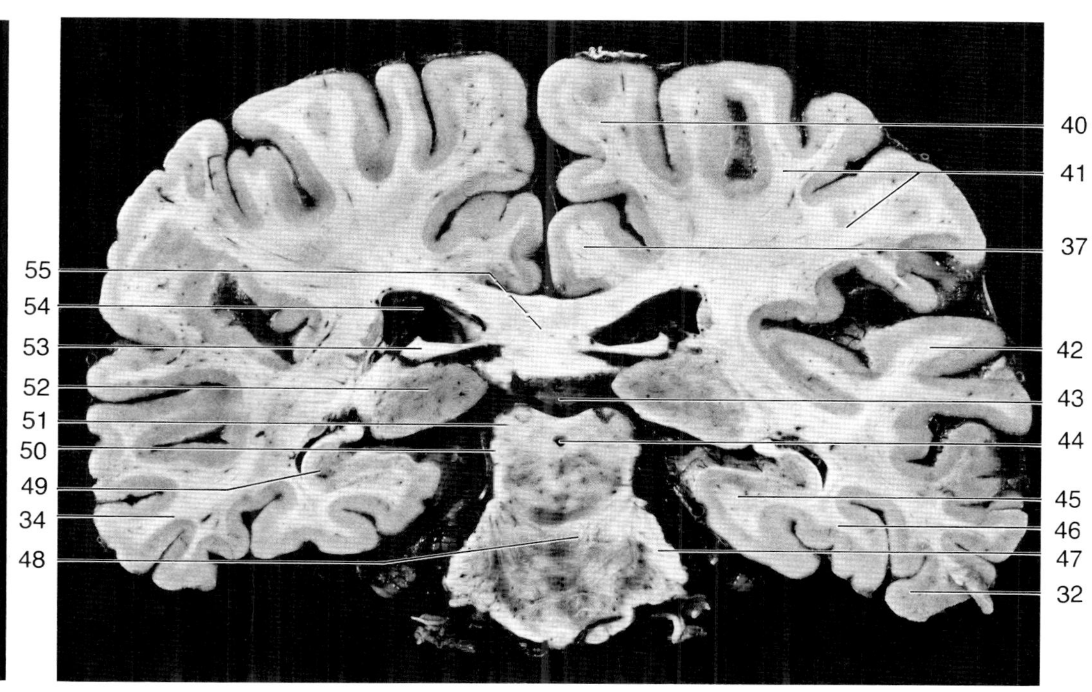

Anatomical section at the level of the pons

2 Superior sagittal sinus
7 Great cerebral vein (of Galen)
8 Posterior horn of the lateral sinus
10 Tentorium of the cerebellum
13 Vermis
13.1 Superior cerebellar cistern
14 Posterior cerebellar notch
22 Semispinalis cervicis muscle
25 Semispinalis capitis muscle
26 Rectus capitis posterior major muscle
27 Sternocleidomastoid muscle
27.1 Calcarine sulcus
27.2 Cerebellar fissures
29 Arbor vitae of the cerebellum
30 Transverse sinus
32 Inferior temporal gyrus
34 Middle temporal gyrus
37 Cingulate gyrus
39 Precuneus
40 Paracentral lobule
41 Postcentral gyrus
42 Superior temporal gyrus
43 Pineal body
44 Aqueduct
45 Hippocampal gyrus
46 Fusiform gyrus
47 Middle cerebellar peduncle
48 Pons
49 Pes hippocampi (Ammon's horn)
50 Inferior colliculus
51 Superior colliculus
52 Pulvinar
53 Fornix
54 Lateral ventricle
55 Corpus callosum

Anatomical Sections and Coronal Reconstructions of the Brain

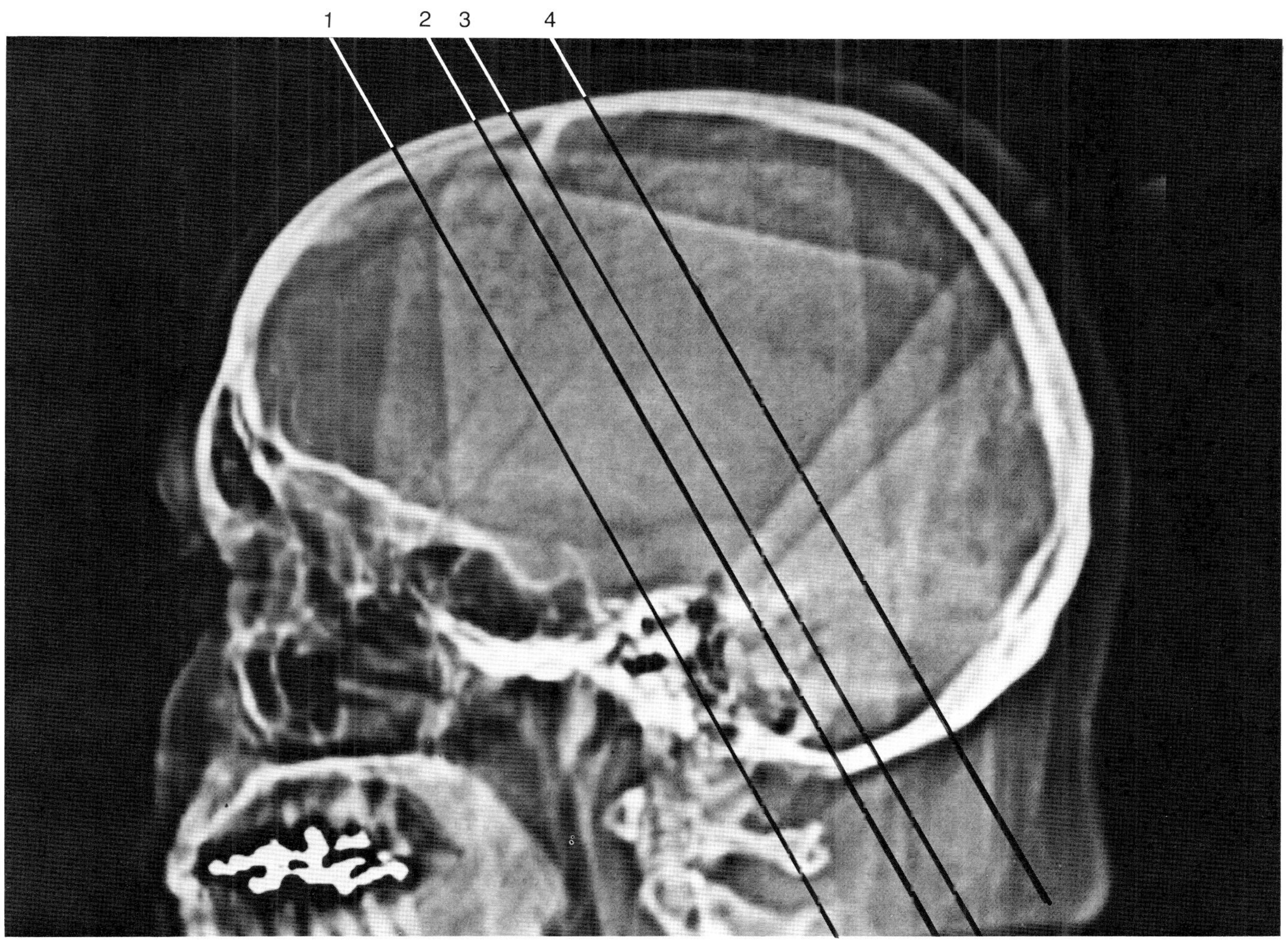

Lateral computed radiograph. Site of coronal reconstructions with 50° angulation from the canthomeatal line at levels no. 1–4. Slice thickness 1 mm.

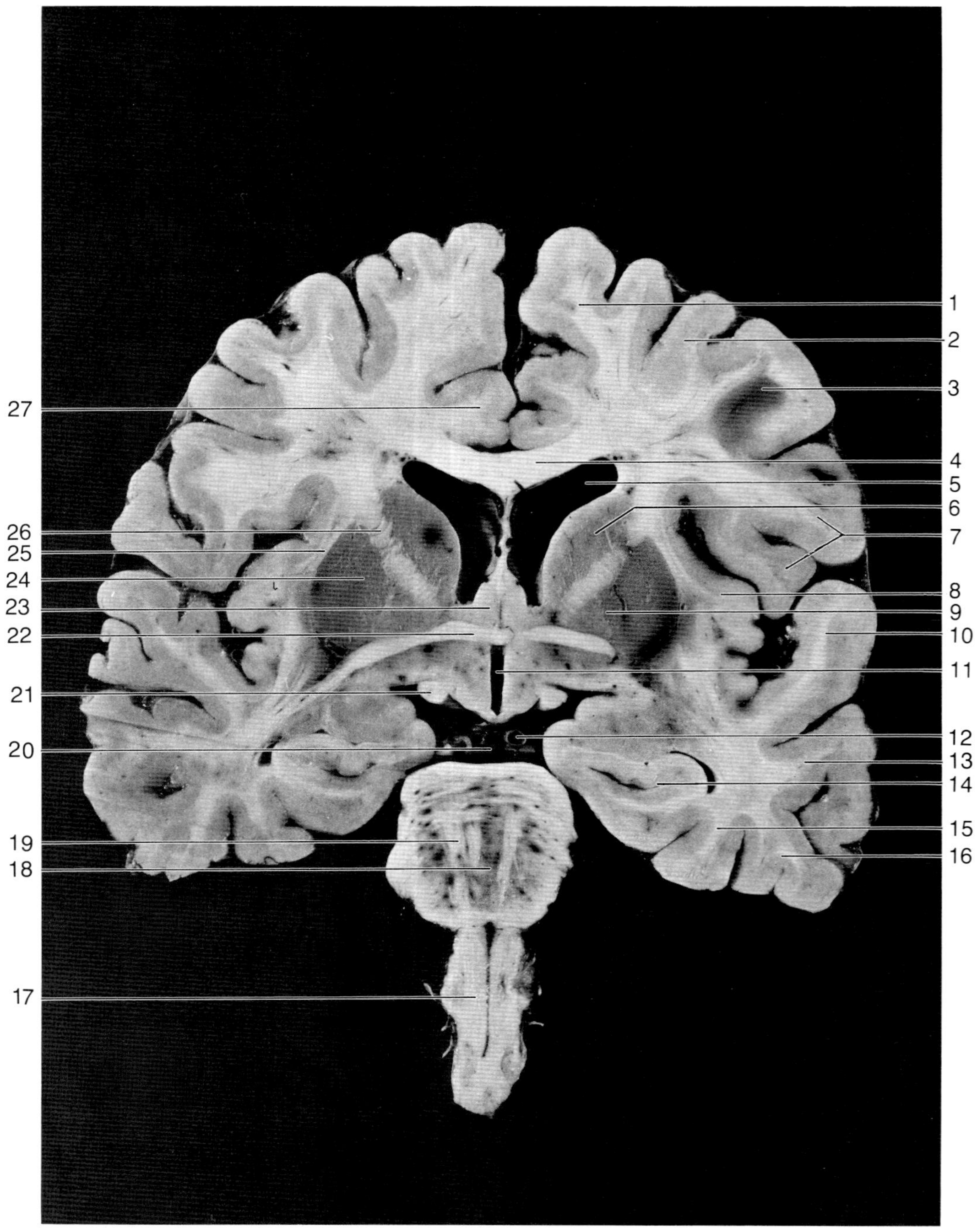

Anatomical section at level 1

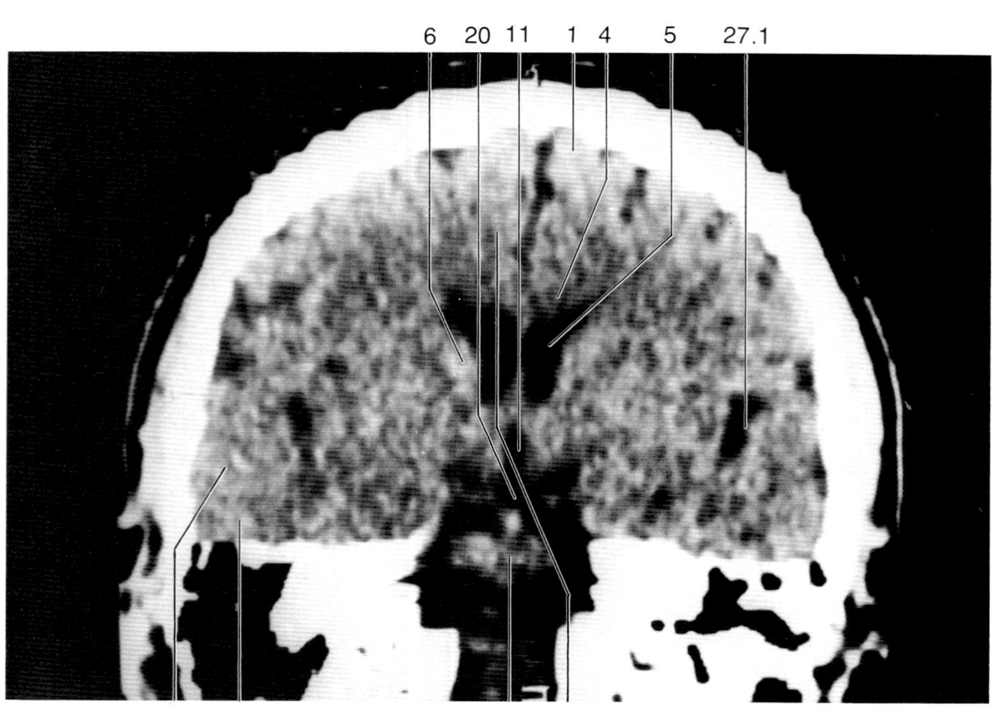

CT, coronal reconstruction, 50° angulation from the canthomeatal line at level 1

1 Superior frontal gyrus
2 Middle frontal gyrus
3 Inferior frontal gyrus
4 Corpus callosum
5 Lateral ventricle
6 Caudate nucleus
7 Frontal operculum
8 Insular cortex
9 Globus pallidus
10 Superior temporal gyrus
11 Third ventricle
12 Superior cerebellar artery
13 Middle temporal gyrus
14 Hippocampal gyrus
15 Fusiform gyrus
16 Inferior temporal gyrus
17 Medulla oblongata
18 Pons
19 Longitudinal fasciculi
20 Interpeduncular cistern
21 Optic tract
22 Anterior commissure
23 Fornix
24 Putamen
25 External capsule
26 Internal capsule
27 Cingulate gyrus
27.1 Lateral fissure

1 Gyrus frontalis superior
2 Gyrus frontalis medius
3 Gyrus frontalis inferior
4 Corpus callosum
5 Ventriculus lateralis
6 Nucleus caudatus
7 Operculum frontale
8 Cortex insulae
9 Globus pallidus
10 Gyrus temporalis superior
11 Ventriculus III
12 A. cerebelli superior
13 Gyrus temporalis medius
14 Gyrus parahippocampalis
15 Gyrus fusiformis
16 Gyrus temporalis inferior
17 Medulla oblongata
18 Pons
19 Fasciculi longitudinales
20 Cisterna interpeduncularis
21 Tractus opticus
22 Fornix
23 Commissura grisea anterior
24 Putamen
25 Capsula externa
26 Capsula interna
27 Gyrus cinguli
27.1 Fissura lateralis

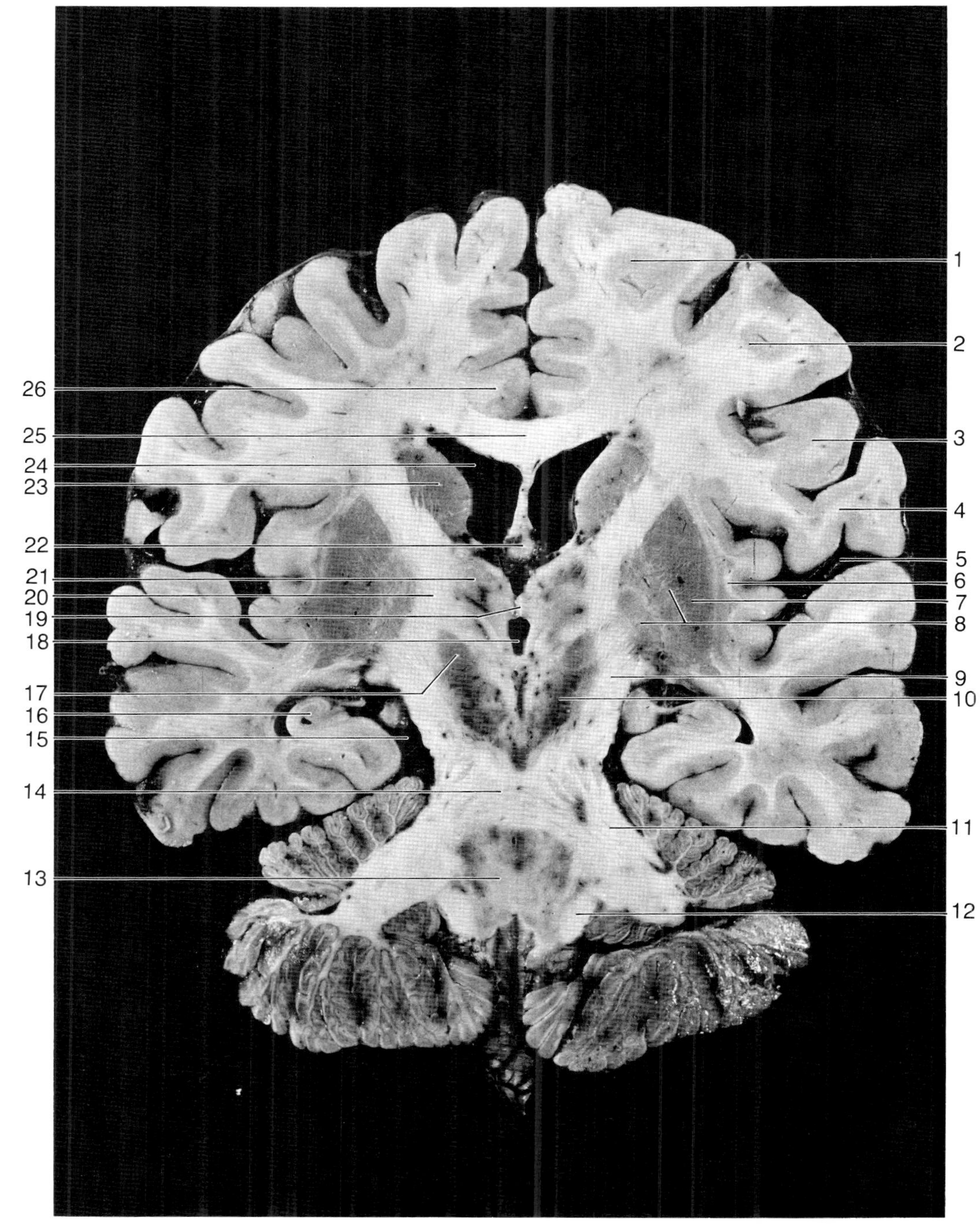

Anatomical section at level 2

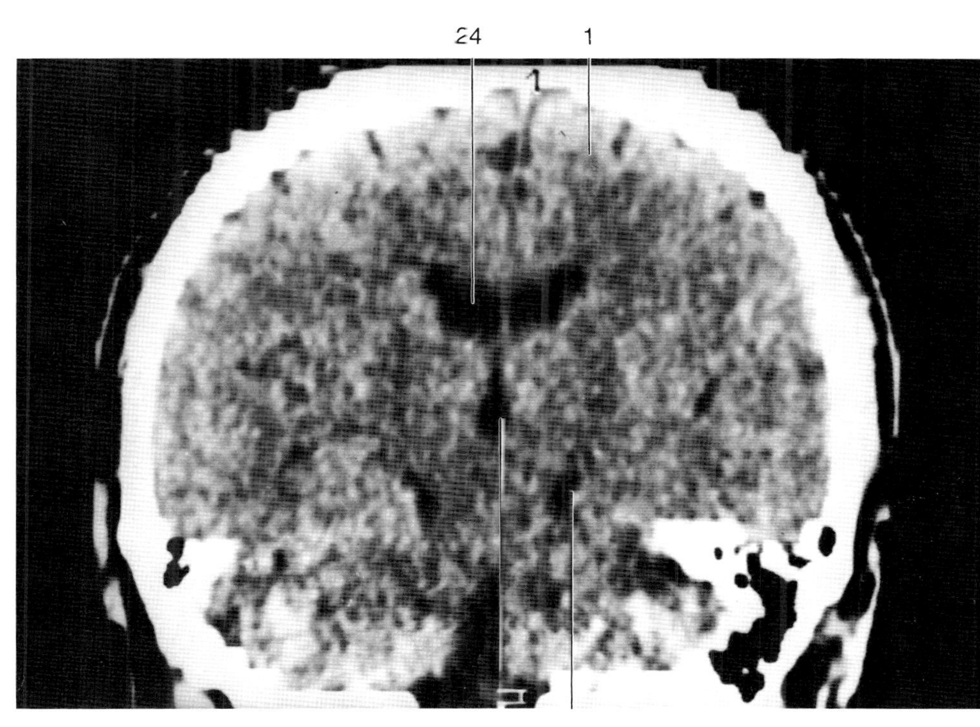

CT, coronal reconstruction, 50° angulation from the canthomeatal line at level 2

1 Superior frontal gyrus
2 Middle frontal gyrus
3 Frontal operculum
4 Parietal operculum
5 Sylvian fissure
6 Claustrum
7 Putamen
8 Globus pallidus
9 Cerebral peduncle
10 Substantia nigra
11 Middle cerebellar peduncle
12 Inferior cerebellar peduncle
13 Pons
14 Tegmentum
15 Ambient cistern
16 Ammon's horn
17 Subthalamic nucleus
18 Third ventricle
19 Massa intermedia
20 Internal capsule
21 Thalamus
22 Fornix
23 Caudate nucleus
24 Lateral ventricle
25 Corpus callosum
26 Cingulate gyrus

1 Gyrus frontalis superior
2 Gyrus frontalis medius
3 Operculum frontale
4 Operculum parietale
5 Fissura cerebri lateralis
6 Claustrum
7 Putamen
8 Globus pallidus
9 Pedunculus cerebri
10 Substantia nigra
11 Pedunculus cerebellaris medius
12 Pedunculus cerebellaris caudalis
13 Pons
14 Tegmentum mesencephali
15 Cisterna ambiens
16 Pes hippocampi (cornu ammonis)
17 Nucleus subthalamicus
18 Ventriculus III
19 Adhaesio interthalamica
20 Capsula interna
21 Thalamus
22 Fornix
23 Nucleus caudatus
24 Ventriculus lateralis
25 Corpus callosum
26 Gyrus cinguli

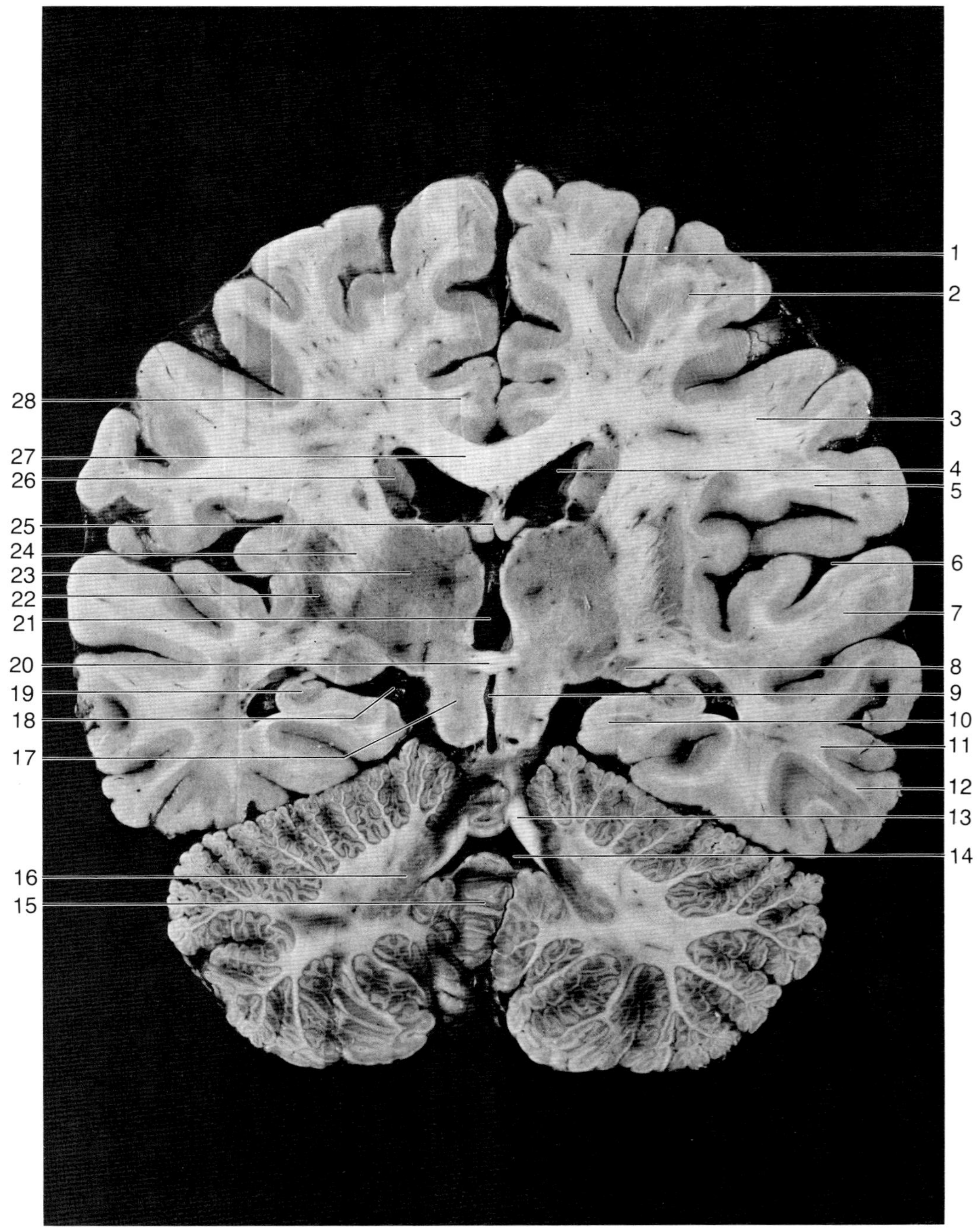

Anatomical section at level 3

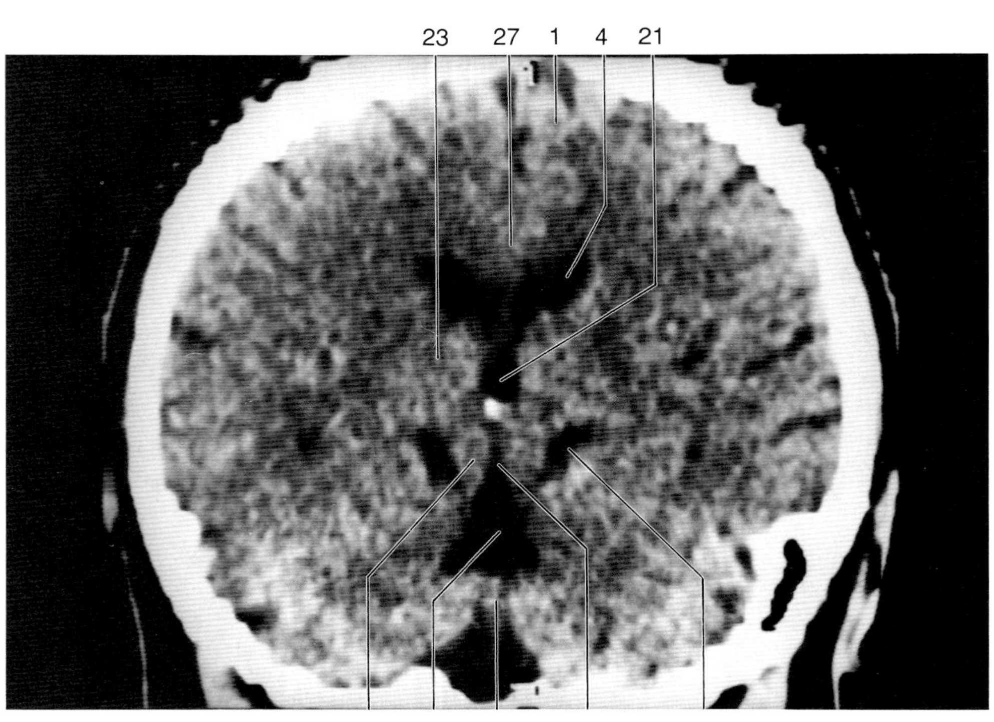

CT, coronal reconstruction, 50° angulation from the canthomeatal line at level 3

1 Superior frontal gyrus
2 Middle frontal gyrus
3 Precentral gyrus
4 Lateral ventricle
5 Parietal operculum
6 Sylvian fissure
7 Superior temporal gyrus
8 Superior temporal sulcus
9 Aqueduct
10 Hippocampal gyrus
11 Middle temporal gyrus
12 Inferior temporal gyrus
13 Superior cerebellar peduncle
14 Fourth ventricle
15 Vermis
16 Dentate nucleus
17 Quadrigeminal plate
18 Ambient cistern
19 Ammon's horn
20 Posterior commissure
21 Third ventricle
22 Putamen
23 Thalamus
24 Internal capsule
25 Fornix
26 Caudate nucleus
27 Corpus callosum
28 Cingulate gyrus

1 Gyrus frontalis superior
2 Gyrus frontalis medius
3 Gyrus praecentralis
4 Ventriculus lateralis
5 Operculum parietale
6 Fissura cerebri lateralis
7 Gyrus temporalis superior
8 Sulcus temporalis superior
9 Aquaeductus Sylvii
10 Gyrus parahippocampalis
11 Gyrus temporalis medius
12 Gyrus temporalis inferior
13 Pedunculus cerebellaris cranialis
14 Ventriculus IV
15 Vermis
16 Nucleus dentatus
17 Lamina quadrigemina
18 Cisterna ambiens
19 Pes hippocampi (Cornu ammonis)
20 Commissura grisea posterior
21 Ventriculus III
22 Putamen
23 Thalamus
24 Capsula interna
25 Fornix
26 Nucleus caudatus
27 Corpus callosum
28 Gyrus cinguli

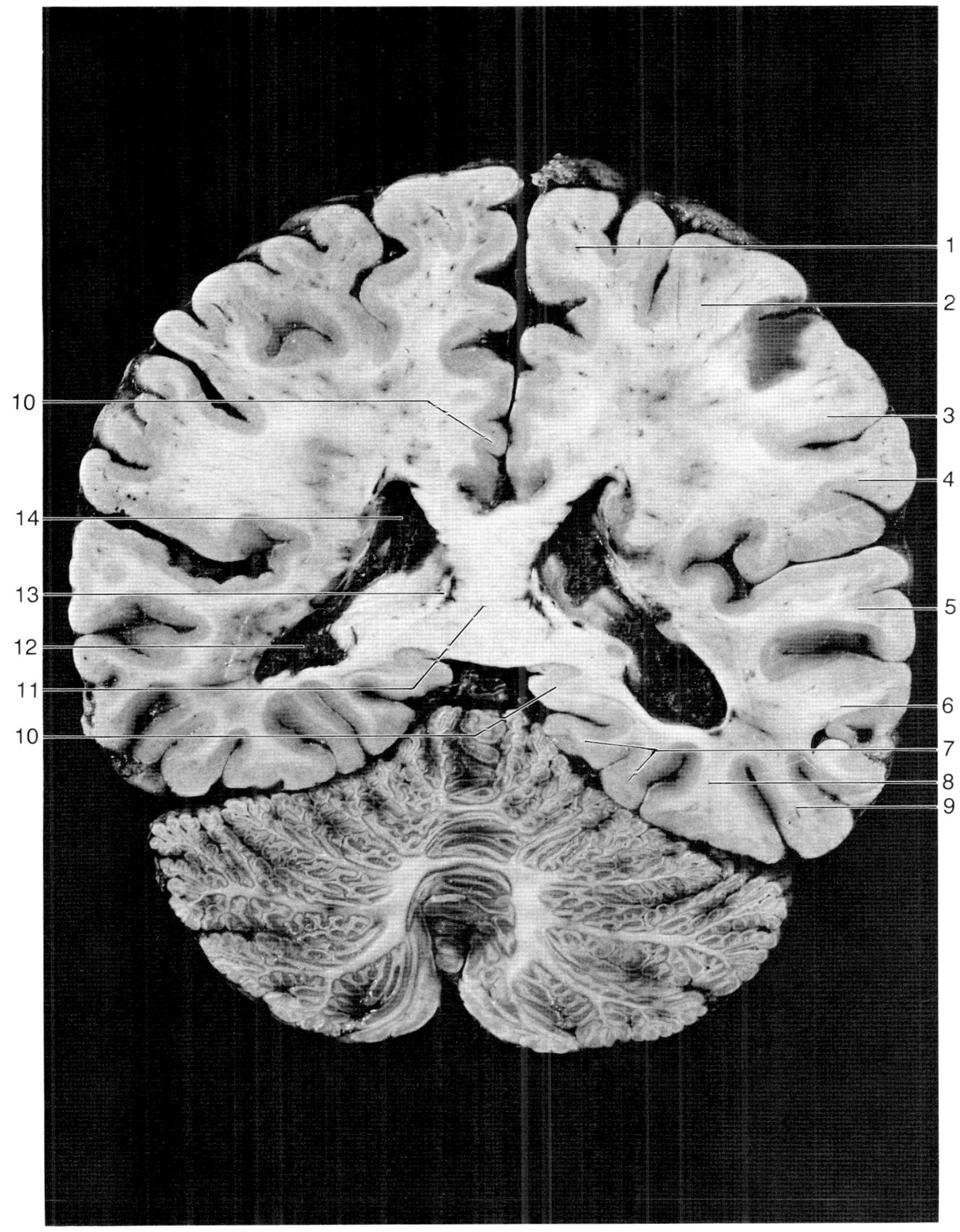

Anatomical section at level 4

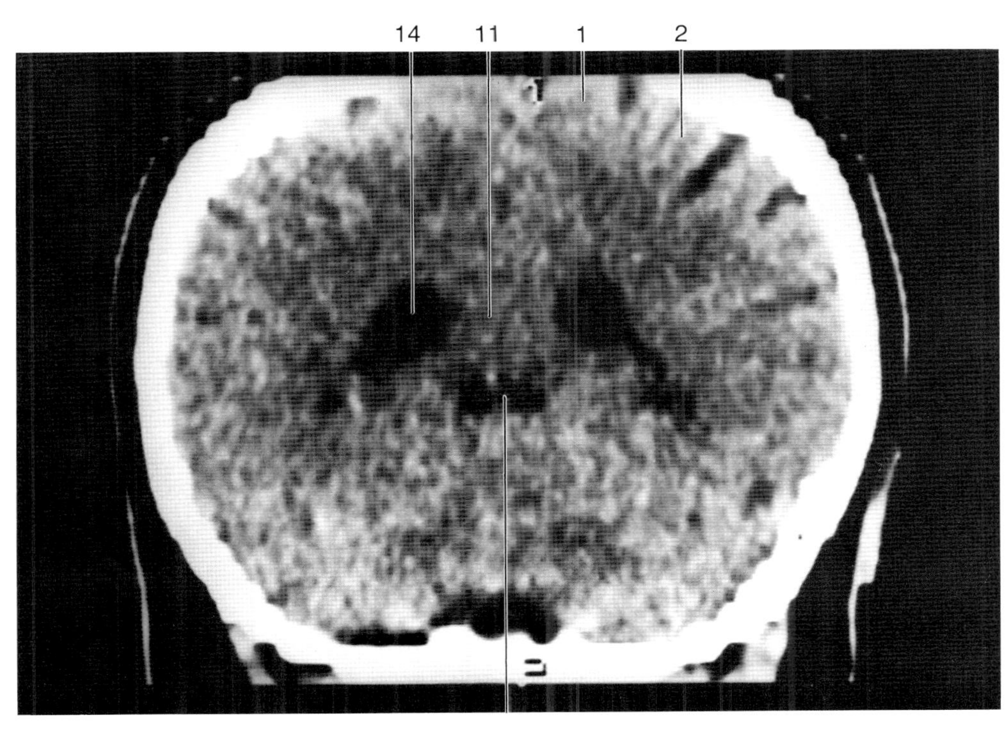

CT, coronal reconstruction, 50° angulation from the canthomeatal line at level 4

1 Superior frontal gyrus
2 Precentral gyrus
3 Postcentral gyrus
4 Supramarginal gyrus
5 Superior temporal gyrus
6 Middle temporal gyrus
7 Hippocampal gyrus
8 Fusiform gyrus
9 Inferior temporal gyrus
10 Cingulate gyrus
10.1 Cistern of the great cerebral vein
11 Splenium of the corpus callosum
12 Posterior horn of the lateral ventricle
13 Hippocampal commissure
14 Trigonum of the lateral ventricle

1 Gyrus frontalis superior
2 Gyrus praecentralis
3 Gyrus postcentralis
4 Gyrus supramarginalis
5 Gyrus temporalis superior
6 Gyrus temporalis medius
7 Gyrus parahippocampalis
8 Gyrus lingualis
9 Gyrus temporalis inferior
10 Gyrus cinguli
10.1 Cisterna v. cerebri magnae
11 Splenium corporis callosi
12 Cornu posterius ventriculi lateralis
13 Commissura hippocampi
14 Trigonum collaterale ventriculi lateralis

Sagittal Sections of the Head

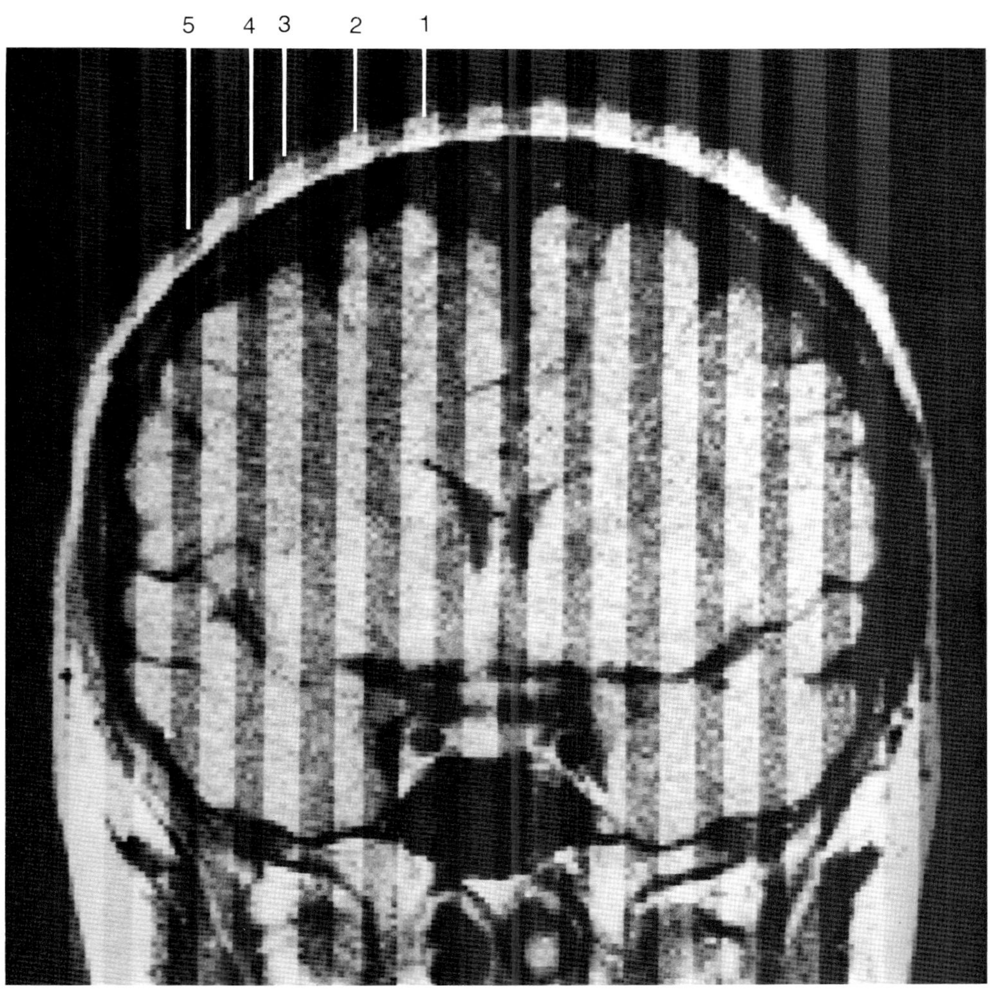

Coronal MRI section. Sagittal slices at levels no 1–5. Slice thickness 5 mm.

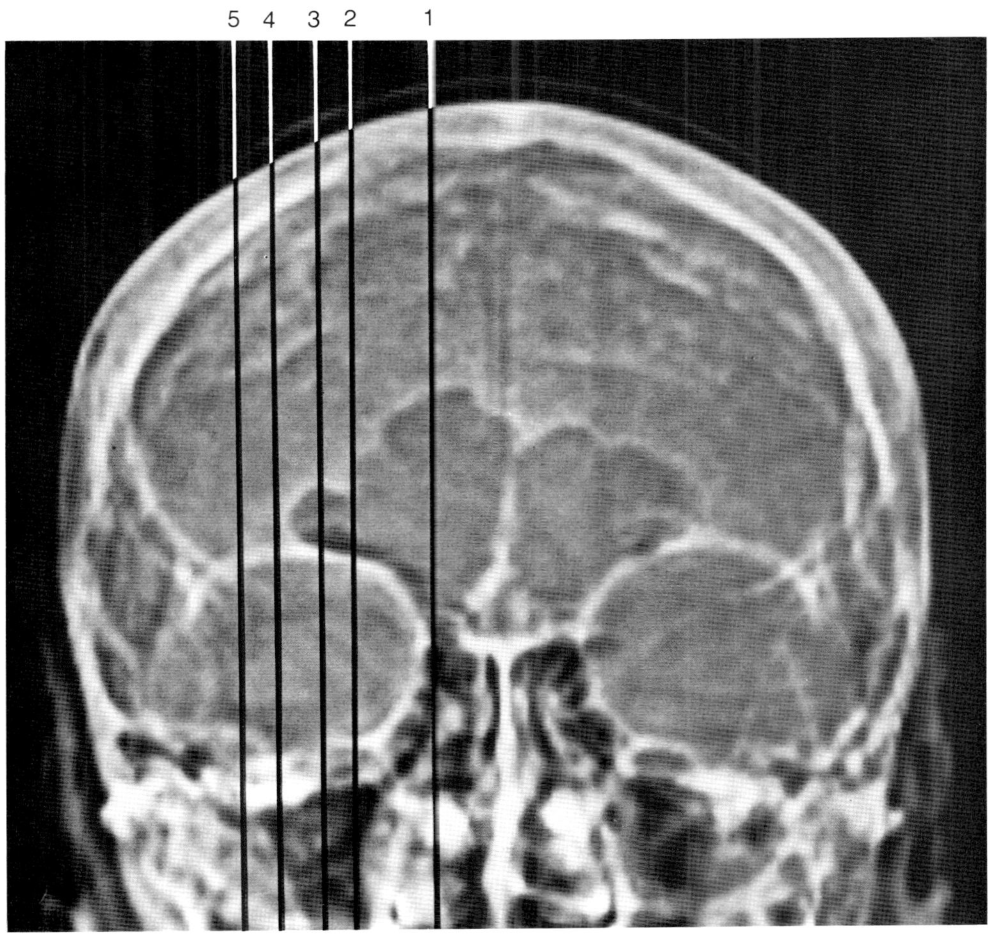

Anterior computed radiograph. Sagittal reconstructions at levels no. 1–5. Slice thickness 4 mm.

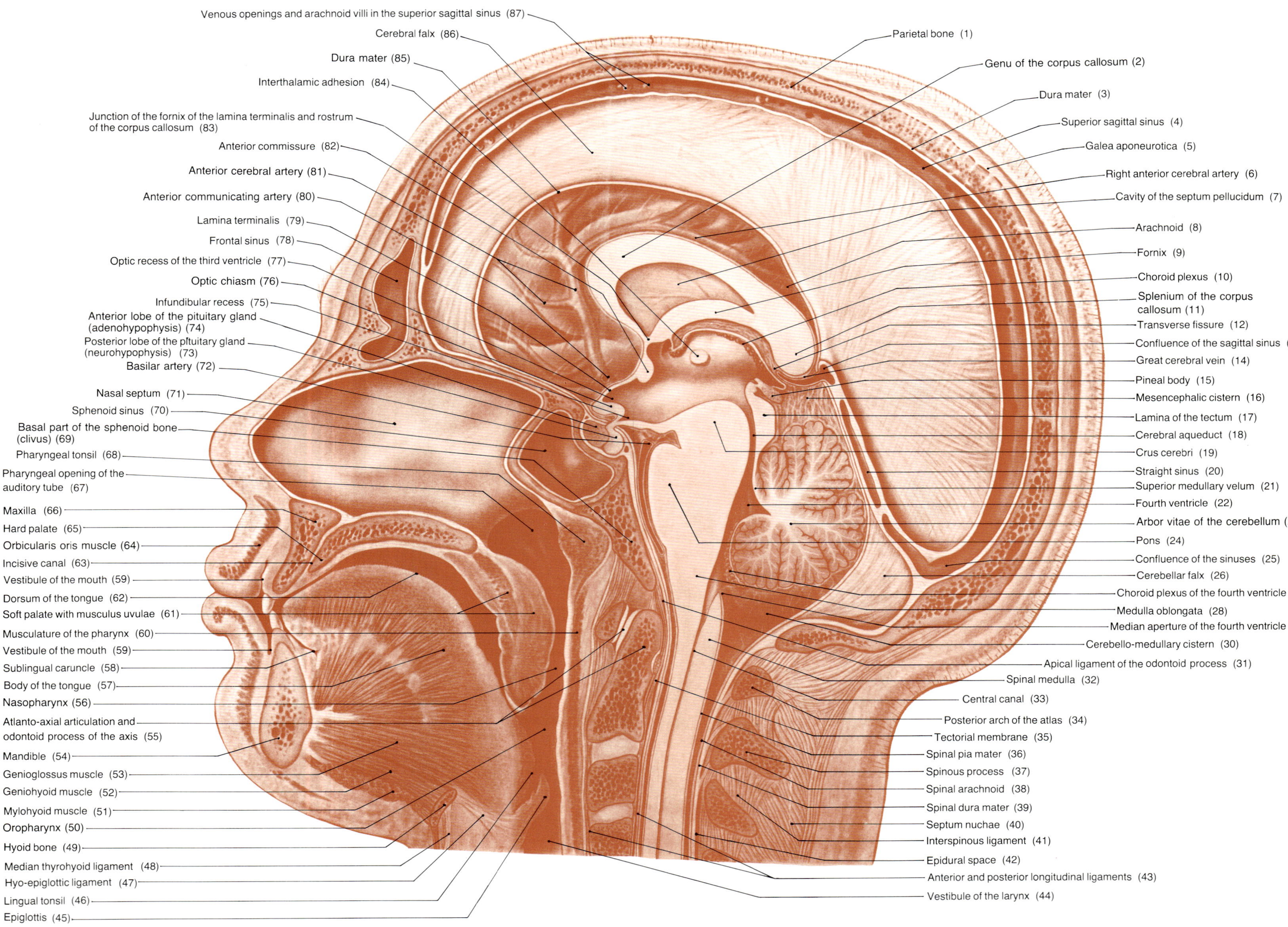

1 Os parietale
2 Genu corporis callosi
2.1 Hypophysis
3 Dura mater
4 Sinus sagittalis superior
5 Galea aponeurotica
6 A. cerebri anterior dextra
7 Cavum septi pellucidi
8 Arachnoidea
9 Fornix
10 Plexus choroideus
11 Splenium corporis callosi
12 Fissura transversa cerebri
13 Sinus sagittalis
14 V. cerebri magna
15 Corpus peneale
16 Cisterna mesencephalica
16.1 V. cerebri magna
16.2 Cisterna quadrigemina
16.3 Cisterna cerebellaris superior
17 Lamina tecti
18 Aquaeductus cerebri
19 Crus cerebri
20 Sinus rectus
21 Velum medullare superius
22 Ventriculus IV
23 Arbor vitae cerebelli
24 Pons
25 Confluens sinuum
26 Falx cerebri
27 Plexus choroideus ventriculi IV
28 Medulla oblongata
29 Apertura mediana ventriculi IV
30 Cisterna cerebellomedullaris
31 Lig. apicis dentis
32 Medulla spinalis
32.1 M. trapezius
32.2 M. splenius capitis
33 Canalis centralis
34 Arcus dorsalis atlantis
35 Membrana tectoria
36 Pia mater spinalis
37 Processus spinosus
38 Arachnoidea spinalis
39 Dura mater spinalis
40 Septum nuchae
41 Lig. interspinale
42 Spatium epidurale
43 Lig. longitudinale anterius et posterius
44 Vestibulum laryngis
45 Epiglottis
46 Tonsilla lingualis
47 Lig. hyoepiglotticum
48 Lig. thyrohyoideum medianum
49 Os hyoideum
50 Pars oralis pharyngis
51 M. mylohyoideus
52 M. geniohyoideus
53 M. genioglossus
54 Mandibula
55 Articulatio atlantoaxialis et Dens axis
56 Pars nasalis pharyngis
57 Corpus linguae
58 Caruncula sublingualis
59 Vestibulum oris
60 M. constrictor pharyngis
61 Palatum molle, M. uvulae
62 Dorsum linguae
63 Canalis incisivus
64 M. orbicularis oris
65 Palatum durum
66 Maxilla
67 Ostium pharyngeum tubae
68 Tonsilla pharyngea
68.1 Cisterna praepontina
69 Pars basilaris ossis sphenoidalis (Clivus)
70 Sinus sphenoidalis
71 Septum nasi
72 A. basilaris
73 Lobus posterior glandulae pituitariae (Neurohypophysis)
74 Lobus anterior glandulae pituitariae (Adenohypophysis)
75 Recessus infundibuli
76 Chiasma opticum
77 Recessus opticus ventriculi tertii
78 Sinus frontalis
79 Lamina terminalis
80 A. communicans anterior
81 A. cerebri anterior
82 Commissura anterior
83 Fornix laminae terminalis, Rostrum corporis callosi
84 Adhaesio interthalamica
85 Dura mater
86 Falx cerebri
87 Apertura venosae et villi arachnoideales sinus sagittalis superior
88 Sulcus cinguli
89 Foramen Monroi
90 Gyri cinguli
91 Thalamus
92 Lobulus paracentralis
93 Praecuneus
94 Culmen
95 Cuneus
96 Sulcus calcarinus
97 Fissura prima
98 Declive
99 Gyrus frontalis superior
100 Gyrus rectus
101 Rostrum corporis callosi
102 Columna anterior fornicis
103 Corpora mamillaria
103.1 Cisterna interpeduncularis
104 Commissura posterior
105 Nodulus cerebelli
106 Uvula cerebelli
107 Tonsilla cerebelli
108 Pyramis
109 Lobulus centralis
110 Fissura pyramidalis
111 Tuber vermis
112 Lobulus semilunaris inferior

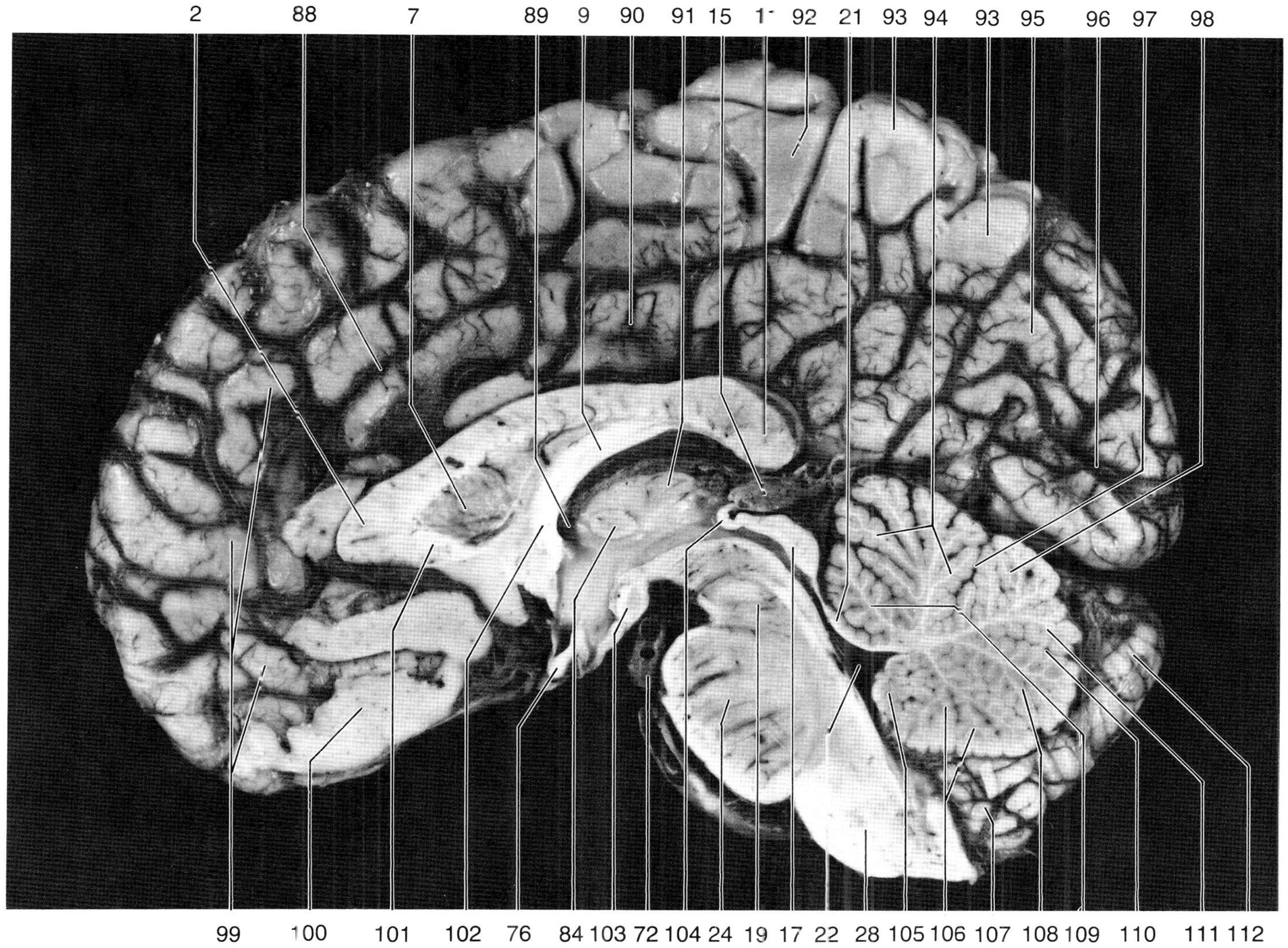

Anatomical section of the medial aspect of the brain

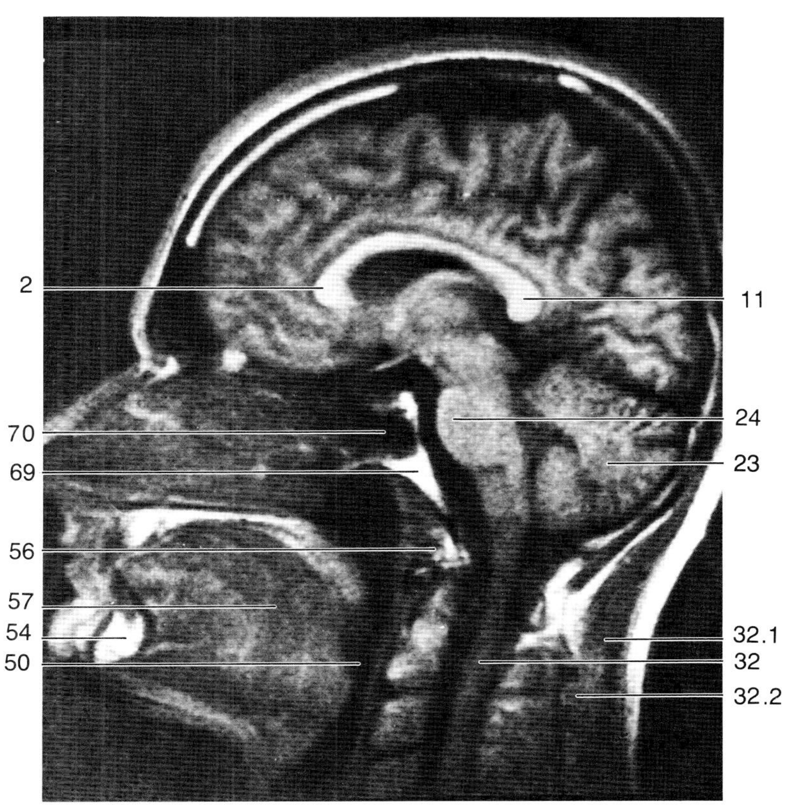

MRI, IR 1400/50

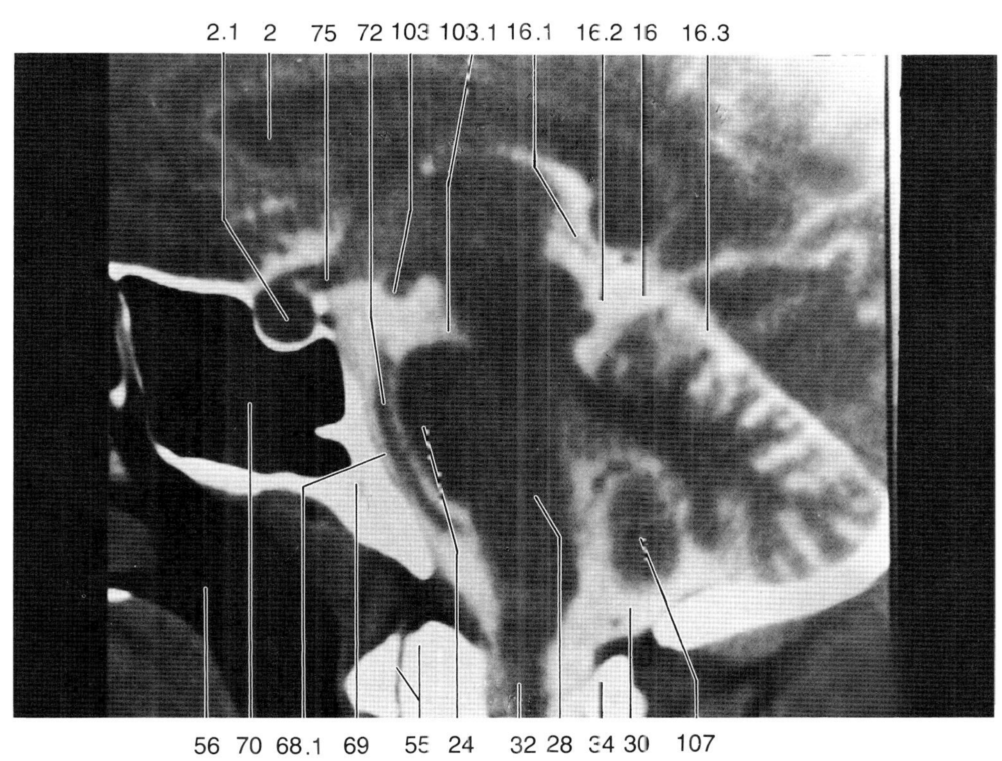

CT with contrast enhancement of the subarachnoid space

2 Genu of the corpus callosum
2.1 Cerebral hypophysis
7 Cavity of the septum pellucidum
9 Fornix
11 Splenium of the corpus callosum
15 Pineal body
16 Mesencephalic cistern
16.1 Great cerebral vein (Galen)
16.2 Quadrigeminal cistern
16.3 Superior cerebral cistern
17 Lamina of the tectum
19 Crus cerebri
21 Superior medullary velum
22 Fourth ventricle
23 Arbor vitae of the cerebellum
24 Pons
28 Medulla oblongata
30 Cerebellomedullary cistern
32 Spinal medulla
32.1 Trapezius muscle
32.2 Splenius capitis muscle
34 Posterior arch of the atlas
50 Oropharynx
54 Mandible
55 Atlanto-axial articulation and odontoid process of the axis
56 Nasopharynx
57 Body of the tongue
68.1 Prepontine cistern
69 Basal part of the sphenoid bone
70 Sphenoid sinus
72 Basilar artery
75 Infundibular recess
76 Optic chiasm
84 Interthalamic adhesion
88 Cingulate sulcus
89 Foramen Monroi
90 Cingulate gyrus
91 Thalamus
92 Paracentral lobule
93 Precuneus
94 Culmen
95 Cuneus
96 Calcarine sulcus
97 Primary fissure
98 Declive
99 Superior frontal gyrus
100 Rectal gyrus
101 Corpus callosum (rostrum)
102 Anterior column of the fornix
103 Mamillary body
103.1 Interpeduncular cistern
104 Posterior commissure
105 Nodule
106 Uvula
107 Cerebellar tonsil
108 Pyramis
109 Central lobule
110 Prepyramidal fissure
111 Tuber vermis
112 Inferior semilunar lobule

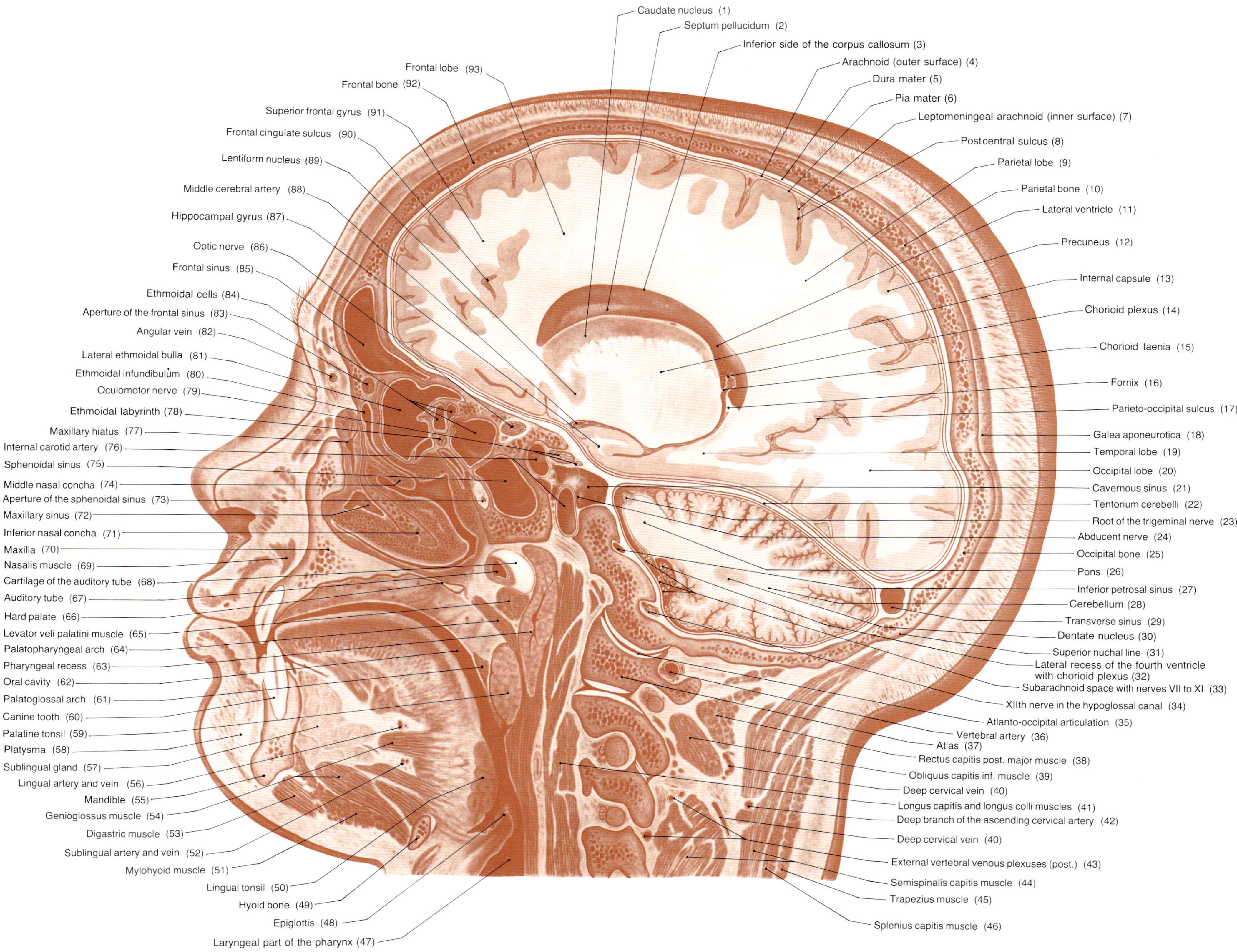

1 Nucleus caudatus
2 Septum pellucidum
3 Margo inferior corporis callosi
4 Arachnoidea, Pars externa
4.1 Lobulus paracentralis
5 Dura mater
6 Pia mater
7 Arachnoidea, Pars interna
8 Sulcus postcentralis
9 Lobus parietalis
10 Os parietale
11 Ventriculus lateralis
12 Praecuneus
13 Capsula interna
14 Plexus chorioideus
14.1 Cisterna ambiens
15 Taenia chorioidea
16 Fornix
17 Sulcus parietooccipitalis
18 Galea aponeurotica
19 Lobus temporalis
20 Lobus occipitalis
21 Sinus cavernosus
22 Tentorium cerebelli
23 N. trigeminus
24 N. abducens
25 Os occipitale
26 Pons
27 Sinus petrosus inferior
28 Cerebellum
29 Sinus transversus
30 Nucleus emboliformis
31 Linea nuchae superior
32 Recessus lateralis ventriculi quarti cum plexu chorioideo
33 Spatium subarachnoideale cum N. VII–XII
34 N. XII, Canalis hypoglossis
35 Articulatio atlantooccipitalis
36 A. vertebralis
37 Atlas
38 M. rectus capitis posterior major
39 M. obliquus capitis inferior
40 V. cervicalis profunda
41 M. longus capitis et longus colli
42 R. profundus a. cervicalis ascendentis
43 Plexus venosi vertebrales externi (posteriores)
44 M. semispinalis capitis
45 M. trapezius
46 M. splenius capitis
47 Pars laryngea pharyngis
48 Epiglottis
49 Os hyoideum
50 Tonsilla lingualis
51 M. mylohyoideus
52 A. et V. sublingualis
53 M. digastricus
54 M. genioglossus
55 Mandibula
56 A. et V. lingualis
57 Glandula sublingualis
58 Platysma
59 Tonsilla palatina
60 Dens caninus
61 Arcus palatoglossus
62 Cavum oris
63 Recessus pharyngeus
64 Arcus palatopharyngeus
65 M. levator veli palatini
66 Palatum durum
67 Tuba auditiva
68 Cartilago tubae auditivae
69 M. nasalis
70 Maxilla
71 Concha nasalis inferior
72 Sinus maxillaris
73 Apertura sinus sphenoidalis
74 Concha nasalis media
75 Sinus sphenoidalis
76 A. carotis interna
77 Hiatus maxillaris
78 Labyrinthus ethmoidalis
79 N. oculomotorius
80 Infundibulum ethmoidale
81 Bulla ethmoidalis lateralis
82 V. angularis
83 Apertura sinus frontalis
84 Cellulae ethmoidales
85 Sinus frontalis
86 N. opticus
87 Gyrus hippocampi
87.1 A. carotis interna
87.2 Gyrus orbitalis
88 A. cerebri media
89 Nucleus lentiformis
90 Sulcus cinguli frontalis
91 Gyrus frontalis superior
92 Os frontale
93 Lobus frontalis
94 Globus pallidus
95 Gyrus cinguli
96 Thalamus
97 Sulcus centralis
98 Putamen
99 Cisterna pontocerebellaris
100 Pedunculus cerebri

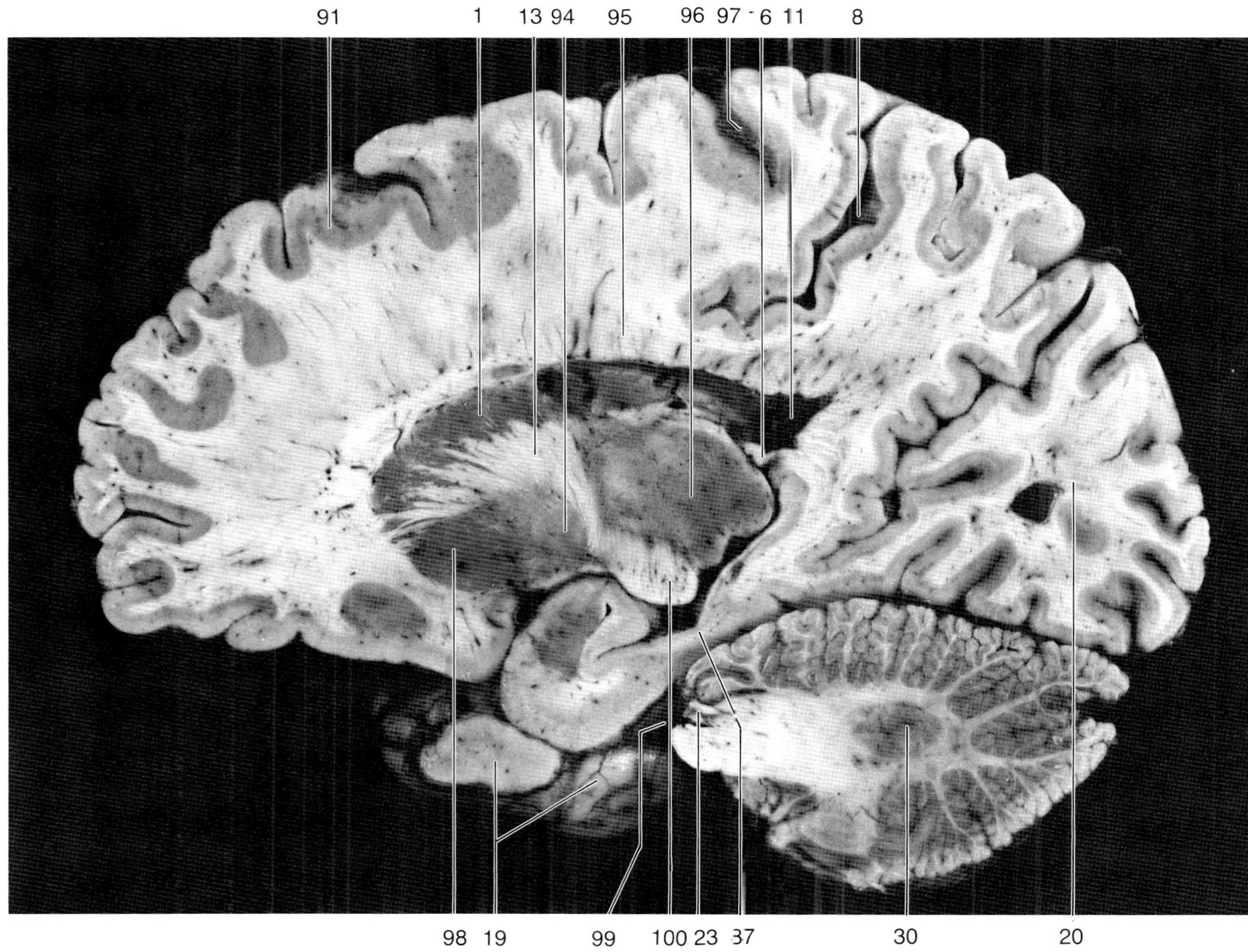

Anatomical section at level 1

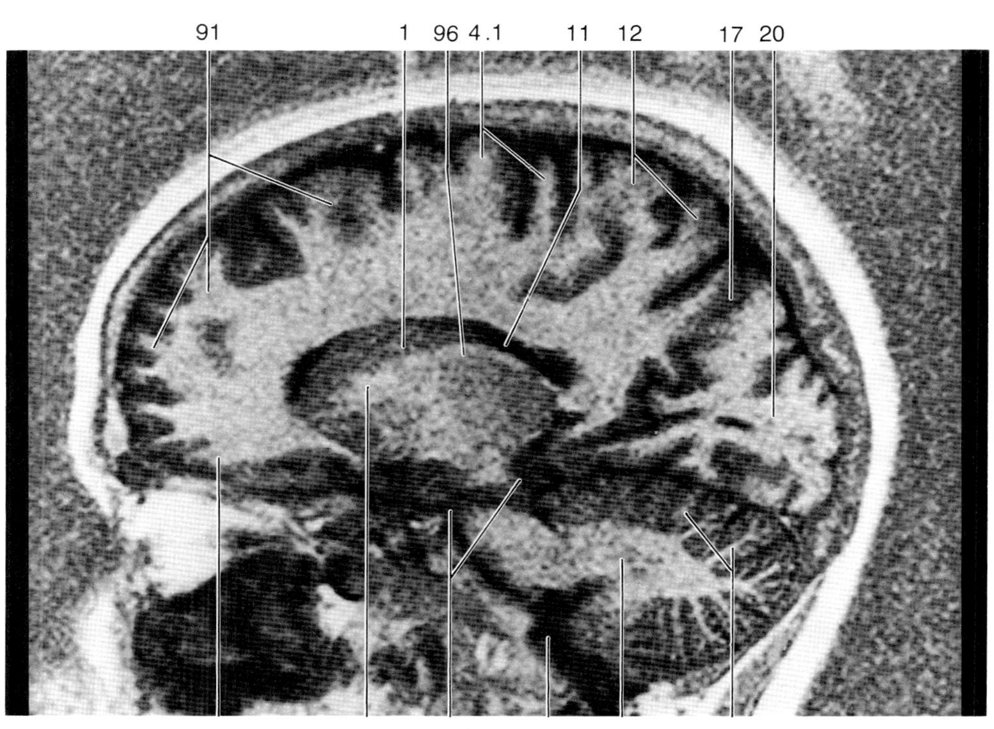

MRI, SI, 1900/400/30, level 1

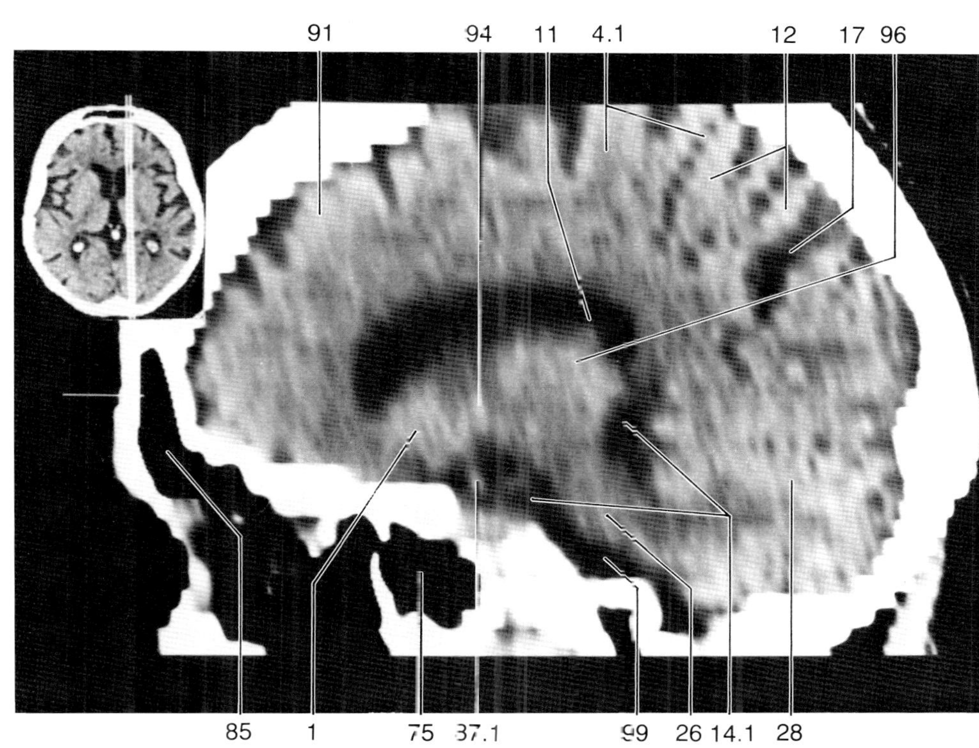

CT, sagittal reconstruction at level 1

- 1 Caudate nucleus
- 4.1 Paracentral lobule
- 8 Postcentral sulcus
- 11 Lateral ventricle
- 12 Precuneus
- 13 Internal capsule
- 14.1 Ambient cistern
- 16 Fornix
- 17 Parietooccipital sulcus
- 19 Temporal lobe
- 20 Occipital lobe
- 23 Root of the trigeminal nerve
- 26 Pons
- 28 Cerebellum
- 30 Dentate nucleus
- 32 Lateral recess of the fourth ventricle with choroid plexus
- 75 Sphenoidal sinus
- 85 Frontal sinus
- 87 Hippocampal gyrus
- 87.1 Internal carotid artery
- 87.2 Orbital gyrus
- 91 Superior frontal sinus
- 94 Globus pallidus
- 95 Cingulate gyrus
- 96 Thalamus
- 97 Central sulcus
- 98 Putamen
- 99 Pontocerebellar cistern
- 100 Cerebral peduncle

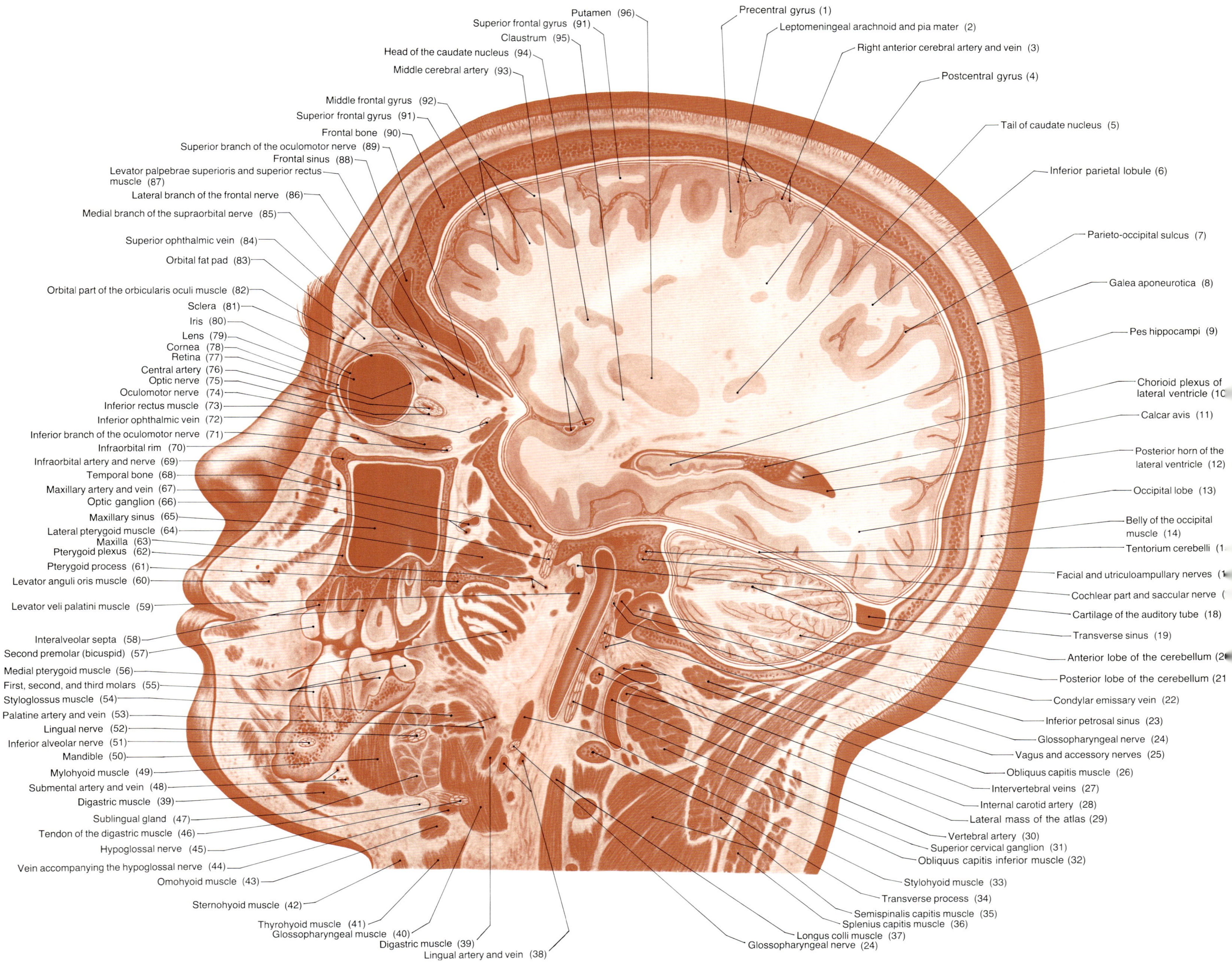

1 Gyrus praecentralis
2 Leptomeninx (Pia mater et Arachnoidea)
3 Rr. a. et v. cerebri anterioris
4 Gyrus postcentralis
5 Cauda nuclei caudati
6 Lobulus parietalis inferior
7 Sulcus parietooccipitalis
8 Galea aponeurotica
9 Pes hippocampi
10 Plexus chorioideus ventriculi lateralis
11 Calcar avis
12 Cornu occipitale ventriculi lateralis
13 Lobus occipitalis
14 Venter m. occipitalis
15 Tentorium cerebelli
16 N. facialis et utriculoampullaris
17 Pars cochlearis et N. saccularis
18 Cartilago tubae auditivae
19 Sinus transversus
20 Lobus anterior cerebelli
21 Lobus posterior cerebelli
22 V. emissaria condyloidea
23 Sinus petrosus inferior
24 N. glossopharyngeus
25 N. vagus et accessorius
26 M. obliquus capitis
27 Vv. intervertebrales
28 A. carotis interna
29 Massa lateralis atlantis
30 A. vertebralis
31 Ganglion cervicale superius
32 M. obliquus capitis inferior
33 M. stylohyoideus
34 Processus transversus
35 M. semispinalis capitis
36 M. splenius capitis
37 M. longus colli
38 A. et V. lingualis
39 M. digastricus
40 M. glossopharyngeus
41 M. thyrohyoideus
42 M. sternohyoideus
43 M. omohyoideus
44 V. comitans n. hypoglossi
45 N. hypoglossus
46 M. digastricus
47 Glandula sublingualis
48 A. et V. submentalis
49 M. mylohyoideus
50 Mandibula
51 N. alveolaris inferior
52 N. lingualis
53 A. et V. palatina
54 M. styloglossus
55 Dentes molares I, II, III
56 M. pterygoideus medialis
57 Dens praemolaris II
58 Septa interalveolaria
59 M. levator veli palatini
60 M. levator anguli oris
61 Processus pterygoideus
62 Plexus pterygoideus
63 Maxilla
64 M. pterygoideus lateralis
65 Sinus maxillaris
66 Ganglion oticum
67 A. et V. maxillaris
68 Os temporale
69 A. et N. infraorbitalis
70 Margo infraorbitalis
70.1 Ala minor ossis sphenoidalis
70.2 Lobus temporalis
70.3 Ala major ossis sphenoidalis
70.4 Foramen lacerum
70.5 Nasopharynx
71 R. inferior n. oculomotorii
72 V. ophthalmica inferior
73 M. rectus inferior
74 N. oculomotorius
75 N. opticus
76 A. centralis
77 Retina
77.1 Corpus vitreum
78 Cornea
79 Lens
80 Iris
81 Sclera
82 Pars orbitalis m. orbicularis oculi
83 Corpus adiposum orbitae
84 V. ophthalmica superior
85 R. medialis n. supraorbitalis
86 R. lateralis n. frontalis
87 M. levator palpebrae superioris et M. rectus superior
88 Sinus frontalis
89 R. superior n. oculomotorii
90 Os frontale
90.1 Pars orbitalis ossis frontalis
91 Gyrus frontalis superior
92 Gyrus frontalis medius
93 A. et V. cerebri media
94 Caput nuclei caudati
95 Claustrum
96 Putamen
97 Lobus frontalis
98 Cortex insulae
98.1 Sulcus postcentralis
98.2 Sulcus praecentralis
98.3 Sulcus centralis
99 Corpus amygdaloideum
100 Hemisphaerium cerebelli
100.1 Cisterna pontocerebellaris

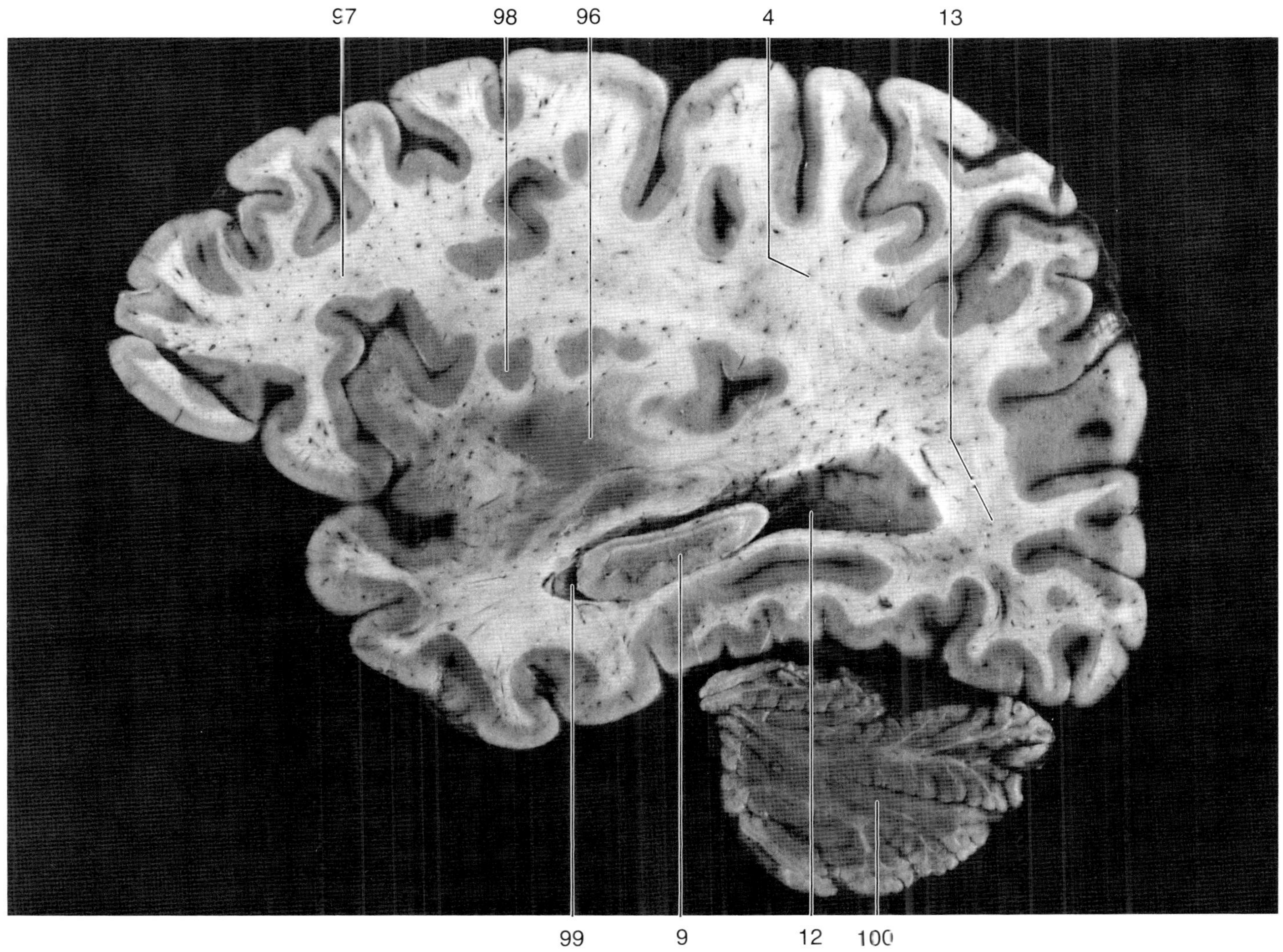

Anatomical section at level 2

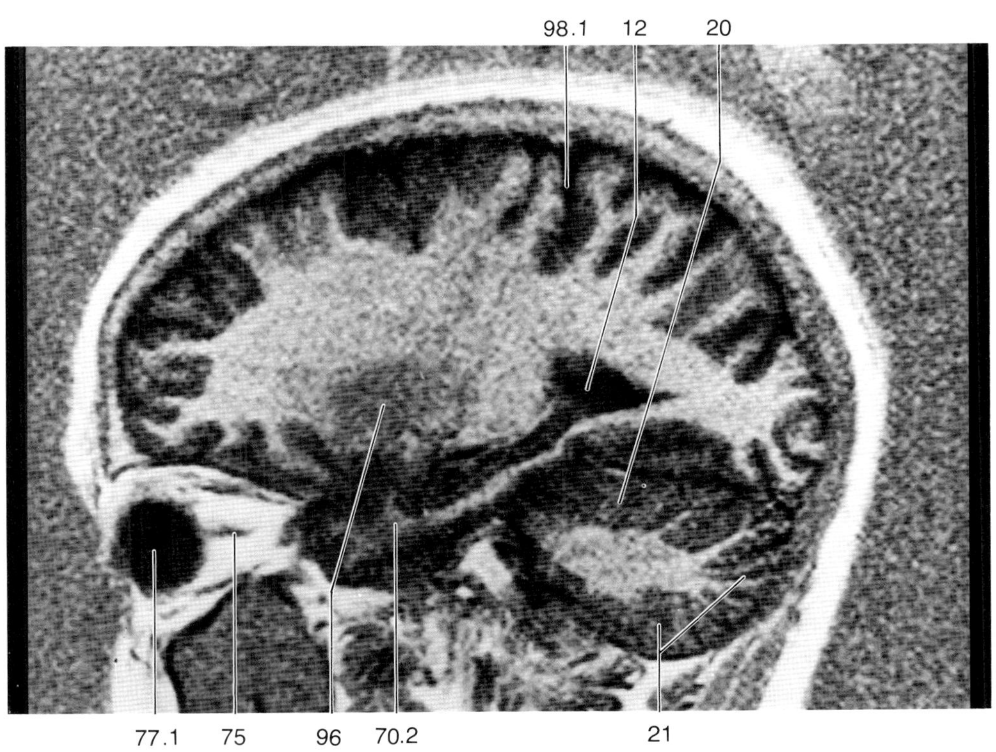

MRI, IR 1900/400/30, level 2

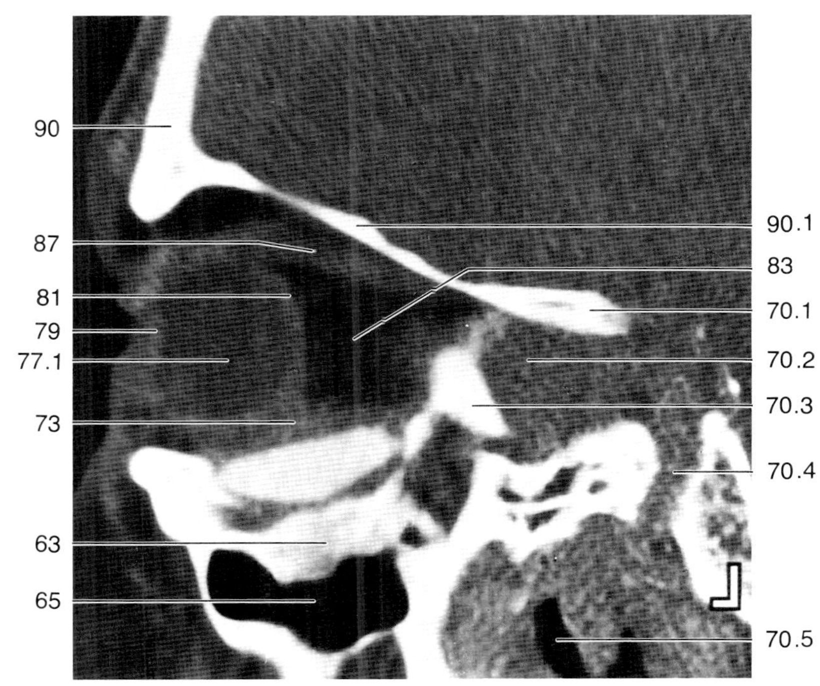

CT, sagittal reconstruction

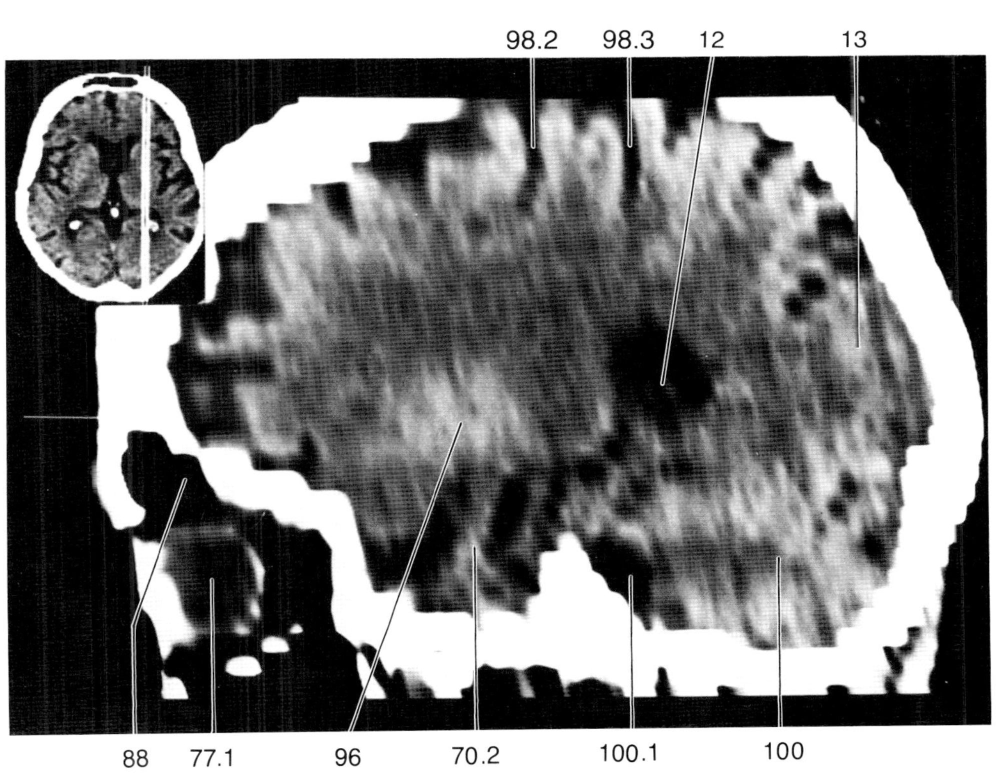

CT, sagittal reconstruction at level 2

4 Parietal lobe
9 Pes hippocampi
12 Lateral ventricle
13 Occipital lobe
20 Anterior lobe of the cerebellum
21 Posterior lobe of the cerebellum
63 Maxilla
65 Maxillary sinus
70.1 Sphenoid bone, lesser wing
70.2 Temporal lobe
70.3 Sphenoid bone, greater wing
70.4 Foramen lacerum
70.5 Nasopharynx
73 Inferior rectus muscle
75 Optic nerve
77.1 Vitreous body
79 Lens
81 Sclera
83 Orbital fat pad
87 Levator palpebrae superioris and superior rectus muscle
88 Frontal sinus
90 Frontal bone
90.1 Orbital part of the frontal bone
96 Putamen
97 Frontal lobe
98 Insular cortex
98.1 Postcentral sulcus
98.2 Precentral sulcus
98.3 Central sulcus
99 Amygdaloid body
100 Cerebellar hemisphere
100.1 Pontocerebellar cistern

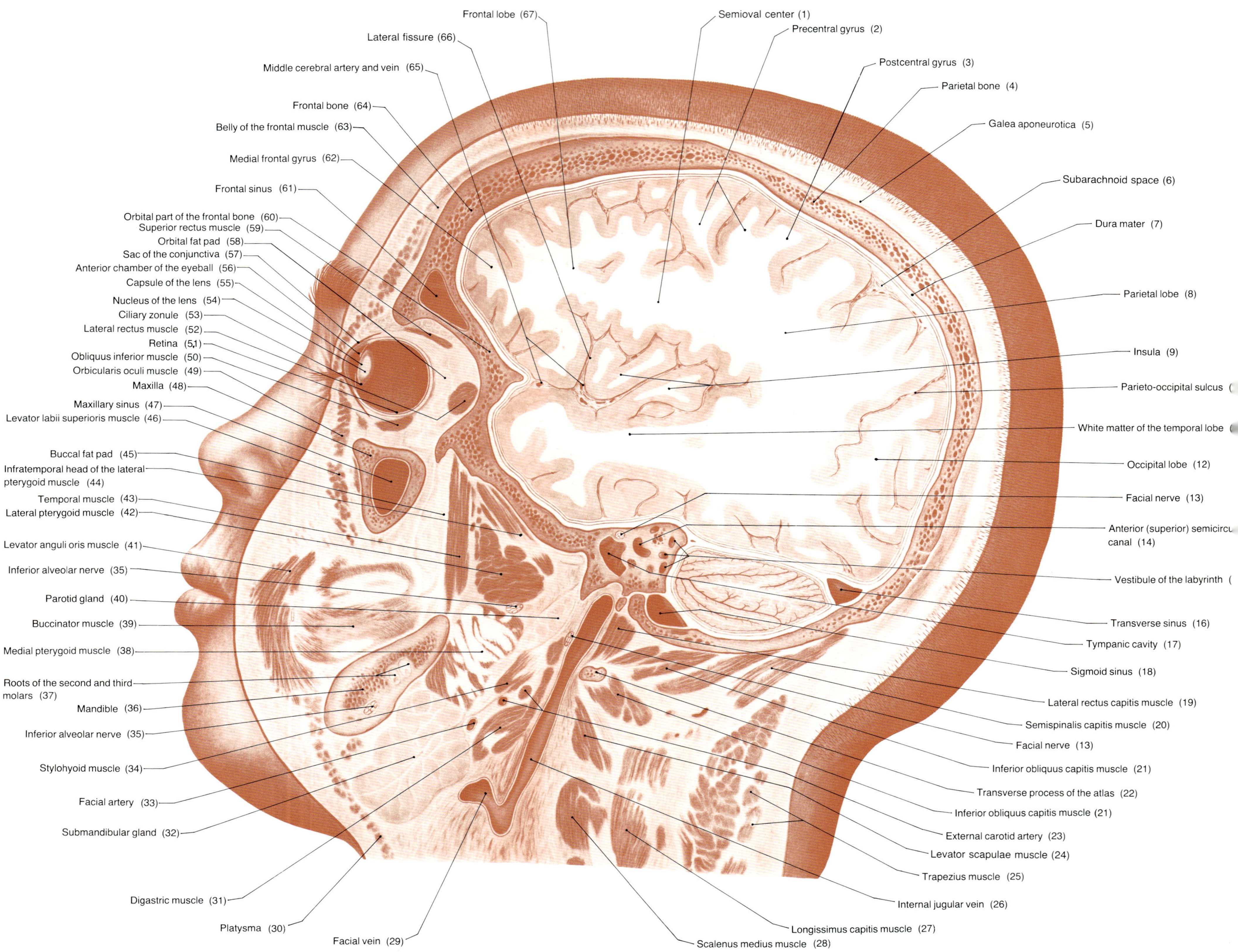

1 Centrum semiovale
2 Gyrus praecentralis
3 Gyrus postcentralis
4 Os parietale
5 Galea aponeurotica
6 Spatium subarachnoideale
7 Dura mater
8 Lobus parietalis
9 Insula
10 Sulcus parietooccipitalis
11 Substantia alba lobi temporalis
11.1 Chorioid plexus
12 Lobus occipitalis
13 N. facialis
14 Canalis semicircularis anterior
15 Vestibulum labyrinthi
16 Sinus transversus
17 Cavum tympani
18 Sinus sigmoideus
19 M. rectus capitis lateralis
20 M. semispinalis capitis
21 M. obliquus capitis inferior
22 Processus transversus atlantis
23 A. carotis externa
24 M. levator scapulae
25 M. trapezius
26 V. jugularis interna
27 M. longissimus capitis
28 M. scalenus medius
29 V. facialis
30 Platysma
31 M. digastricus
32 Glandula submandibularis
33 A. facialis
34 M. stylohyoideus
35 N. alveolaris inferior
36 Mandibula
37 Radices dentium molarium II, III
38 M. pterygoideus medialis
39 M. buccinator
40 Glandula parotis
41 M. levator anguli oris
42 M. pterygoideus lateralis
43 M. temporalis
44 Caput infratemporale m. pterygoidei lateralis
45 Corpus adiposum buccae
46 M. levator labii superioris
47 Sinus maxillaris
48 Maxilla
49 M. orbicularis oculi
50 M. obliquus inferior
51 Retina
52 M. rectus lateralis
53 Zonula ciliaris
54 Nucleus lentis
54.1 Vitreous body
55 Capsula lentis
56 Camera anterior bulbi
57 Saccus conjunctivae
58 Corpus adiposum orbitae
59 M. rectus superior
60 Pars orbitalis ossis frontalis
61 Sinus frontalis
62 Gyrus frontalis medius
63 Venter m. frontalis
64 Os frontale
65 A. et V. cerebri media
66 Fissura lateralis cerebri
67 Lobus frontalis
68 Sulcus centralis
69 Gyrus supramarginalis
70 Cornu temporale ventriculi lateralis
71 Hemisphaerium cerebelli

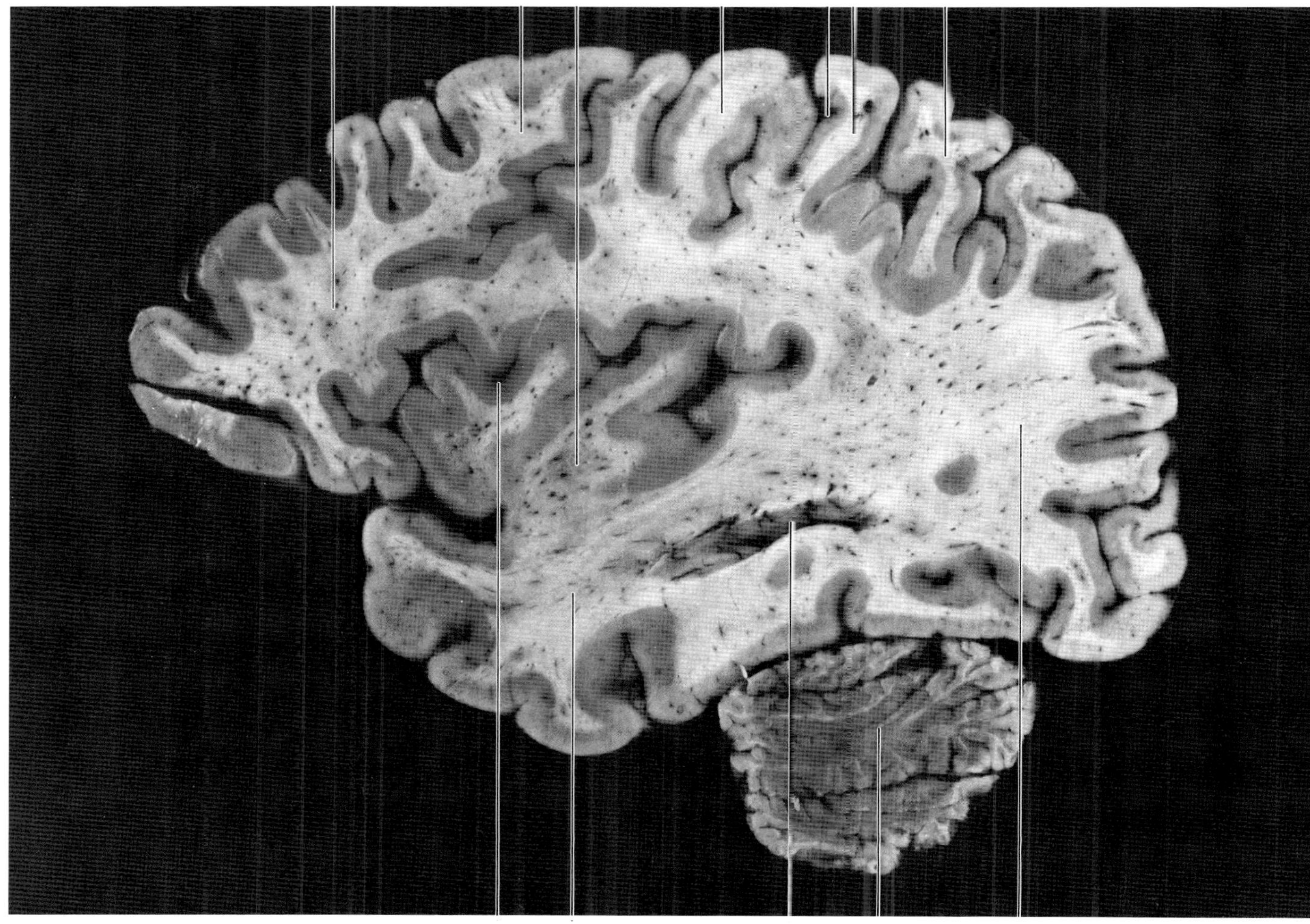

Anatomical section at level 3

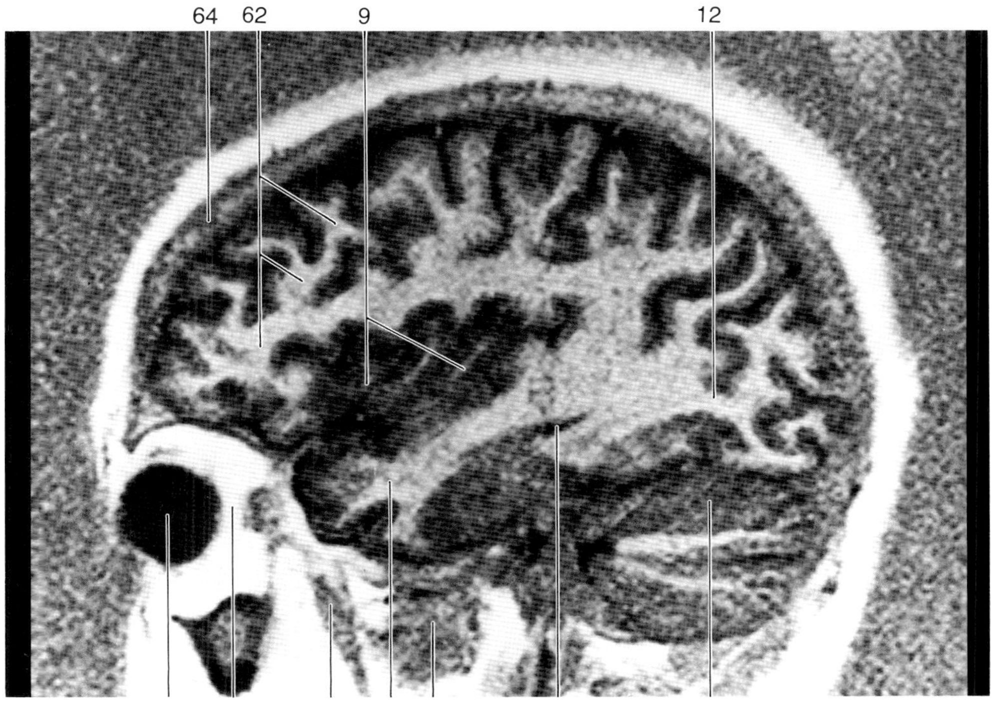

MRI, IR 1900/400/30, level 3

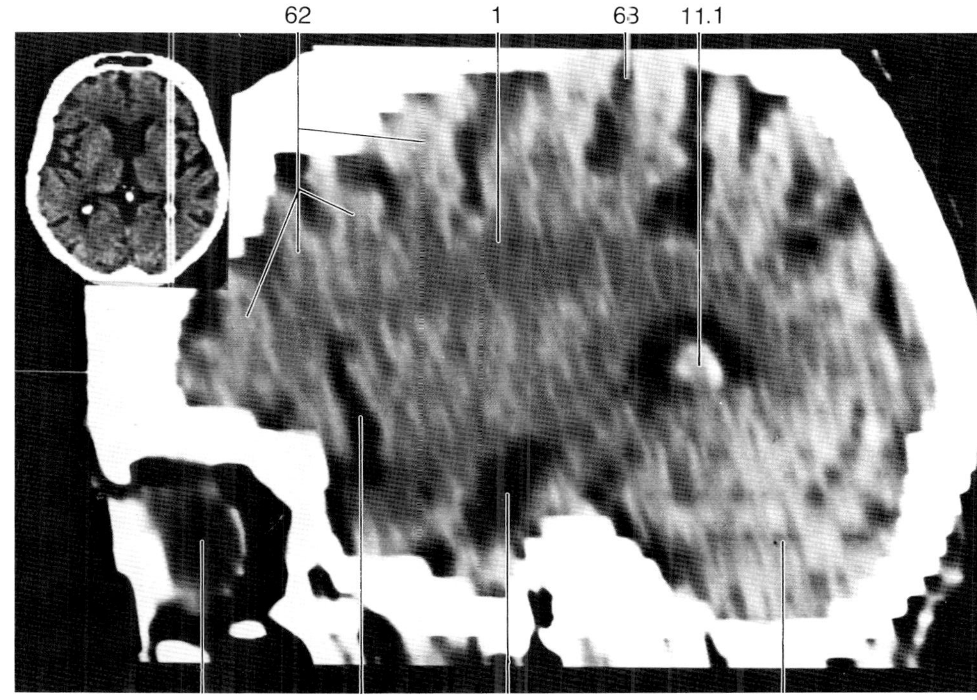

CT, sagittal reconstruction at level 3

1	Semioval center	58	Orbital fat pad
2	Precentral gyrus	62	Medial frontal gyrus
3	Postcentral gyrus	64	Frontal bone
9	Insula	66	Lateral fissure
11	White matter of the temporal lobe	67	Frontal lobe
		68	Central sulcus
11.1	Chorioid plexus	69	Supramarginal gyrus
12	Occipital lobe	70	Temporal horn of the lateral ventricle
42	Lateral pterygoid muscle		
43	Temporal muscle	71	Cerebellar hemisphere
54.1	Vitreous body		

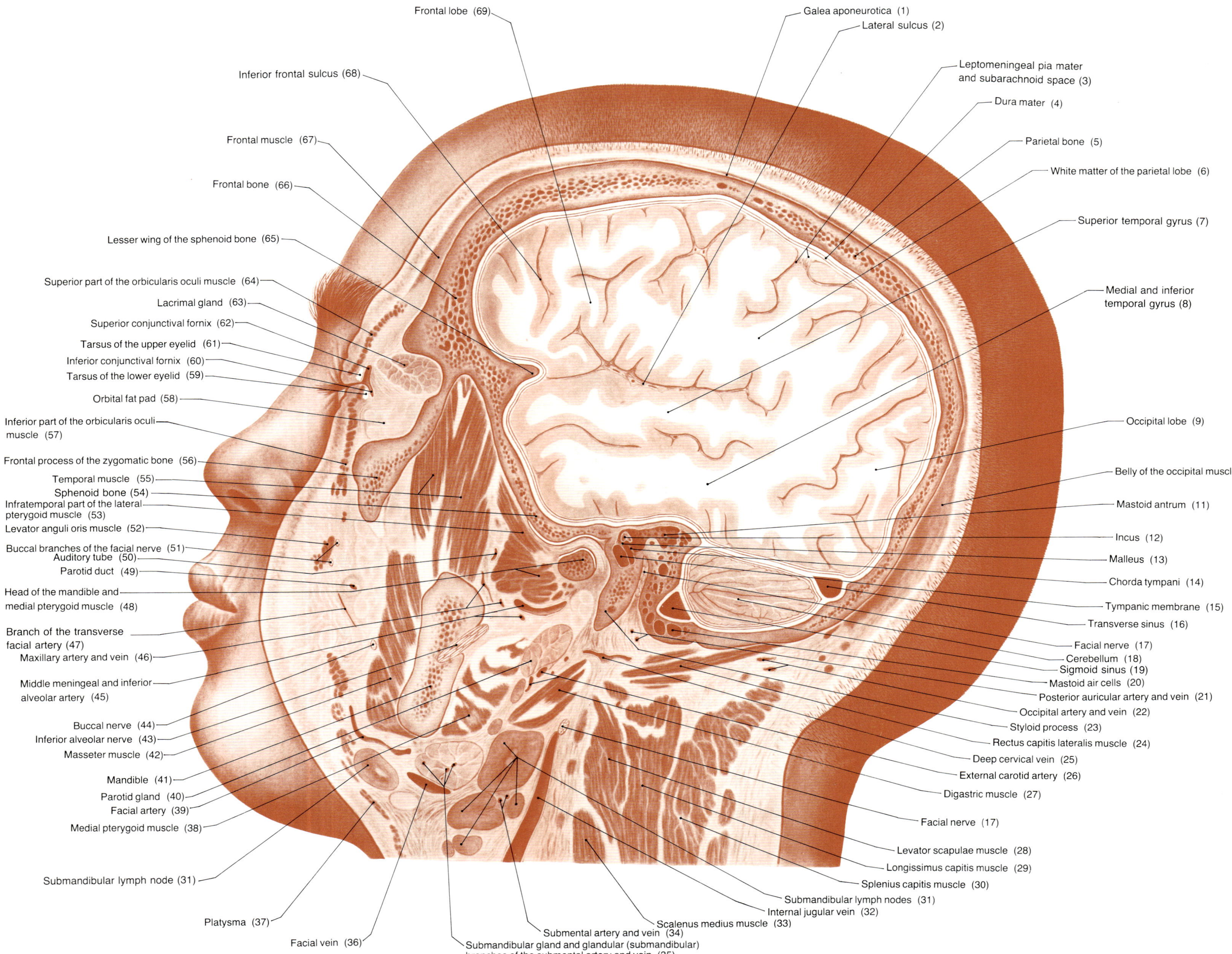

1 Galea aponeurotica
2 Sulcus lateralis
3 Pia mater et spatium subarachnoideale
4 Dura mater
5 Os parietale
6 Substantia alba lobi parietalis
7 Gyrus temporalis superior
7.1 Sulcus temporalis superior
7.2 Sulcus praecentralis
7.3 Sulcus centralis
7.4 Sulcus postcentralis
7.5 Cornu temporale ventriculi lateralis
8 Gyrus temporalis medius et inferior
9 Lobus occipitalis (Gyri occipitotemporalis)
10 Venter m. occipitalis
11 Antrum mastoideum
12 Incus
13 Malleus
14 Chorda tympani
15 Membrana tympani
16 Sinus transversus
17 N. facialis
18 Cerebellum
19 Sinus sigmoideus
20 Cellulae mastoideae
21 A. et V. auricularis posterior
22 A. et V. occipitalis
23 Processus styloideus
24 M. rectus capitis lateralis
25 V. cervicalis profunda
26 A. carotis externa
27 M. digastricus
28 M. levator scapulae
29 M. longissimus capitis
30 M. splenius capitis
31 Nodus lymphaticus submandibularis
32 V. jugularis interna
33 M. scalenus medius
34 A. et V. submentalis
35 Glandula submandibularis et Rr. glandulares (submand.) A. et V. submandibularis
36 V. facialis
37 Platysma
38 M. pterygoideus medialis
39 A. facialis
40 Glandula parotis
41 Mandibula
42 M. masseter
43 N. alveolaris inferior
44 N. buccalis
45 A. meningea media et A. alveolaris inferior
46 A. et V. maxiallaris
47 R. a. transversa facialis
48 Caput mandibulae et M. pterygoideus medialis
49 Ductus parotideus
50 Tuba auditiva
51 Rr. buccales n. facialis
52 M. levator anguli oris
53 Pars infratemporalis m. pterygoidei lateralis
54 Os sphenoidale
55 M. temporalis
56 Processus frontalis (oss. zyg.)
57 M. orbicularis oculi inferior
58 Capsula adiposa orbitae
59 Tarsus inferior palpebrae
60 Fornix conjunctivae inferior
61 Tarsus superior palpebrae
62 Fornix conjunctivae superior
63 Glandula lacrimalis
64 M. orbicularis oculi superior
65 Ala minor (oss. sphen.)
66 Os frontale
67 M. frontalis
68 Sulcus frontalis inferior
69 Lobus frontalis
70 Insula
71 Sulcus circularis insulae

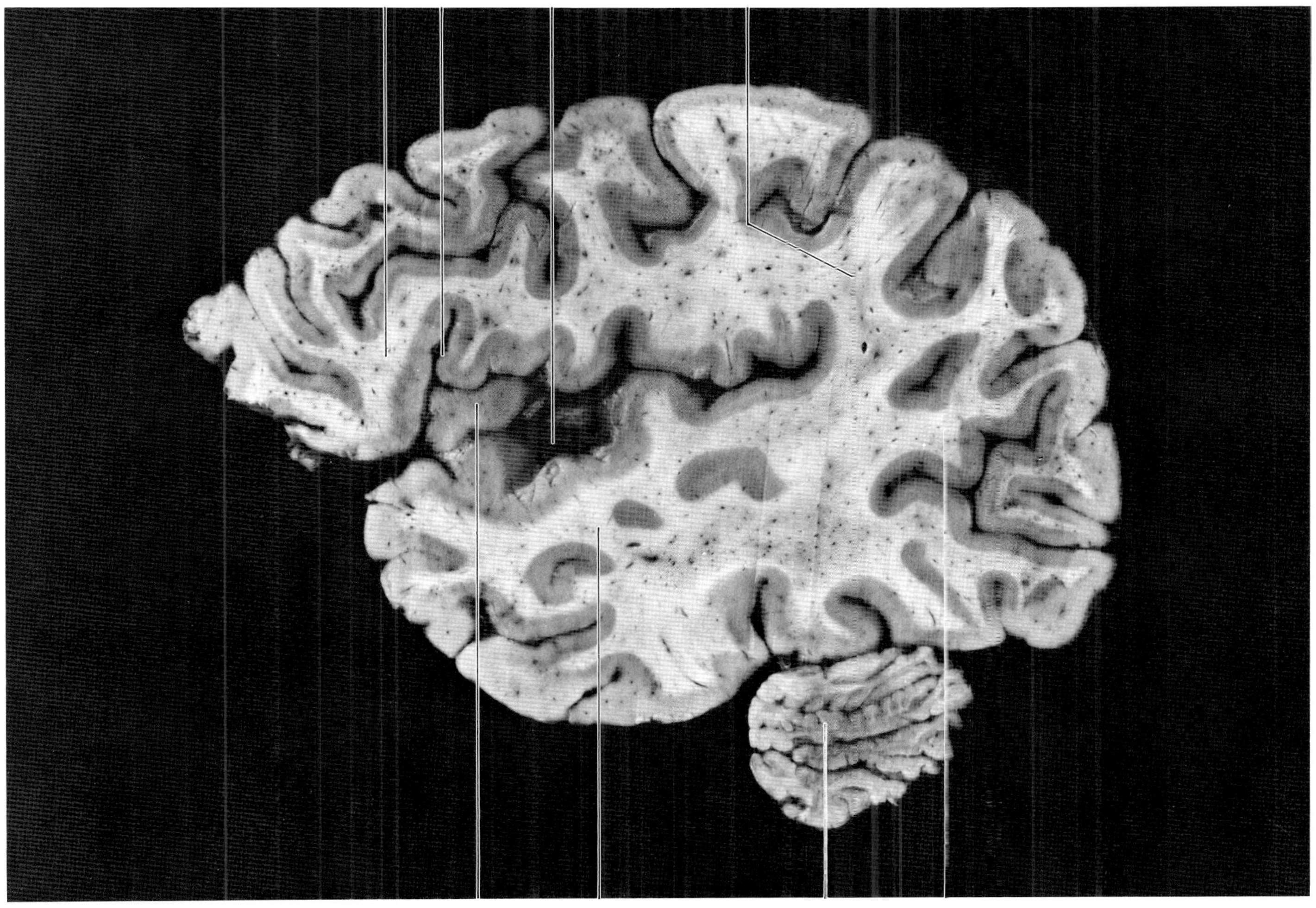

Anatomical section at level 4

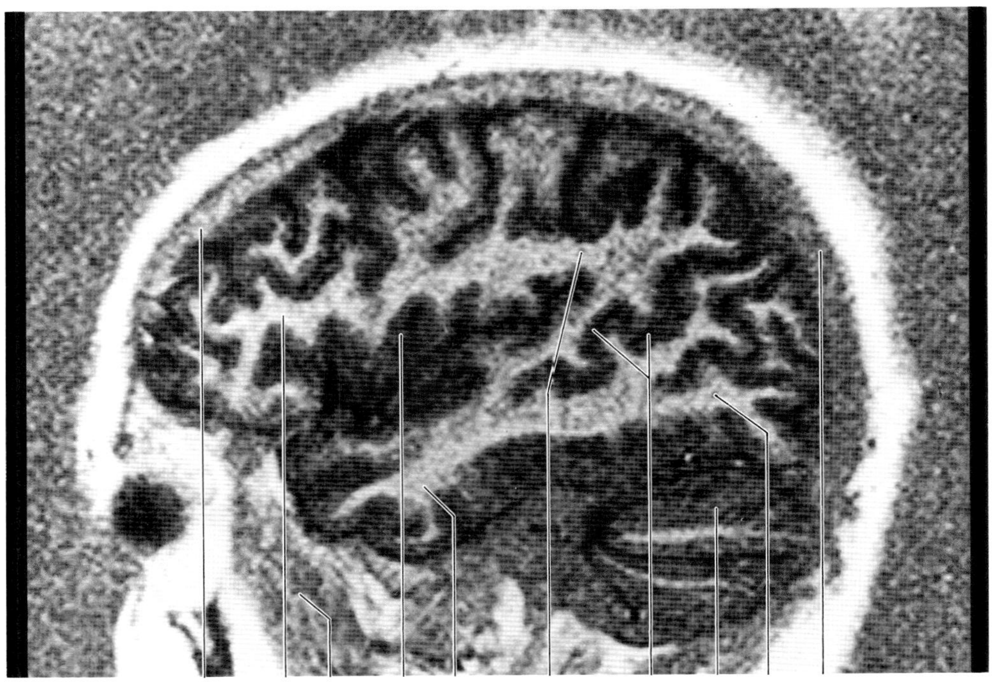

MRI IR 1900/400/300, level 4

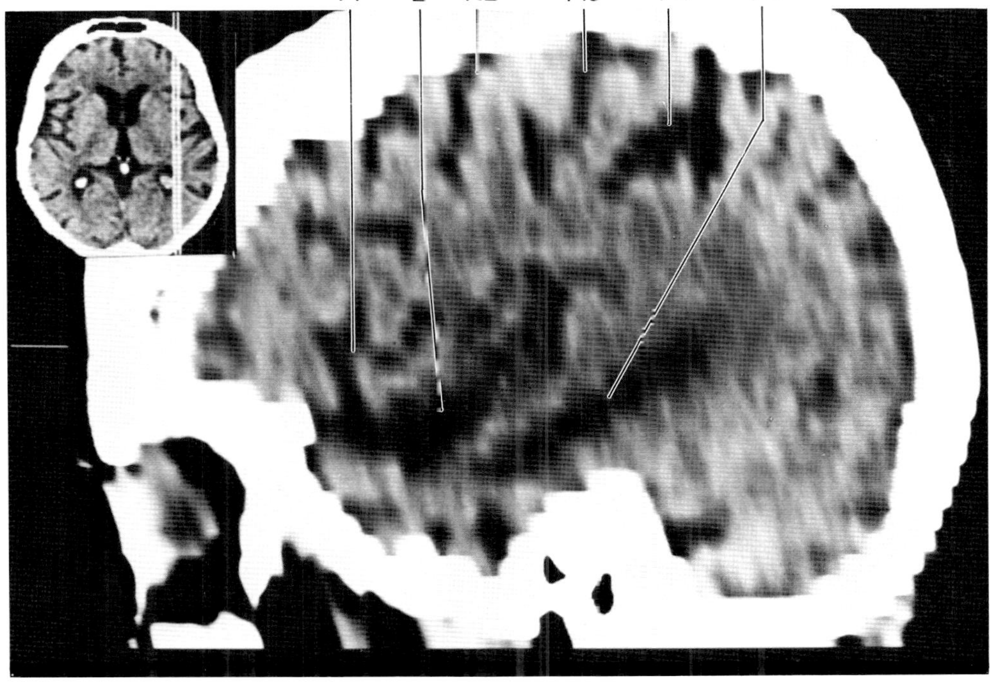

CT, sagittal reconstruction at level 4

2 Lateral fissure
5 Parietal bone
6 White matter of the parietal lobe
7 Superior temporal gyrus
7.1 Superior temporal sulcus
7.2 Precentral sulcus
7.3 Central sulcus
7.4 Postcentral sulcus
7.5 Temporal horn of the lateral ventricle
8 Parietooccipital sulcus
9 Occipital lobe (occipitotemporal gyrus)
18 Cerebellum
55 Temporal muscle
66 Frontal bone
69 Frontal lobe
70 Insula
71 Circular sulcus

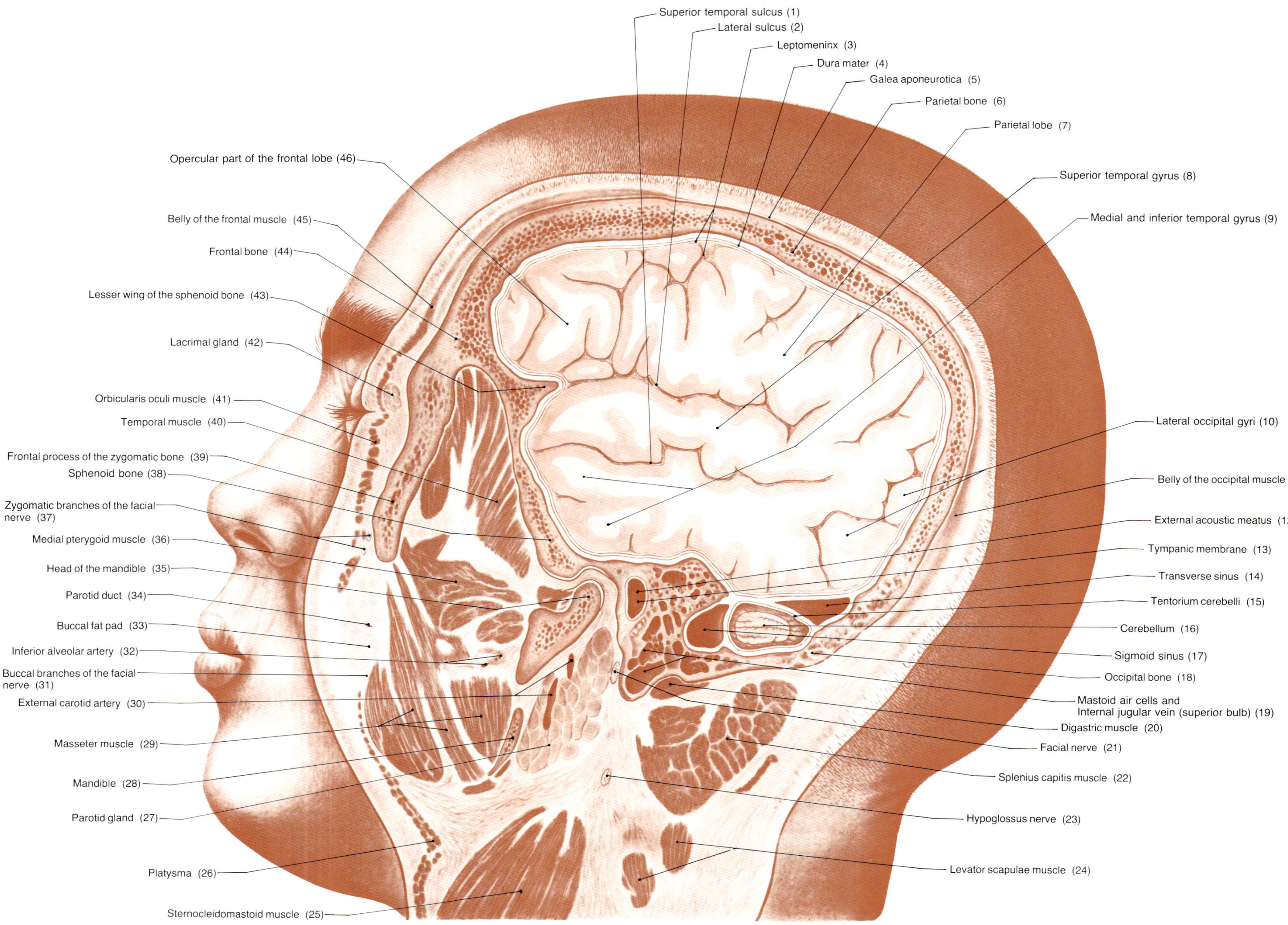

1 Sulcus temporalis superior
2 Fissura lateralis
3 Leptomeninx
4 Dura mater
5 Galea aponeurotica
6 Os parietale
7 Lobus parietalis
8 Gyrus temporalis superior
9 Gyrus temporalis medius et inferior
10 Gyri orbitales laterales
11 Venter m. occipitalis
12 Meatus acusticus externus
13 Membrana tympani
14 Sinus transversus
15 Tentorium cerebelli
16 Cerebellum
17 Sinus sigmoideus
18 Os occipitale
19 Cellulae mastoideae et Bulbus v. jugularis superius
20 M. digastricus
21 N. facialis
22 M. splenius capitis
23 N. hypoglossus
24 M. levator scapulae
25 M. sternocleidomastoideus
26 Platysma
27 Glandula parotis
28 Mandibula
29 M. masseter
30 A. carotis externa
31 Rr. buccales n. faciales
32 A. alveolaris inferior
33 Corpus adiposum buccae
34 Ductus parotideus
35 Caput mandibulae
36 M. pterygoideus medialis
37 Rr. zygomatici n. facialis
38 Os sphenoidale
39 Processus frontalis (oss. zyg.)
40 M. temporalis
41 M. orbicularis oculi
42 Glandula lacrimalis
43 Ala minor (oss. sphen.)
44 Os frontale
45 Venter m. frontalis
46 Lobus frontalis (pars opercularis)
46.1 Sulcus praecentralis
46.2 Sulcus centralis
46.3 Sulcus postcentralis
46.4 Gyrus supramarginalis

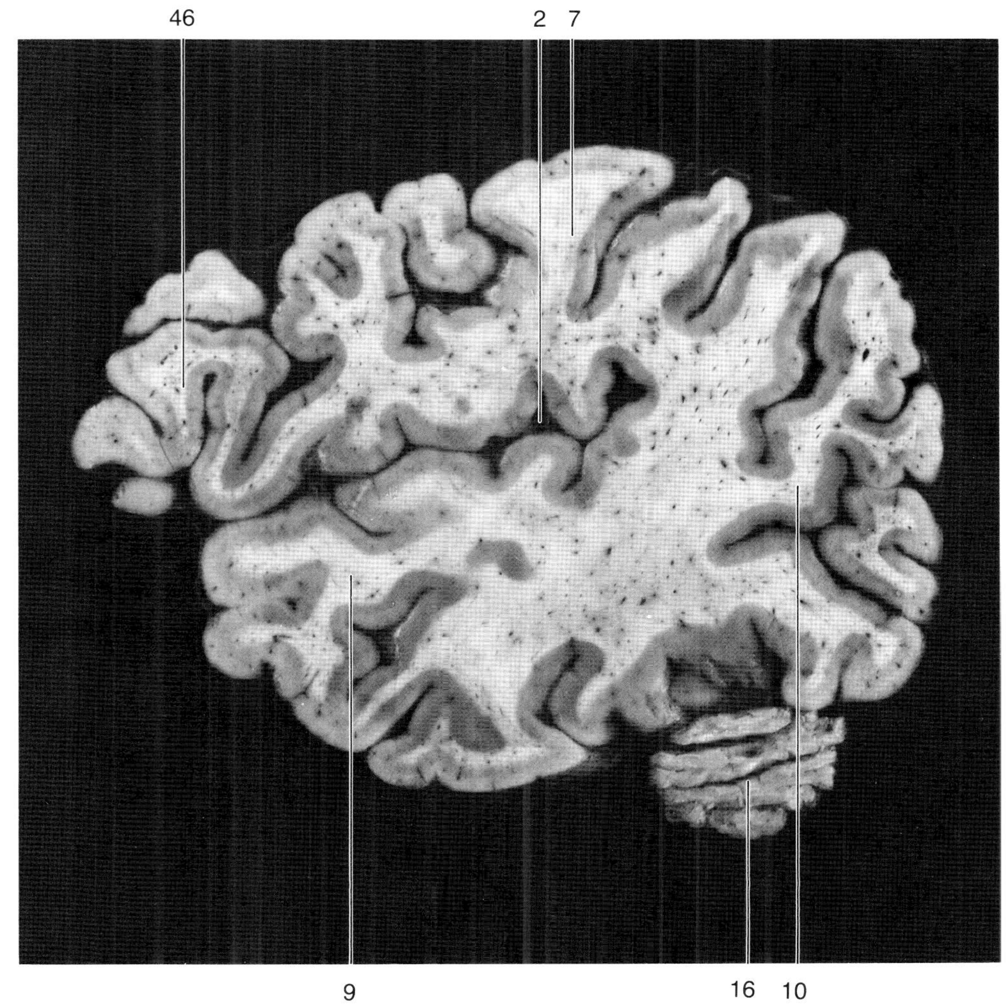

Anatomical section at level 5

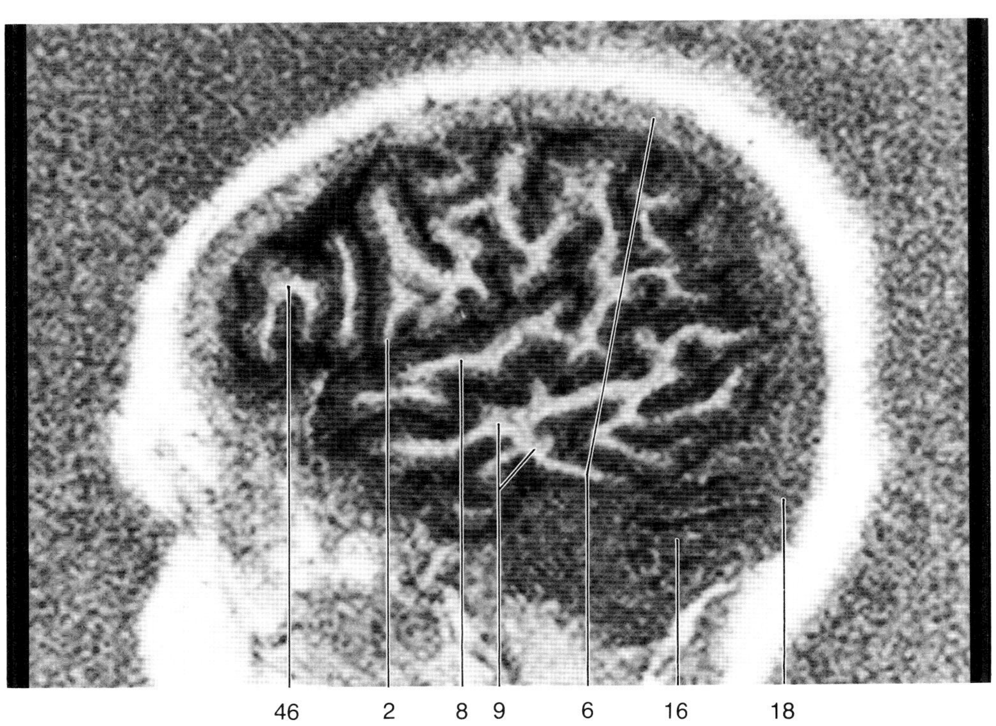

MRI, IR 1900/400/300, level 5

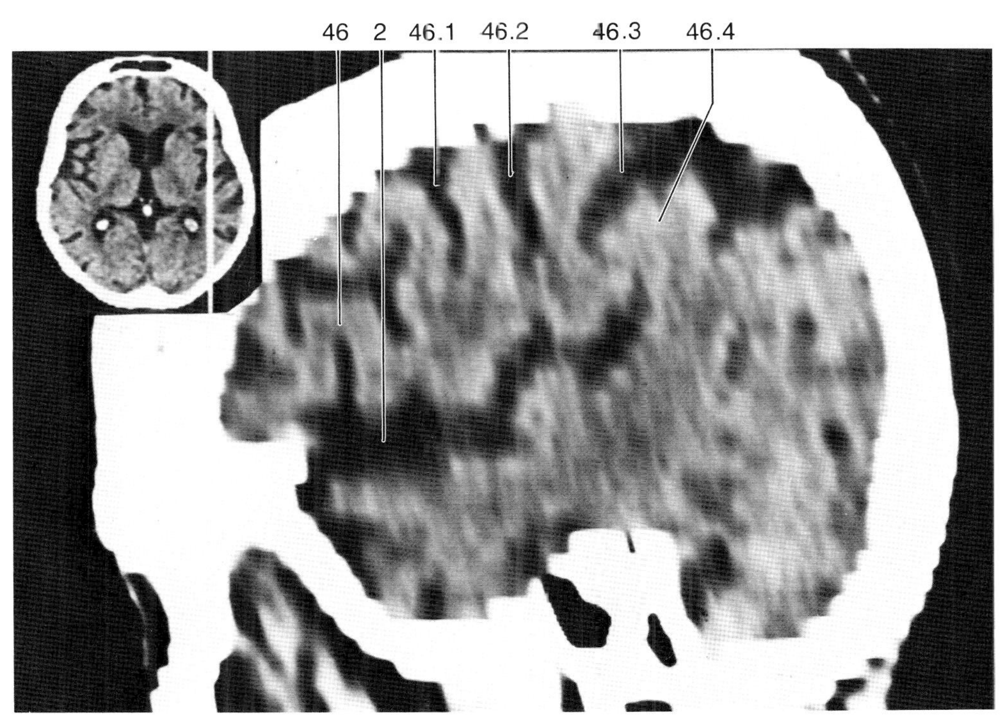

CT, sagittal reconstruction at level 5

2	Lateral fissure
6	Parietal bone
7	Parietal lobe
8	Superior temporal gyrus
9	Medial and inferior temporal gyrus
10	Occipital lobe
16	Cerebellum
18	Occipital bone
46	Opercular part of the frontal lobe
46.1	Precentral sulcus
46.2	Central sulcus
46.3	Postcentral sulcus
46.4	Supramarginal gyrus

Axial Sections of the Brain and Head

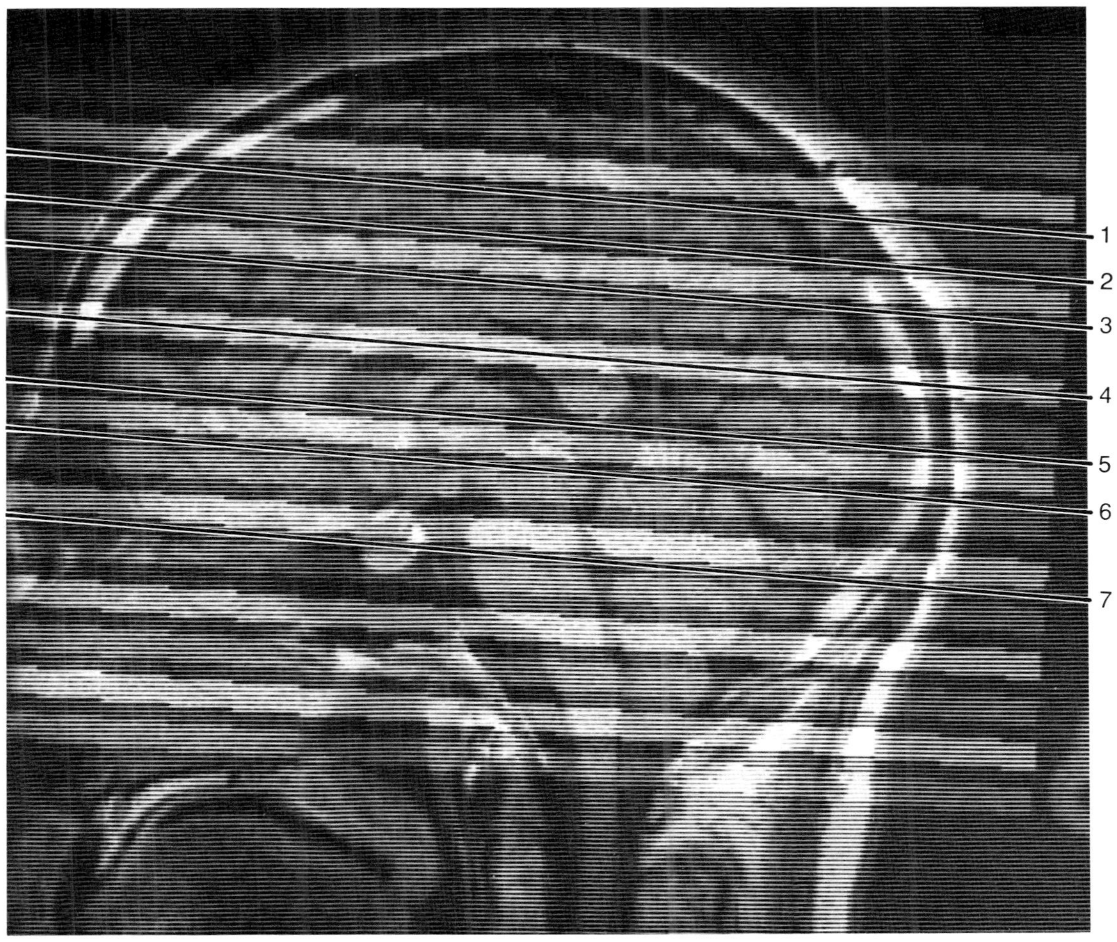

Sagittal MRI section. Axial slices at levels no. 1–7. Slice thickness 5 mm.

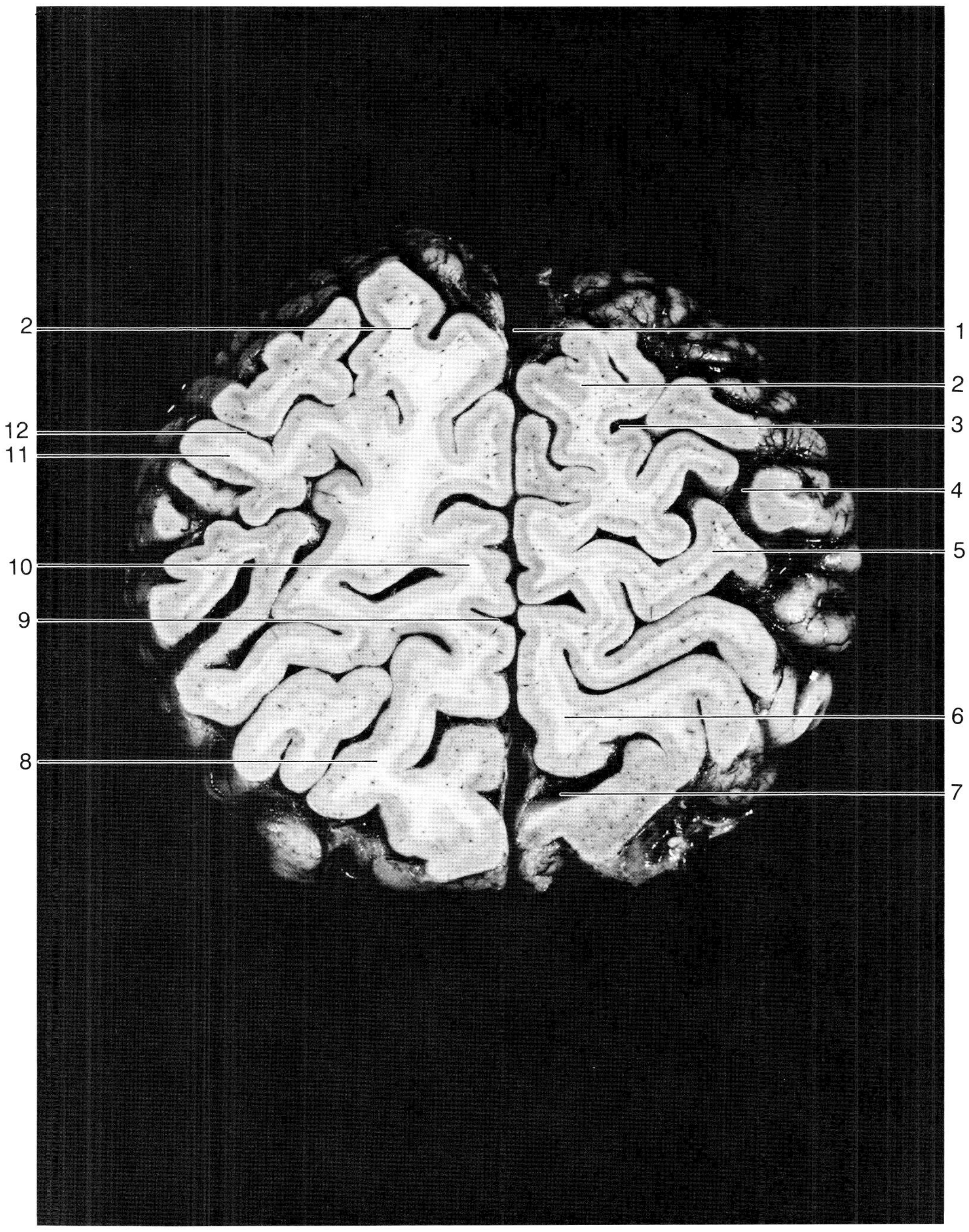

Anatomical section at level 1

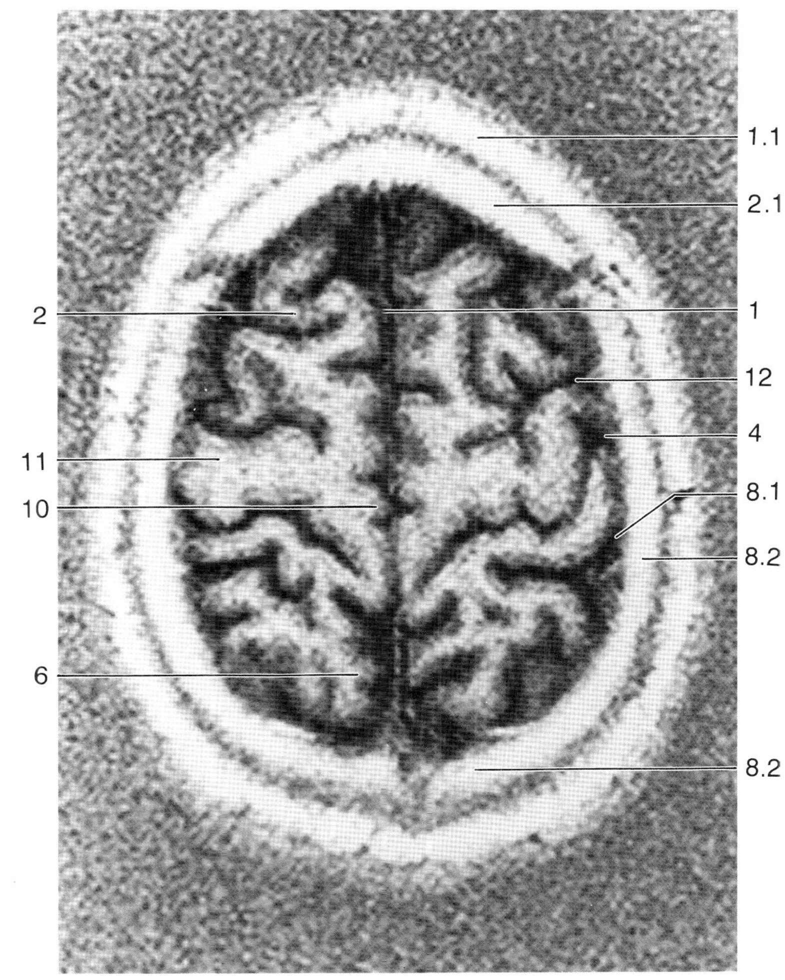

MRI section at level 1, IR 1800/400/30

1	Longitudinal cerebral fissure	1	Fissura longitudinalis cerebri
1.1	Korium and galea aponeurotica	1.1	Corium et galea aponeurotica
2	Superior frontal gyrus	2	Gyrus frontalis superior
2.1	Frontal bone	2.1	Os frontale
3	Superior frontal sulcus	3	Sulcus frontalis superior
4	Central sulcus	4	Sulcus centralis
5	Postcentral gyrus	5	Gyrus postcentralis
6	Precuneus	6	Praecuneus
7	Parieto-occipital sulcus	7	Sulcus parieto-occipitalis
8	Superior parietal lobule	8	Lobulus parietalis superior
8.1	Postcentral sulcus	8.1	Sulcus postcentralis
8.2	Parietal bone	8.2	Os parietale
9	Cingulate sulcus	9	Sulcus cinguli
10	Paracentral lobule	10	Lobulus paracentralis
11	Precentral gyrus	11	Gyrus praecentralis
12	Precentral sulcus	12	Sulcus praecentralis

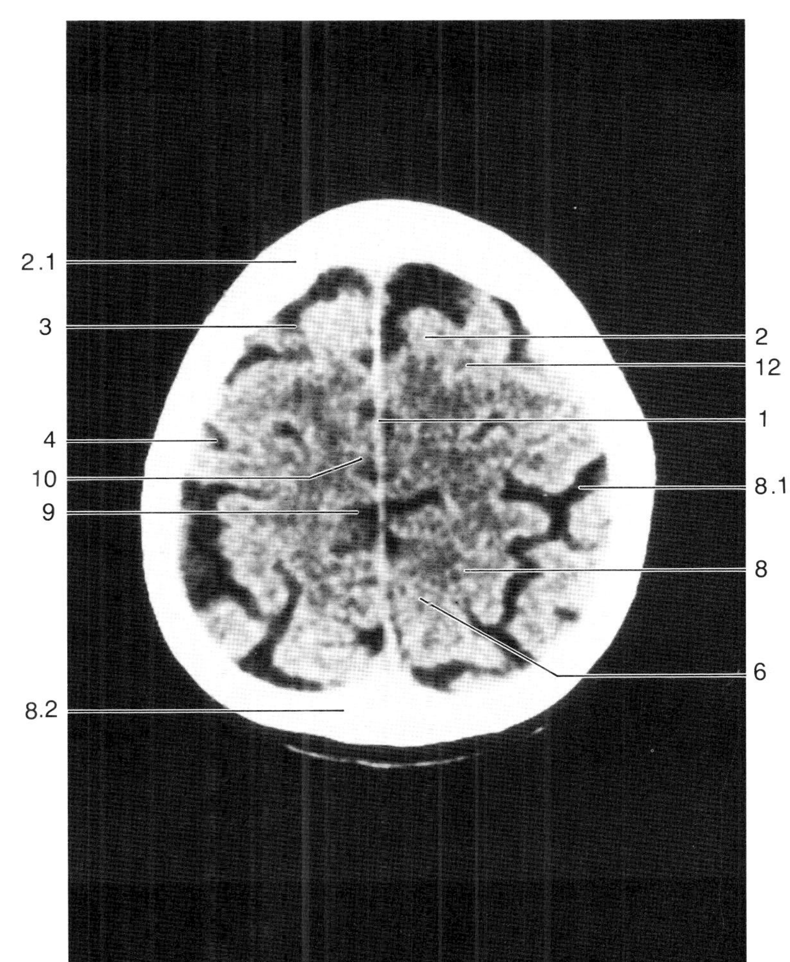

CT scan at level 1

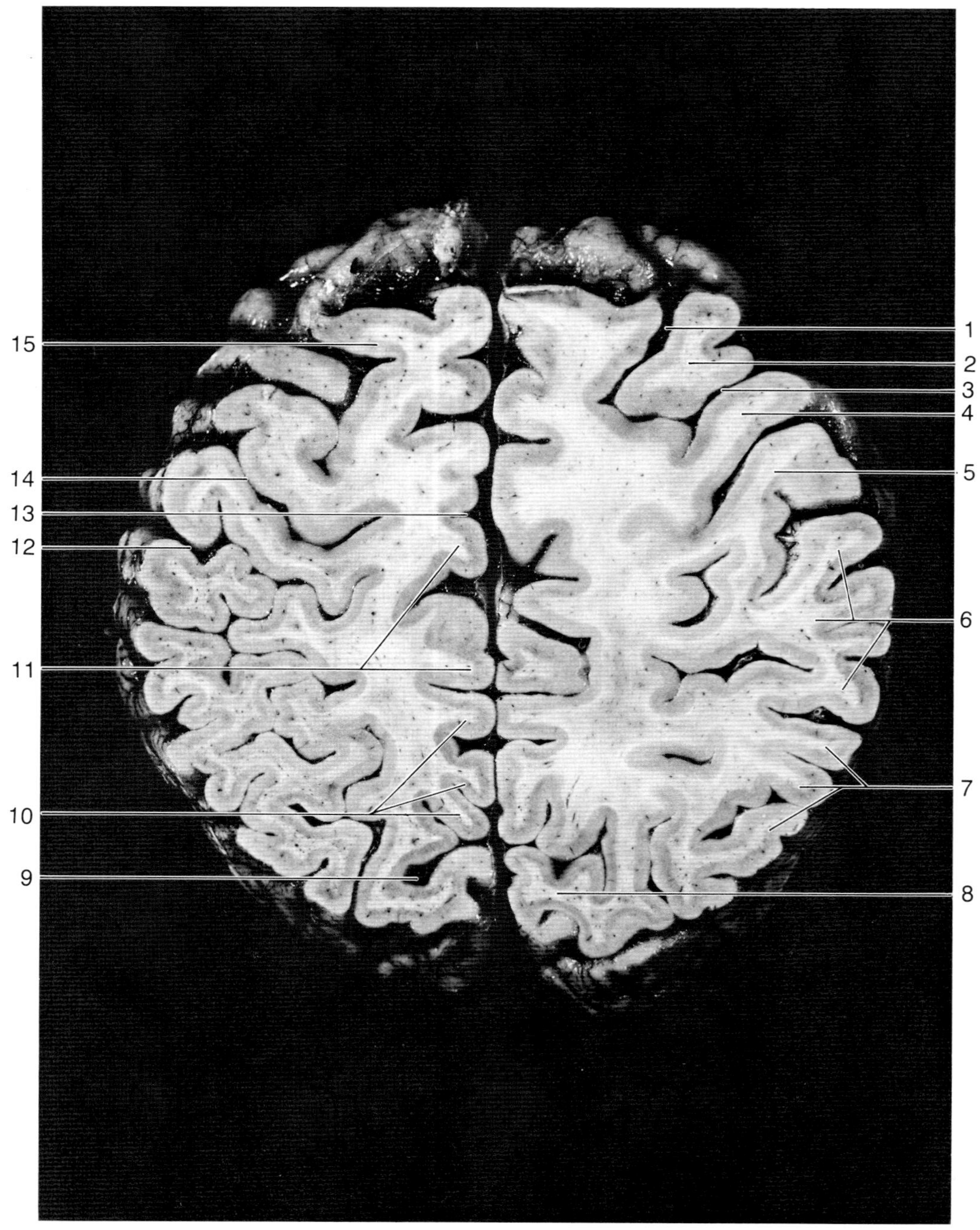

Anatomical section at level 2

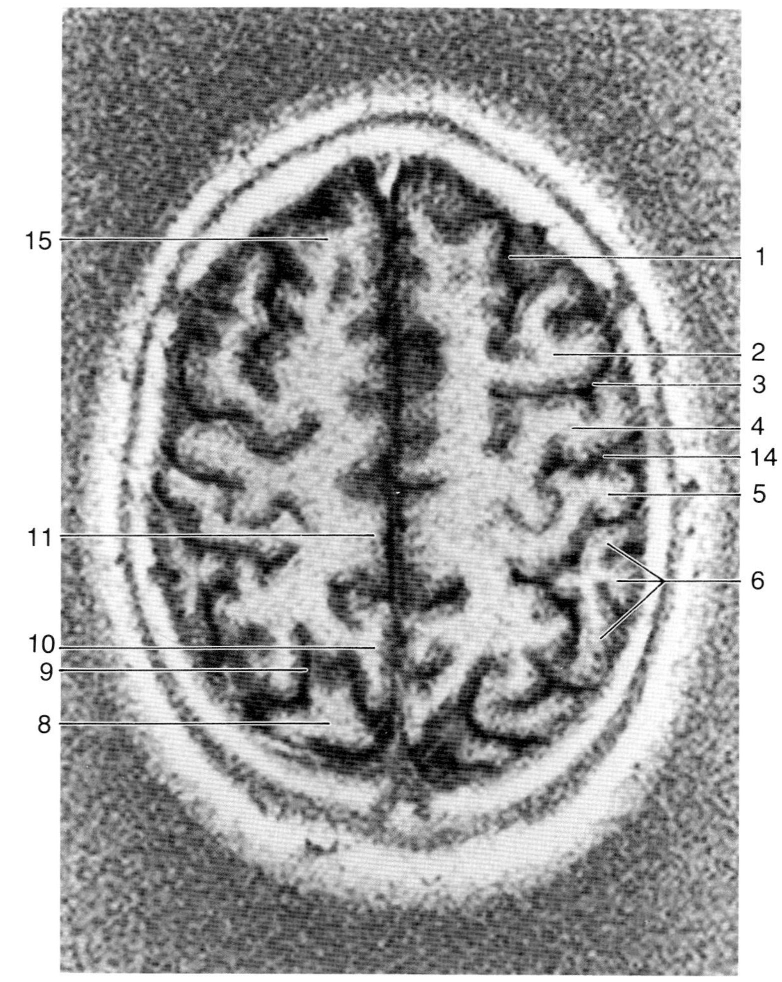

MRI section at level 2, IR 1800/400/30

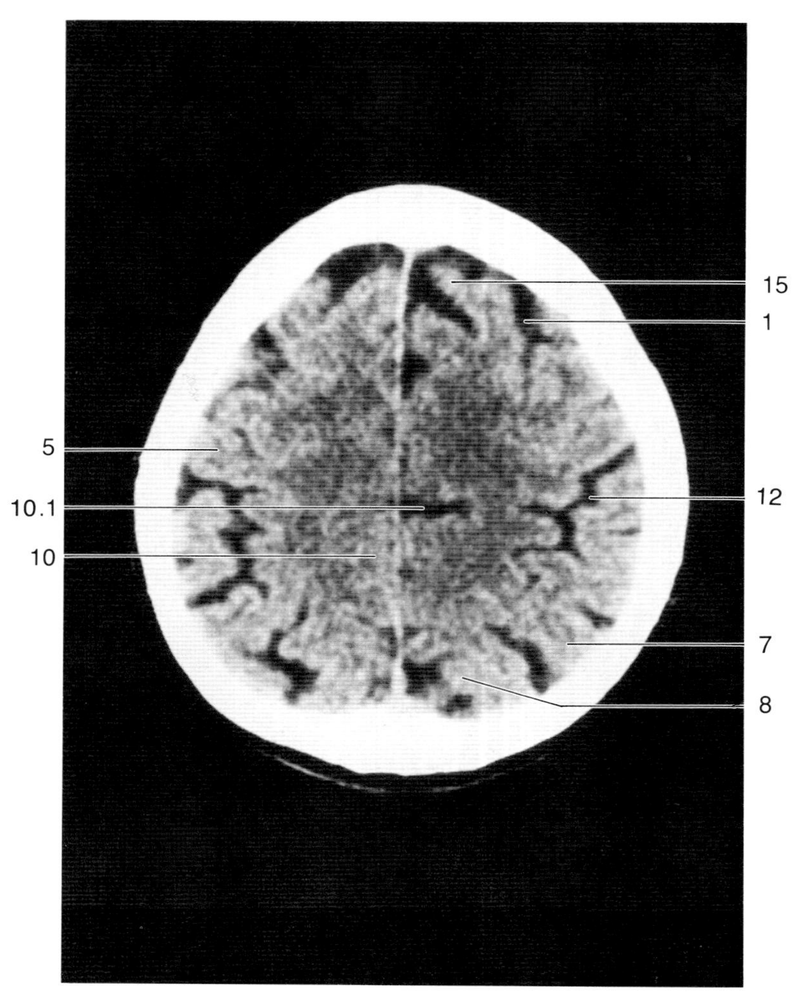

CT scan at level 2

1	Superior frontal sulcus	1	Sulcus frontalis superior
2	Middle frontal gyrus	2	Gyrus frontalis medius
3	Precentral sulcus	3	Sulcus praecentralis
4	Precentral gyrus	4	Gyrus praecentralis
5	Postcentral gyrus	5	Gyrus postcentralis
6	Supramarginal gyrus	6	Gyrus supramarginalis
7	Angular gyrus	7	Gyrus angularis
8	Occipital lobe	8	Lobus occipitalis
9	Parieto-occipital sulcus	9	Sulcus parieto-occipitalis
10	Precuneus	10	Praecuneus
10.1	Cingulate sulcus	10.1	Sulcus cinguli
11	Paracentral lobule	11	Lobulus paracentralis
12	Postcentral sulcus	12	Sulcus postcentralis
13	Paracentral sulcus	13	Sulcus paracentralis
14	Central sulcus	14	Sulcus centralis
15	Superior frontal gyrus	15	Gyrus frontalis superior

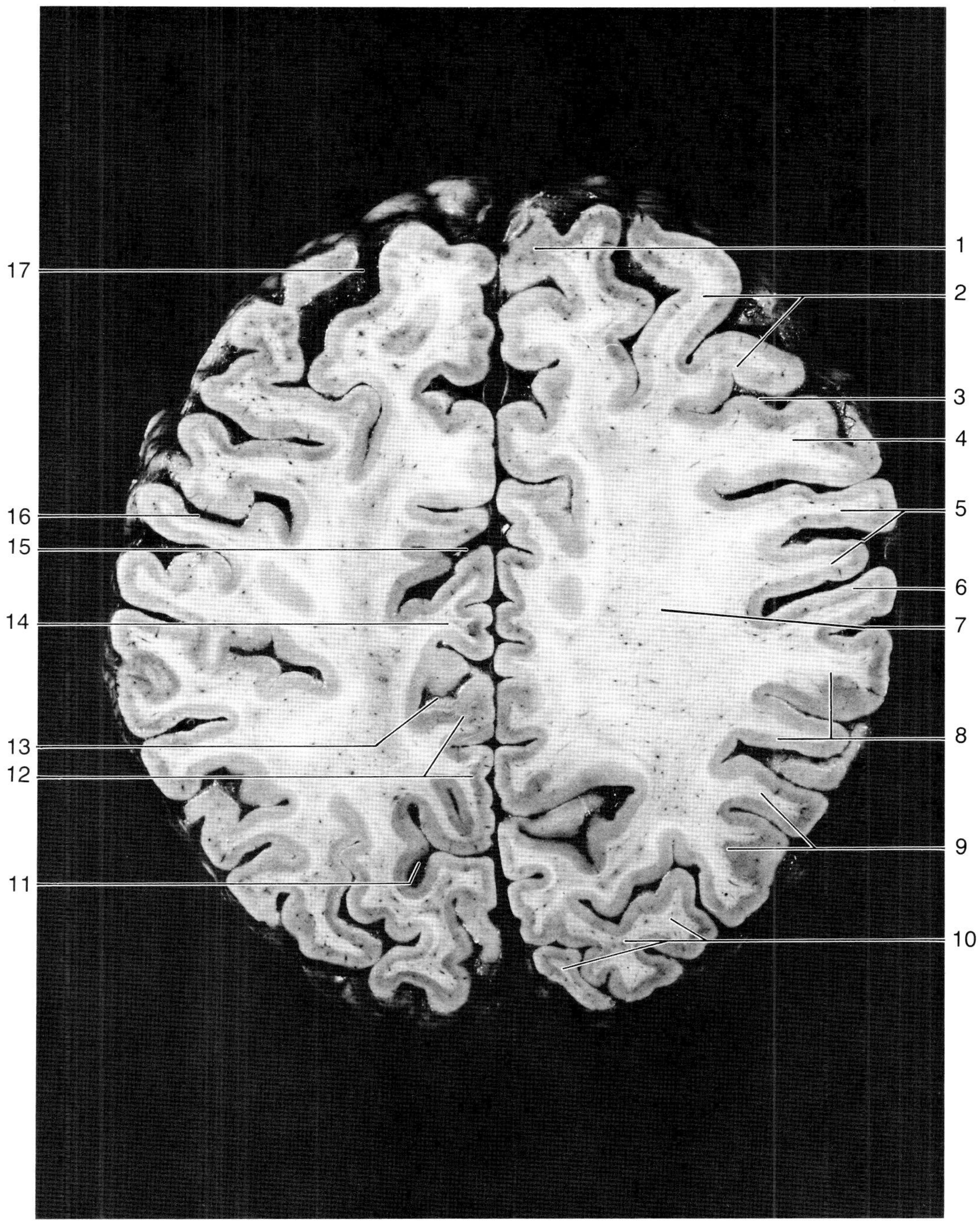

Anatomical section at level 3

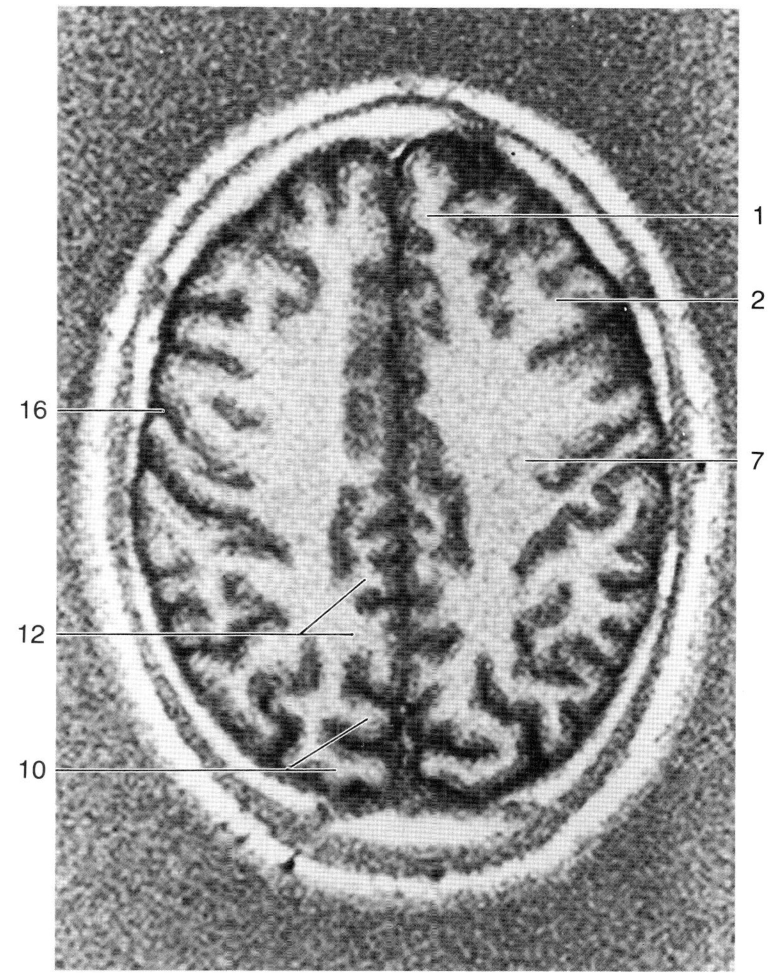

MRI section at level 3, IR 1800/400/30

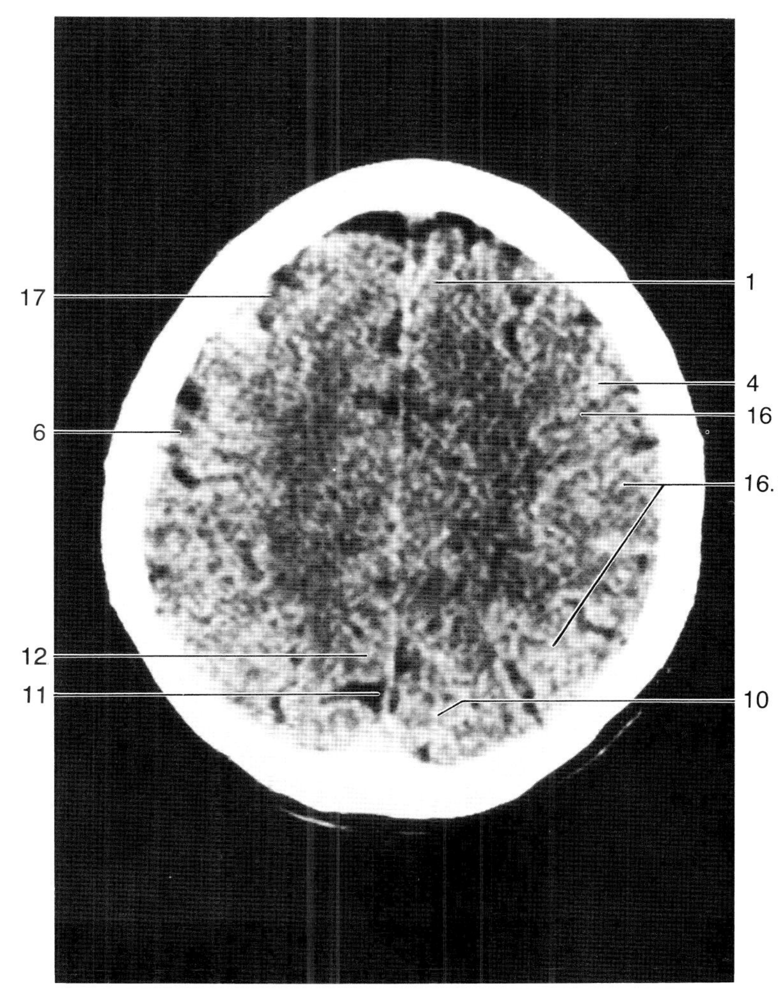

CT scan at level 3

1	Superior frontal gyrus	1	Gyrus frontalis superior
2	Middle frontal gyrus	2	Gyrus frontalis medius
3	Precentral sulcus	3	Sulcus praecentralis
4	Precentral gyrus	4	Gyrus praecentralis
5	Postcentral gyrus	5	Gyrus postcentralis
6	Postcentral sulcus	6	Sulcus postcentralis
7	Semioval center	7	Centrum semiovale
8	Supramarginal gyrus	8	Gyrus supramarginalis
9	Angular gyrus	9	Gyrus angularis
10	Occipital gyri	10	Gyri occipitales
11	Parieto-occipital sulcus	11	Sulcus parieto-occipitalis
12	Precuneus	12	Praecuneus
13	Subparietal sulcus	13	Sulcus subparietalis
14	Cingulate gyrus	14	Gyrus cinguli
15	Cingulate sulcus	15	Sulcus cinguli
16	Central sulcus	16	Sulcus centralis
16.1	Inferior parietal lobule	16.1	Lobulus parietalis inferior
17	Superior frontal sulcus	17	Sulcus frontalis superior

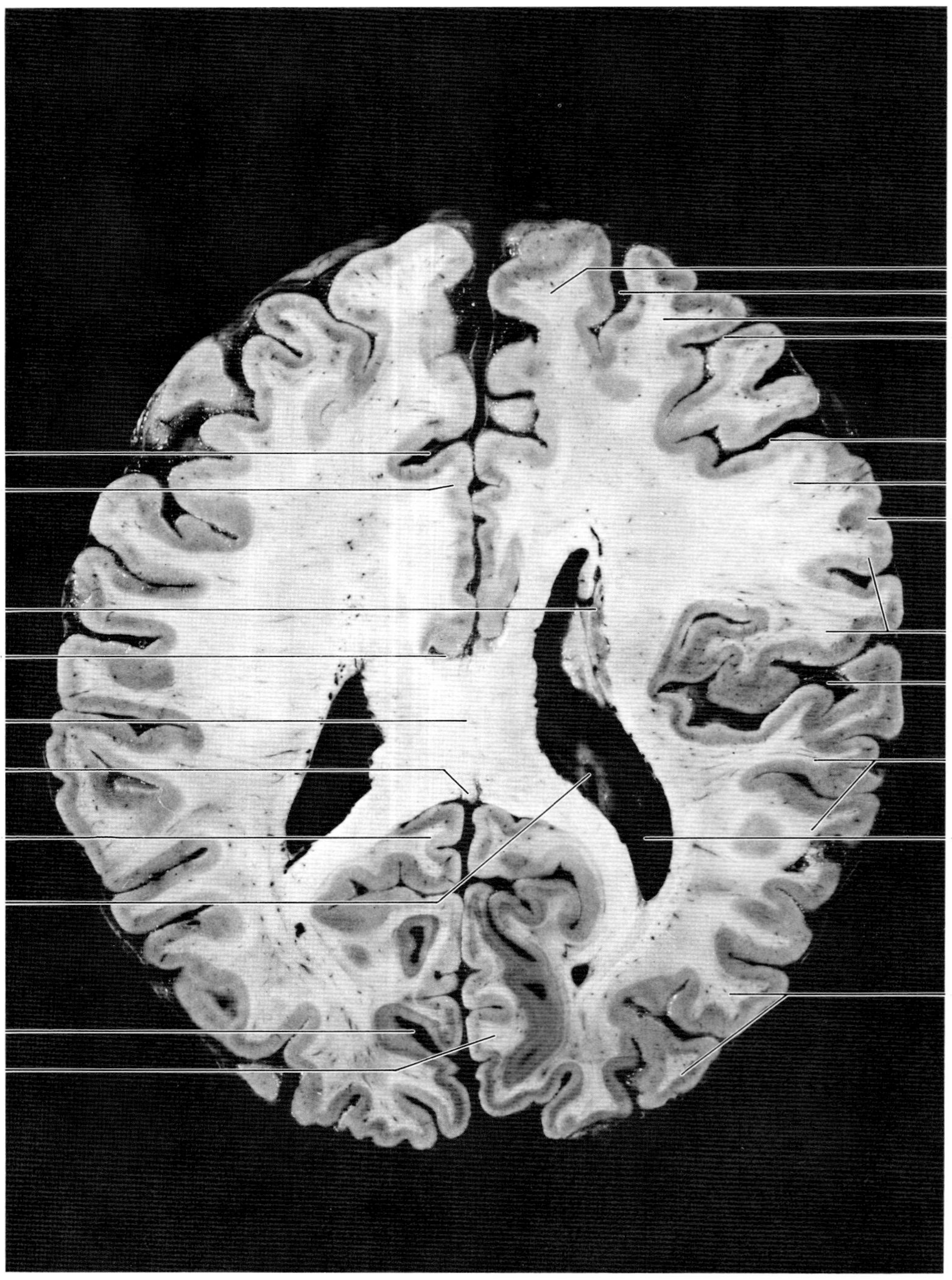

Anatomical section at level 4

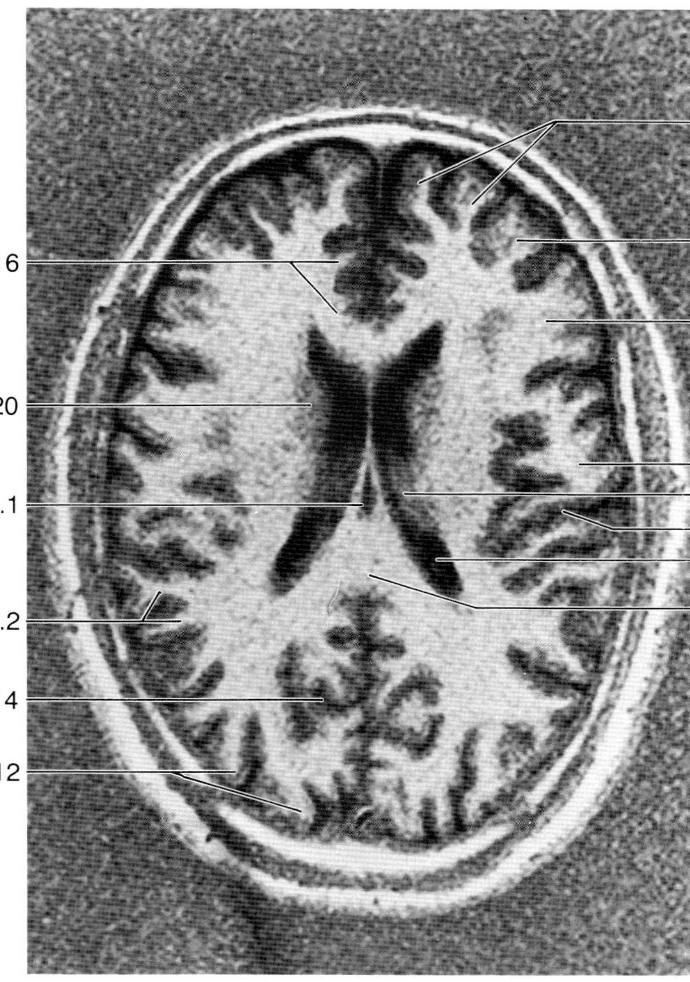

MRI section at level 4, IR 1800/400/30

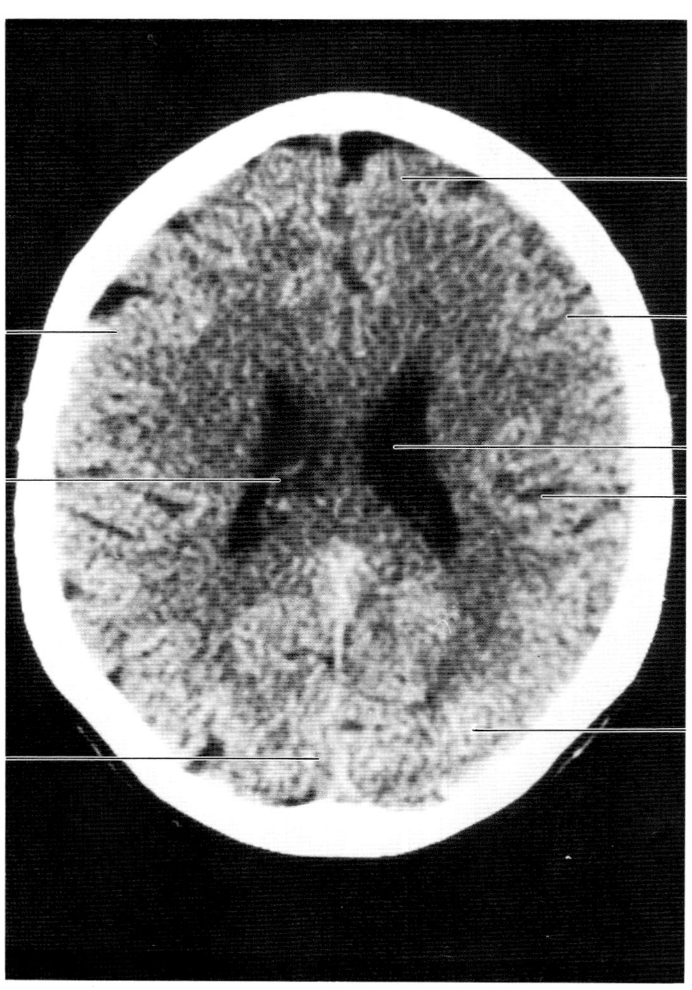

CT scan at level 4

1 Superior frontal gyrus
2 Superior frontal sulcus
3 Middle frontal gyrus
4 Inferior frontal sulcus
4.1 Inferior frontal gyrus
5 Precentral sulcus
6 Precentral gyrus
7 Central sulcus
8 Postcentral gyrus
9 Lateral fissure
10 Superior temporal gyrus
11 Lateral ventricle
12 Lateral occipital gyri
13 Lingual gyrus
14 Calcarine sulcus
15 Choroid plexus
16 Cingulate gyrus
17 Splenium of the corpus callosum
18 Body of the corpus callosum
19 Callosal sulcus
20 Caudate nucleus
20.1 Cistern of the velum interpositum
20.2 Inferior parietal lobule
21 Cingulate sulcus

1 Gyrus frontalis superior
2 Sulcus frontalis superior
3 Gyrus frontalis medius
4 Sulcus frontalis inferior
4.1 Gyrus frontalis inferior
5 Sulcus praecentralis
6 Gyrus praecentralis
7 Sulcus centralis
8 Gyrus postcentralis
9 Fissura lateralis
10 Gyrus temporalis superior
11 Ventriculus lateralis
12 Gyri occipitales laterales
13 Gyrus lingualis
14 Sulcus calcarinus
15 Plexus choroideus
16 Gyrus cinguli
17 Splenium corporis callosi
18 Truncus corporis callosi
19 Sulcus callosus
20 Nucleus caudatus
20.1 Cisterna veli interpositi
20.2 Lobulus parietalis inferior
21 Sulcus cinguli

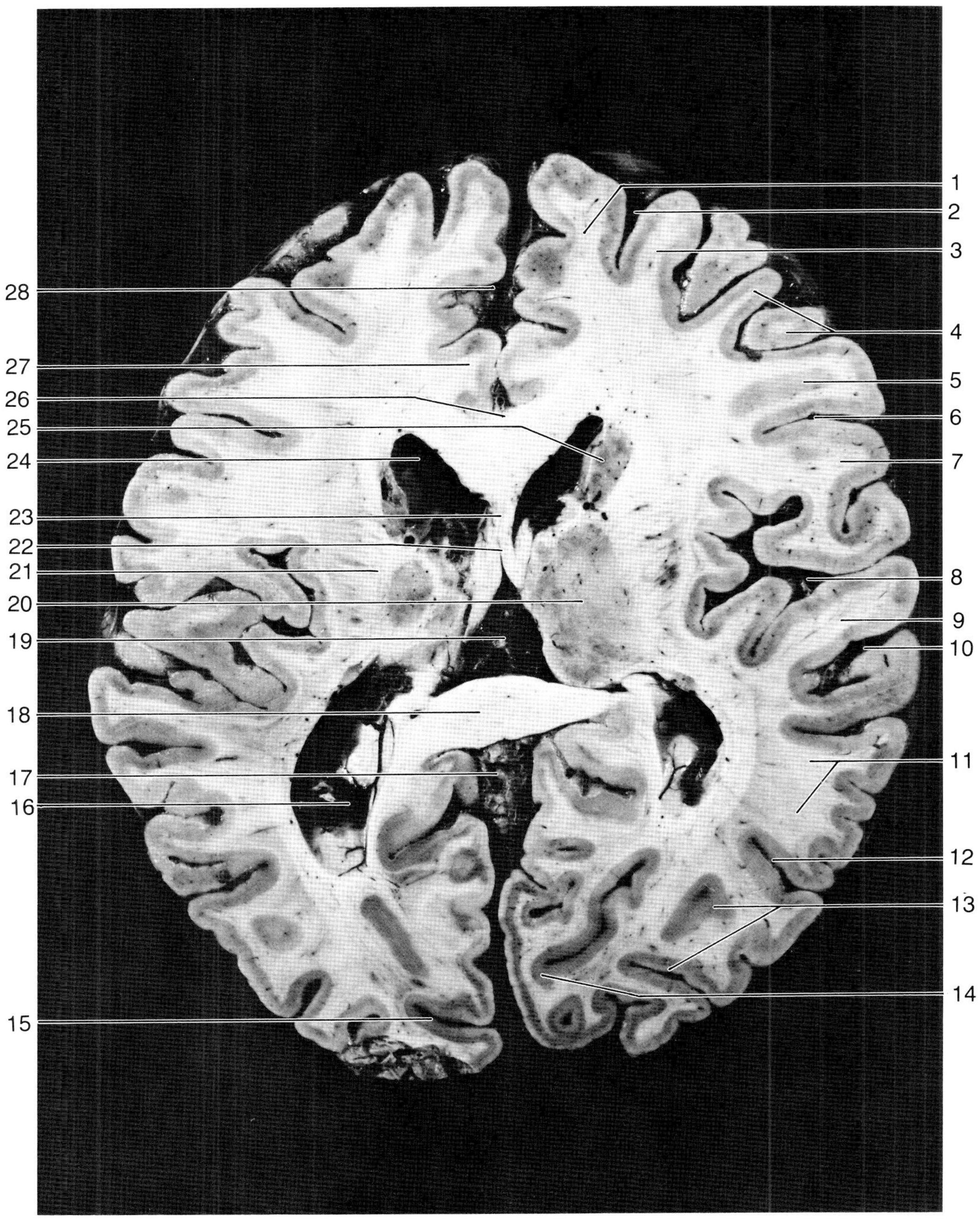

Anatomical section at level 5

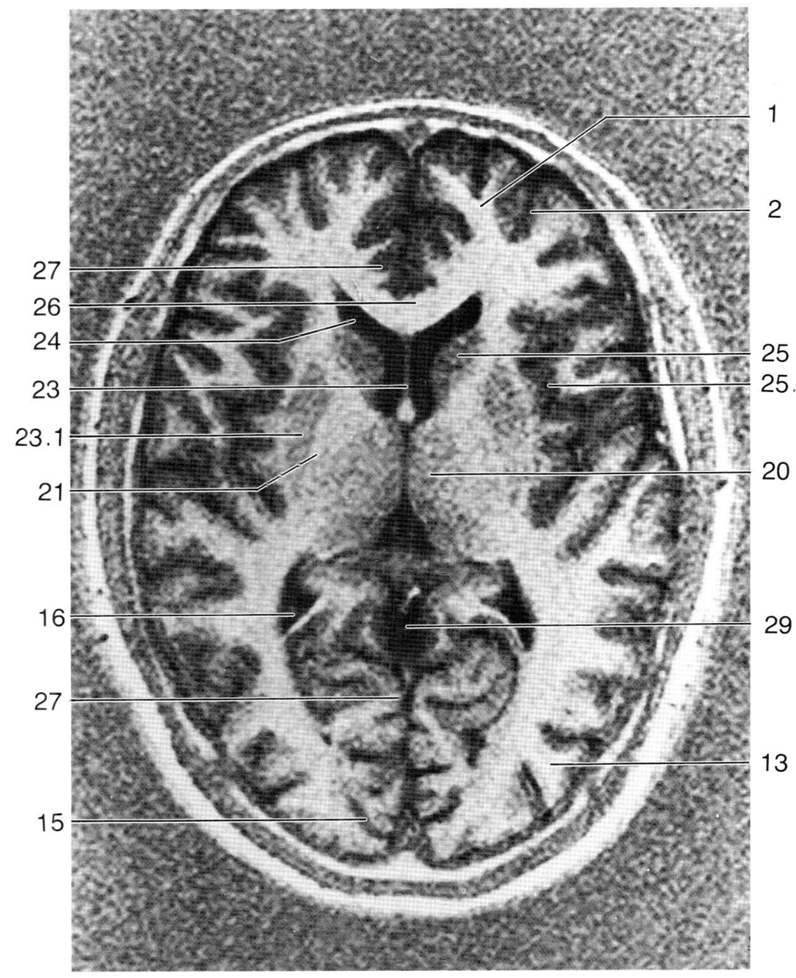

MRI section at level 5, IR 1800/400/30

1	Superior frontal gyrus	Gyrus frontalis superior
2	Superior frontal sulcus	Sulcus frontalis superior
3	Middle frontal gyrus	Gyrus frontalis medius
4	Inferior frontal gyrus	Gyrus frontalis inferior
5	Precentral gyrus	Gyrus praecentralis
6	Central sulcus	Sulcus centralis
7	Postcentral gyrus	Gyrus postcentralis
8	Lateral fissure	Fissura lateralis
9	Superior temporal gyrus	Gyrus temporalis superior
10	Superior temporal sulcus	Sulcus temporalis superior
11	Middle temporal gyrus	Gyrus temporalis medius
12	Middle temporal sulcus	Sulcus temporalis medius
13	Lateral occipital gyrus	Gyrus occipitalis lateralis
14	Lingual gyrus	Gyrus lingualis
15	Calcarine sulcus	Sulcus calcarinus
16	Trigonum of the lateral ventricle	Trigonum ventriculi lateralis
16.1	Posterior horn of the lateral ventricle	Cornu posterius ventriculi lateralis
17	Vermis of the cerebellum	Vermis cerebelli
18	Splenium of the corpus callosum	Splenium corporis callosi
18.1	Superior cerebellar cistern	Cisterna cerebelli superior
19	Third ventricle	Ventriculus III
20	Thalamus	Thalamus
21	Internal capsule	Capsula interna
22	Fornix	Fornix
23	Septum pellucidum	Septum pellucidum
23.1	Putamen	Putamen
24	Anterior horn of lateral ventricle	Cornu anterius ventriculi lateralis
25	Head of the caudate nucleus	Caput nuclei caudati
25.1	Insular cortex	Cortex insulae
26		Genu corporis callosi
27		Gyrus cinguli
28		Sulcus cinguli

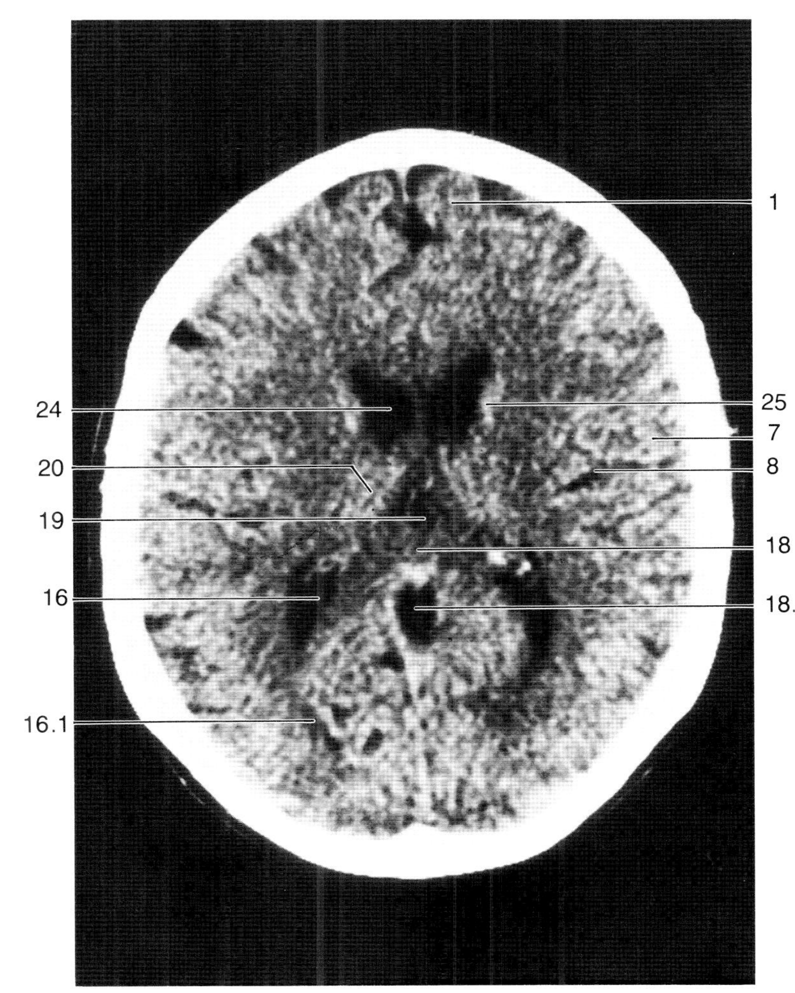

CT scan at level 5

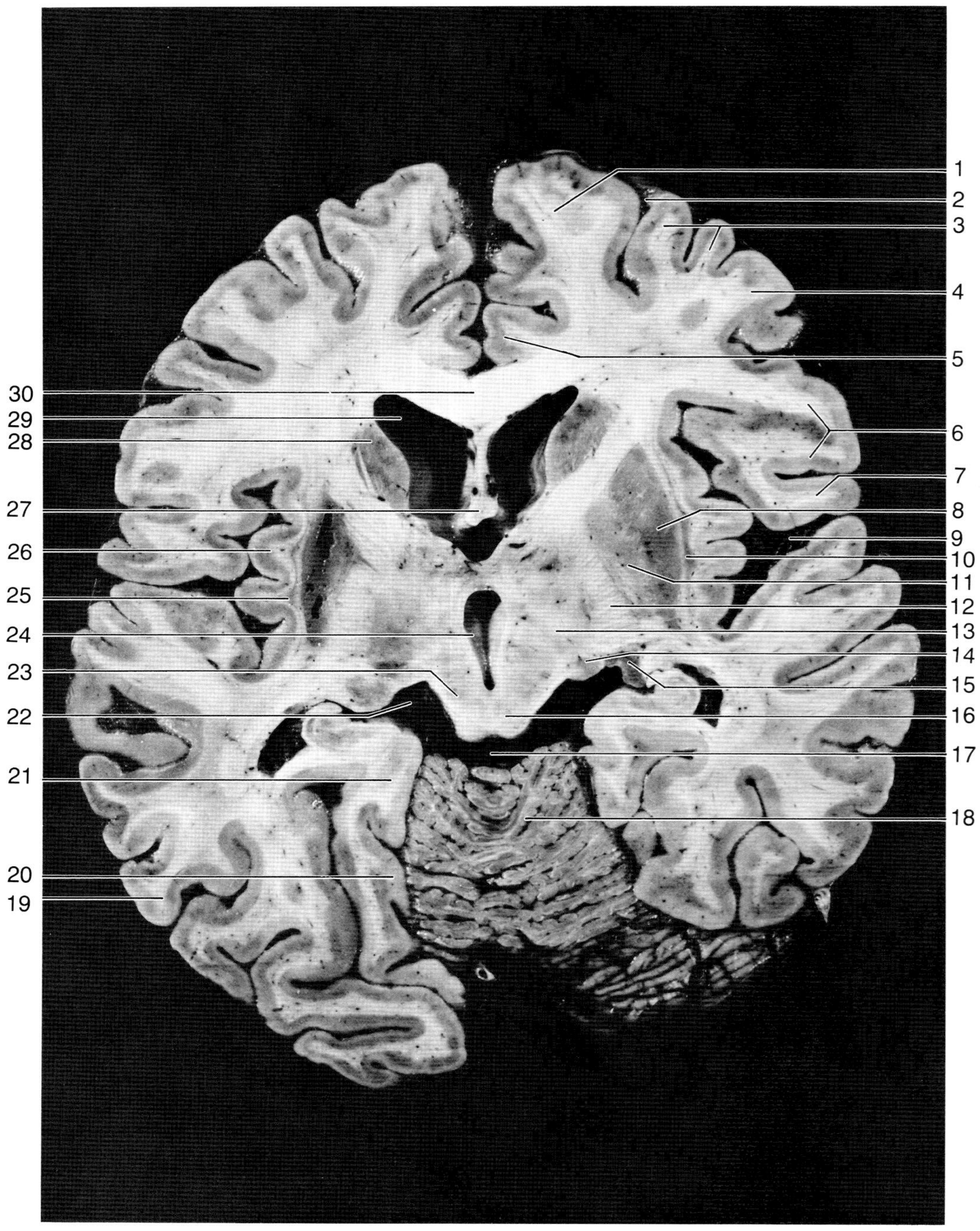

Anatomical section at level 6

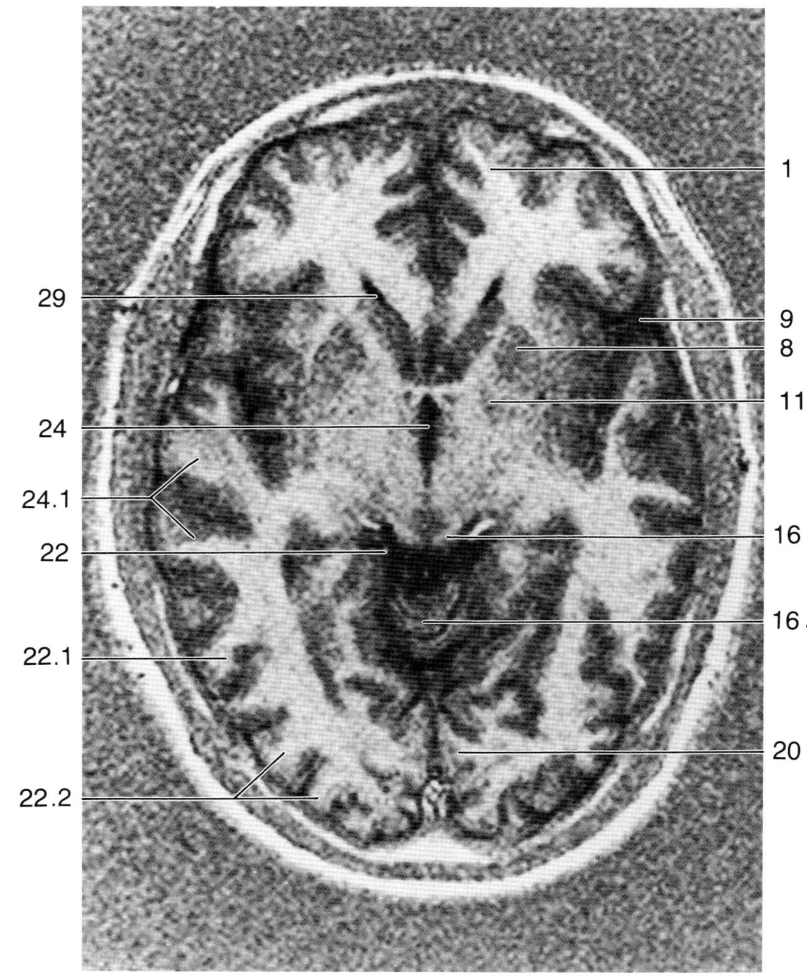

MRI section at level 6, IR 1800/400/30

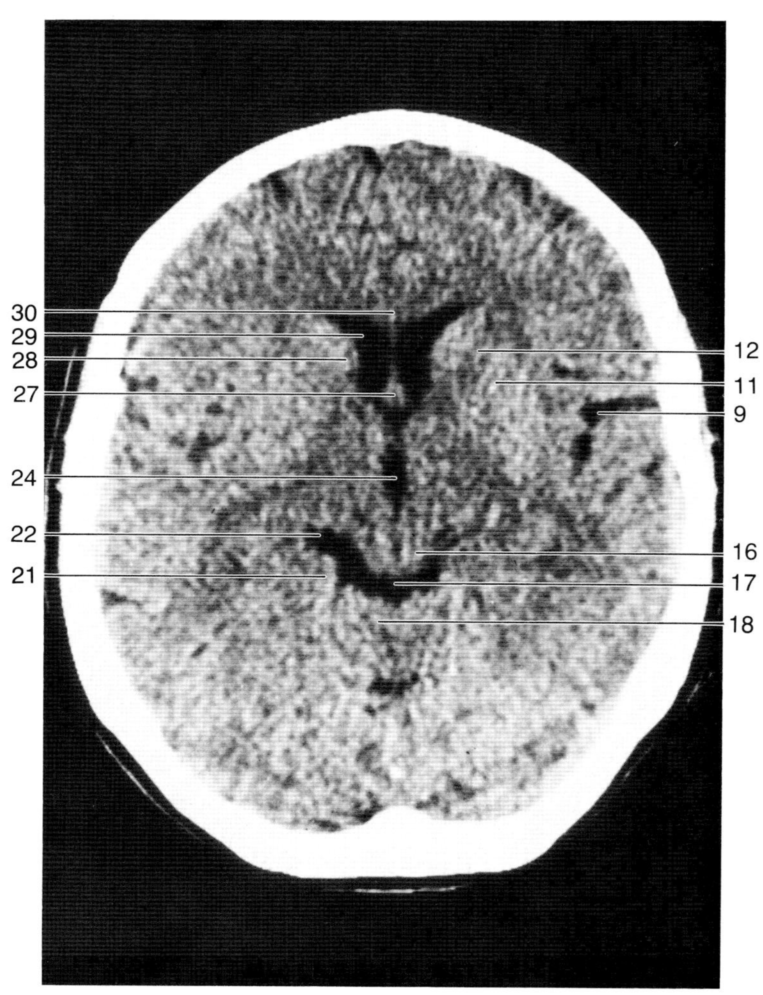

CT scan at level 6, IR 1000/400/75

1	Superior frontal gyrus	Gyrus frontalis superior
2	Superior frontal sulcus	Sulcus frontalis superior
3	Middle frontal gyrus	Gyrus frontalis medius
4	Inferior frontal gyrus	Gyrus frontalis inferior
5	Cingulate gyrus	Gyrus cinguli
6	Inferior frontal gyrus	Gyrus frontalis inferior
7	Precentral gyrus	Gyrus praecentralis
8	Putamen	Putamen
9	Lateral fissure	Fissura lateralis
10	External capsule	Capsula externa
11	Globus pallidus	Globus pallidus
12	Internal capsule	Capsula interna
13	Subthalamus	Subthalamus
14	Medial geniculate body	Corpus geniculatum mediale
15	Lateral geniculate body	Corpus geniculatum laterale
16	Inferior colliculus	Colliculus superior
16.1	Vermis of the cerebellum	Vermis cerebelli
17	Quadrigeminal cistern	Cisterna laminae quadrigeminae
18	Cerebellum	Cerebellum
19	Inferior temporal gyrus	Gyrus temporalis inferior
20	Fusiform gyrus	Gyrus fusiformis
21	Hippocampal gyrus	Gyrus hippocampi
22	Ambient cistern	Cisterna ambiens
22.1	Middle temporal gyrus	Gyrus temporalis medius
22.2	Occipital gyri	Gyri occipitales
23	Pretectal area	Area praetectalis
24	Third ventricle	Ventriculus III
24.1	Superior temporal gyrus	Gyrus temporalis superior
25	Claustrum	Claustrum
26	Insula	Insula
27	Fornix	Fornix
28	Head of the caudate nucleus	Nucleus caudatus
29	Anterior horn of the lateral ventricle	Cornu anterius ventriculi lateralis
30	Genu of the corpus callosum	Corpus callosum

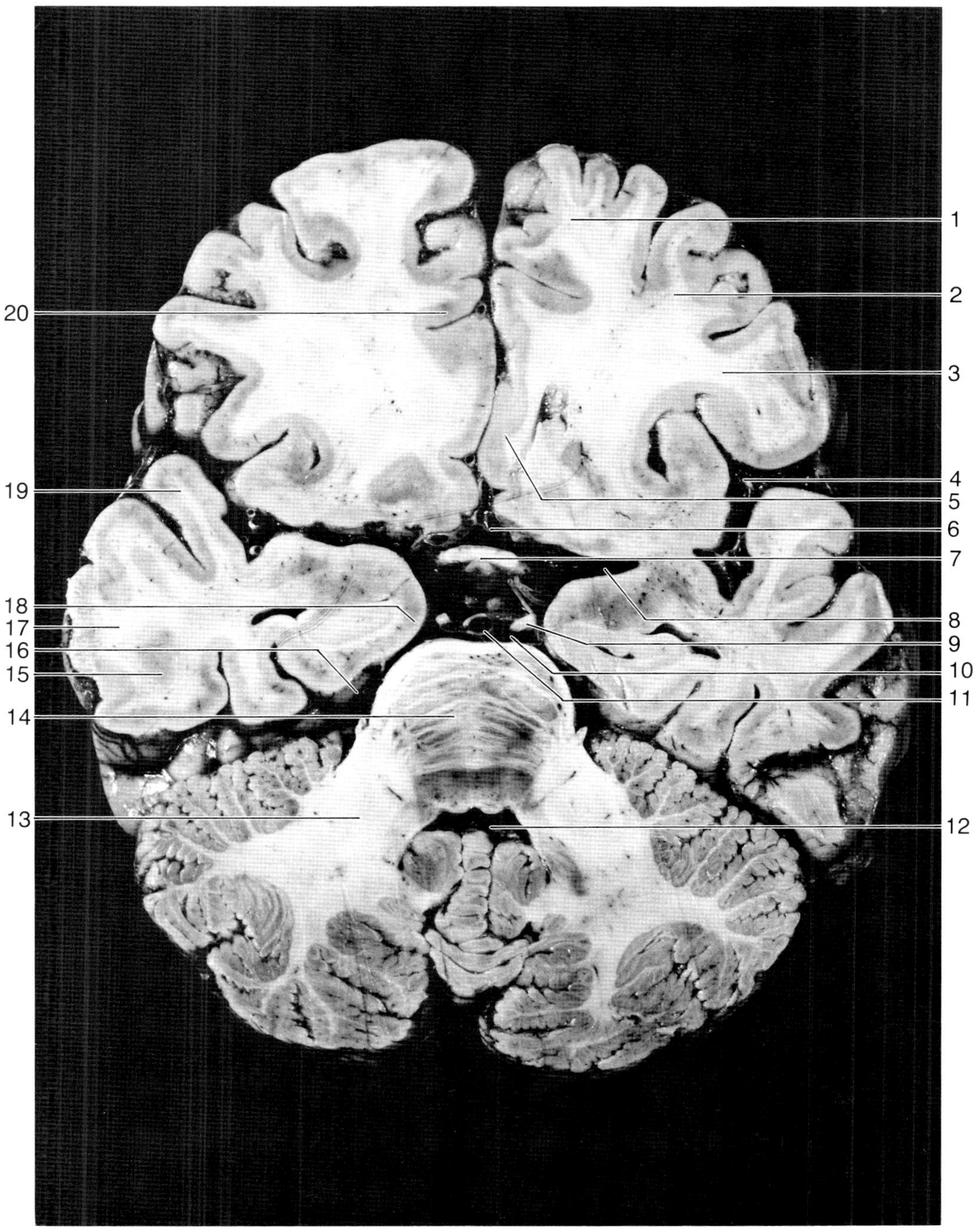

Anatomical section at level 7

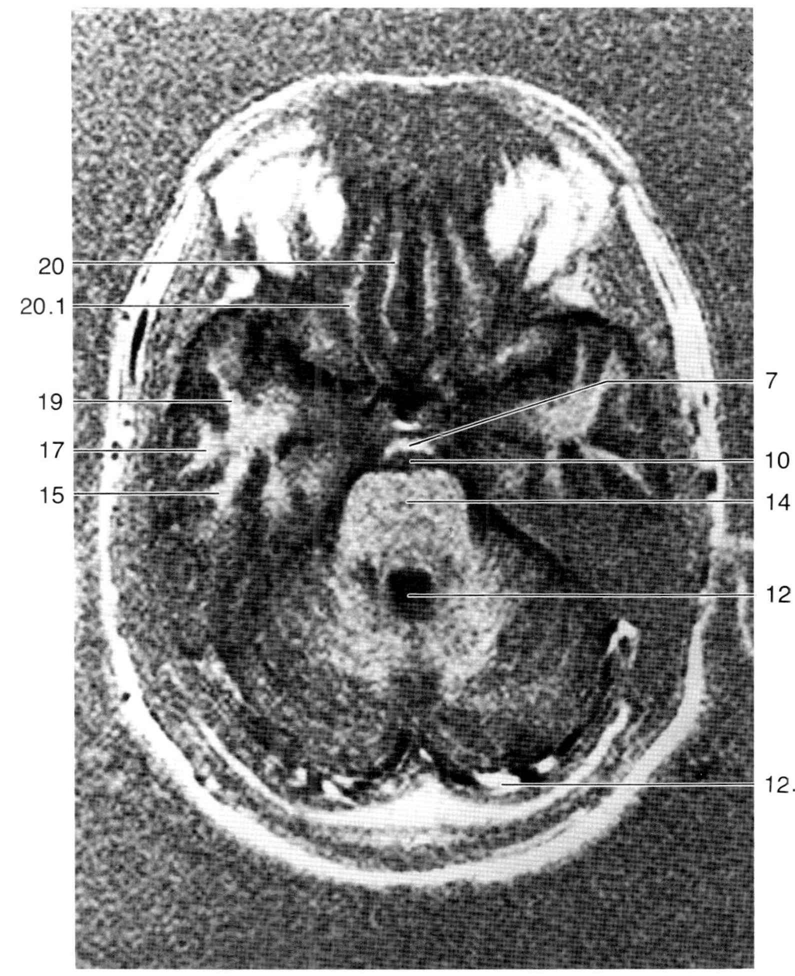

MRI section at level 7, IR 1800/400/30

1	Superior frontal gyrus	1	Gyrus frontalis superior
2	Middle frontal gyrus	2	Gyrus frontalis medius
3	Inferior frontal gyrus	3	Gyrus frontalis inferior
4	Lateral fissure	4	Fissura lateralis
5	Cingulate gyrus	5	Gyrus cinguli
6	Chiasmatic cistern	6	Cisterna chiasmatis
7	Optic chiasm	7	Chiasma opticum
8	Vallecula of the cerebral cistern	8	Cisterna valleculae cerebri
9	Oculomotor nerve	9	N. oculomotorius
10	Pontine cistern	10	Cisterna pontis
11	Basilar artery	11	A. basilaris
12	Fourth ventricle	12	Ventriculus IV
12.1	Transverse sinus	12.1	Sinus transversus
13	Middle cerebellar peduncle	13	Pedunculus cerebellaris medius
14	Pons	14	Pons
15	Inferior temporal gyrus	15	Gyrus temporalis inferior
16	Pontocerebellar cistern	16	Cisterna pontocerebellaris
17	Middle temporal gyrus	17	Gyrus temporalis medius
18	Hippocampal gyrus	18	Gyrus hippocampalis
19	Superior temporal gyrus	19	Gyrus temporalis superior
20	Rectal gyrus	20	Gyrus rectus
20.1	Orbital gyrus	20.1	Gyrus orbitalis

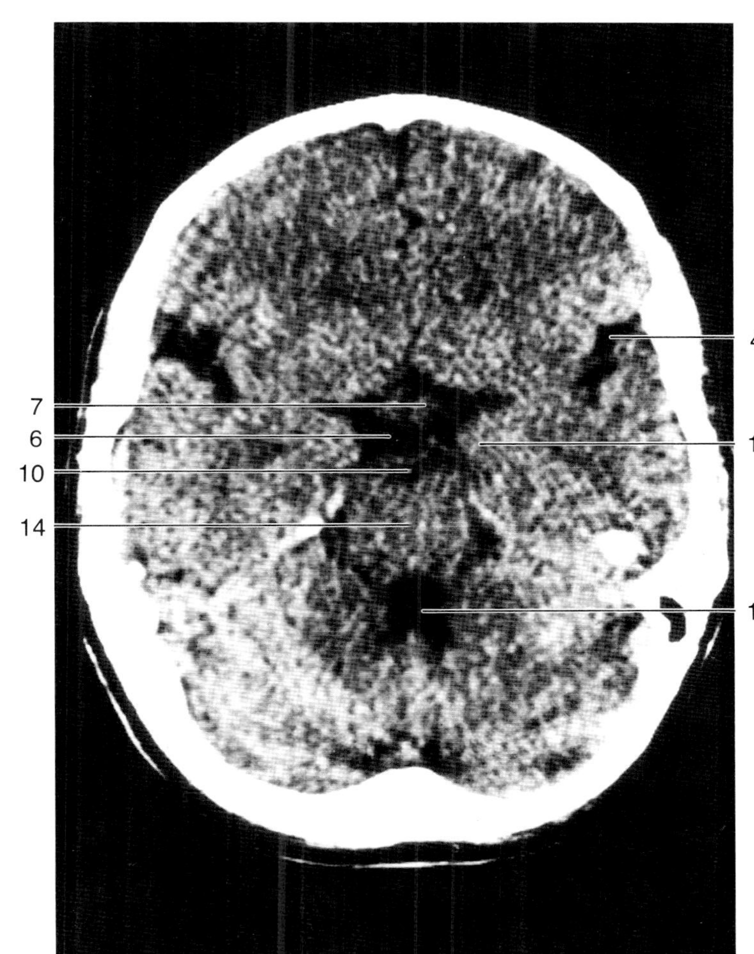

CT scan at level 7

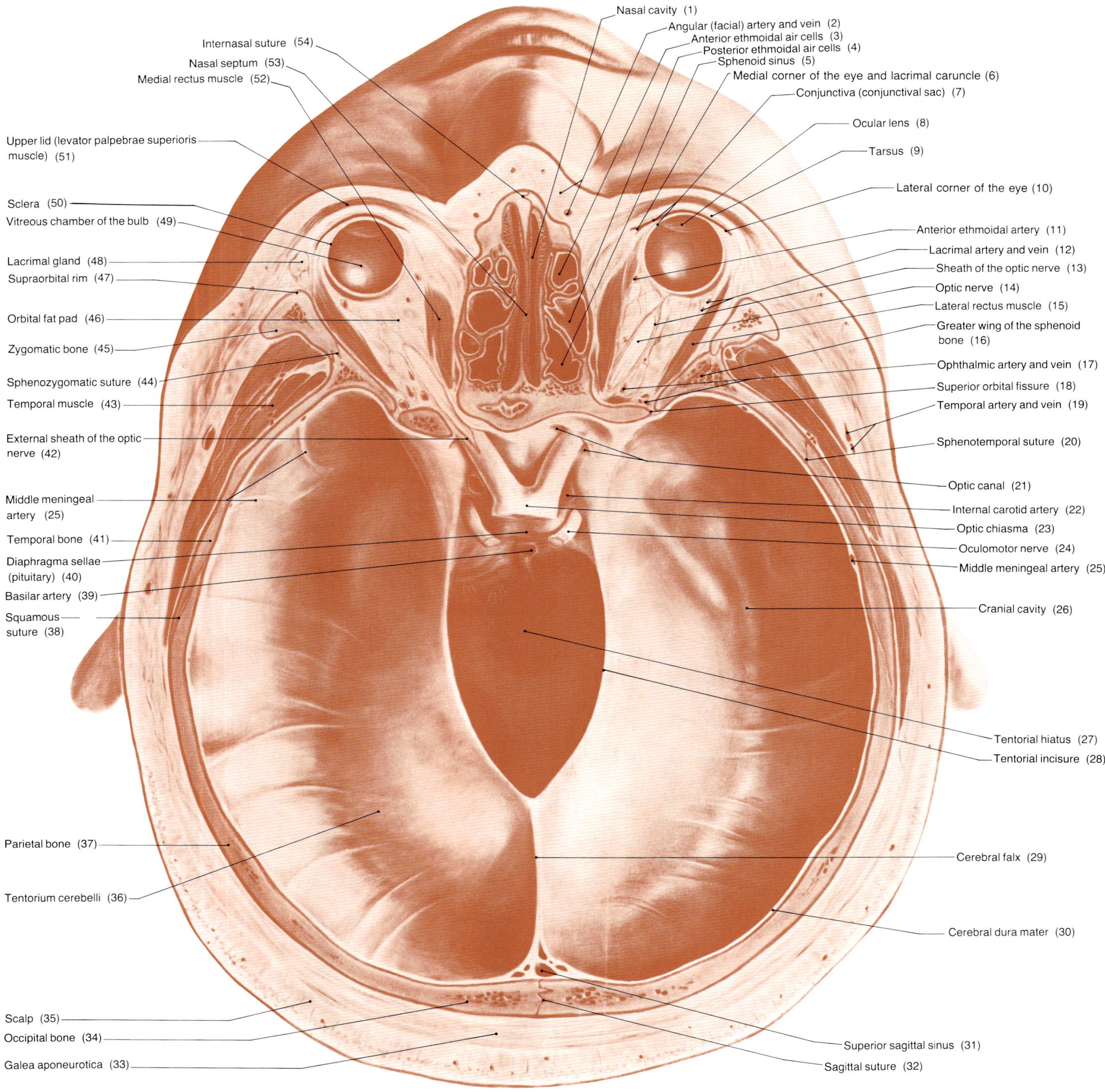

1 Cavum nasi proprium
2 A. et V. angularis (facialis)
3 Cellulae ethmoidales anteriores
4 Cellulae ethmoidales posteriores
5 Sinus sphenoidalis
6 Angulus oculi medialis et Caruncula lacrimalis
7 Conjunctiva (Saccus conjunctivae)
8 Cornea
9 Tarsus
10 Angulus oculi lateralis
11 A. ethmoidalis anterior
12 A. et V. lacrimalis
13 Vagina n. optici
14 N. opticus
15 M. rectus lateralis
16 Ala major (oss. sphen.)
17 A. et V. ophthalmica
18 Fissura orbitalis superior
19 A. et V. temporalis
20 Sutura sphenotemporalis
21 Canalis opticus
22 A. carotis interna
22.1 A. cerebri media
22.2 A. communicans posterior
22.3 A. cerebri posterior
23 Chiasma opticum
24 N. oculomotorius
25 A. meningea media
26 Cavum cranii
26.1 Lobus temporalis
27 Hiatus tentorii
28 Incisura tentorii
28.1 Plexus chorioideus
28.2 Sinus rectus
29 Falx cerebri
29.1 Pons
30 Dura mater encephali
31 Sinus sagittalis superior
32 Sutura sagittalis
33 Galea aponeurotica
34 Os occipitale
35 Epicranium
36 Tentorium cerebelli
36.1 Cisterna suprasellaris
36.2 Cisterna supracerebellaris
36.3 Ventriculus IV
36.4 Cerebellum
37 Os parietale
38 Sutura squamosa
39 A. basilaris
40 Diaphragma sellae (Hypophysis)
41 Os temporale
42 Vagina externa n. optici
43 M. temporalis
44 Sutura sphenozygomatica
45 Os zygomaticum
45.1 Ala minor ossis sphenoidalis
46 Corpus adiposum orbitae
47 Margo supraorbitalis
48 Glandula lacrimalis
49 Camera vitrea bulbi
50 Sclera
51 Palpebra superior (M. levator palpebrae superioris)
52 M. rectus medialis
53 Septum nasi
54 Sutura internasalis

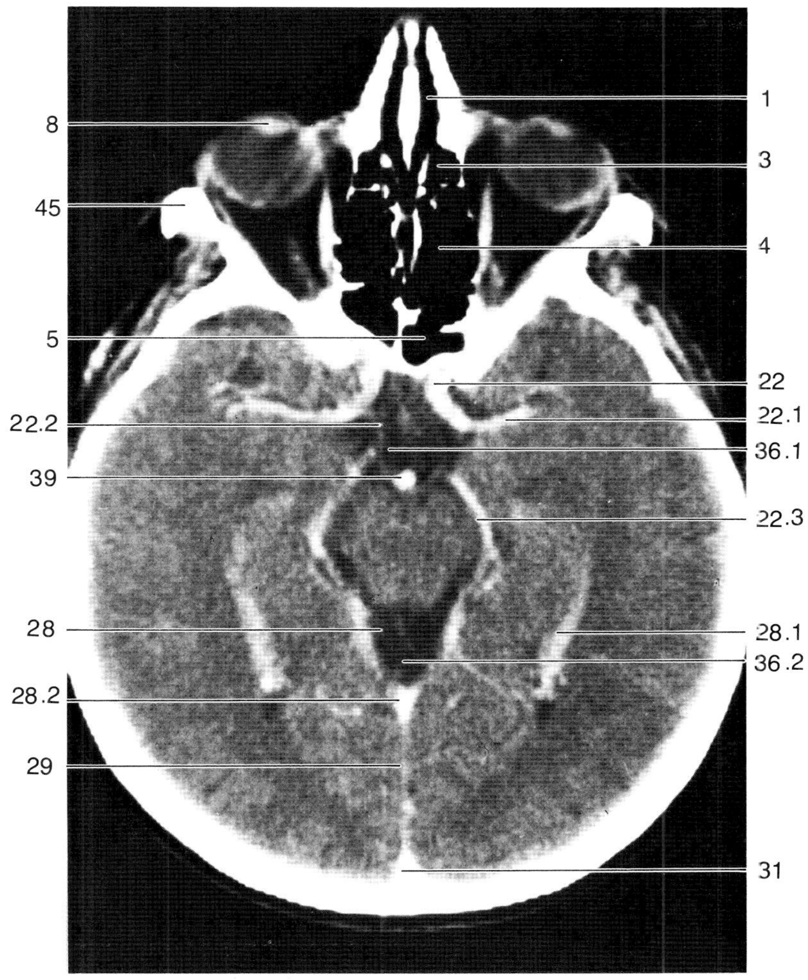

CT enhanced after bolus injection of contrast medium

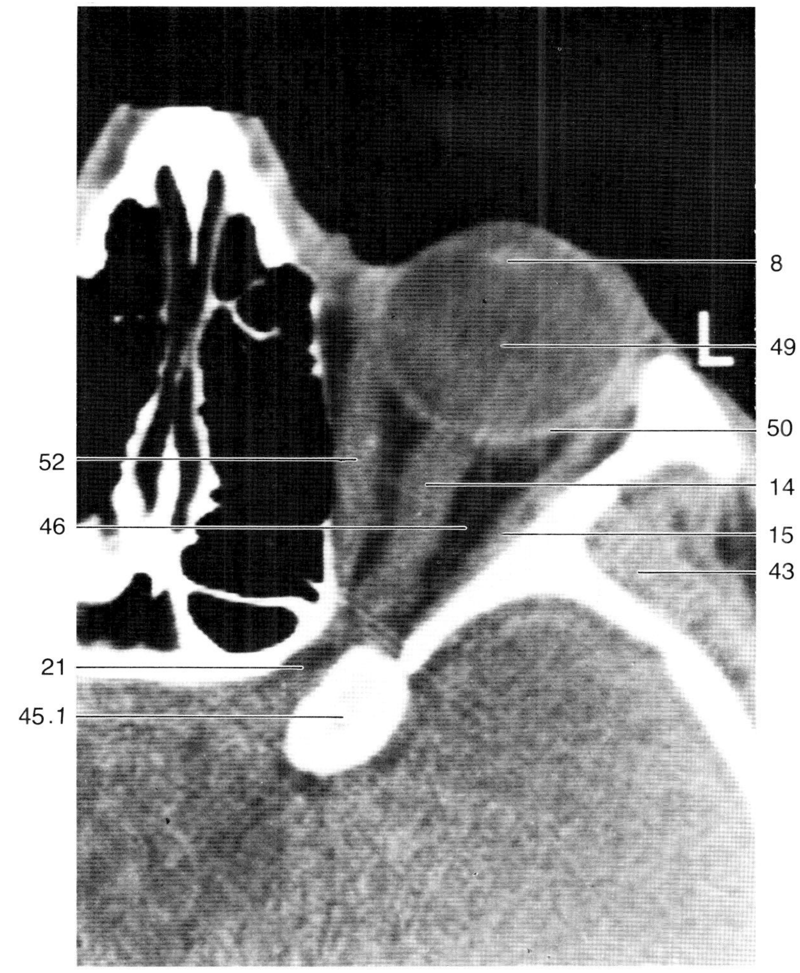

CT scan, unenhanced

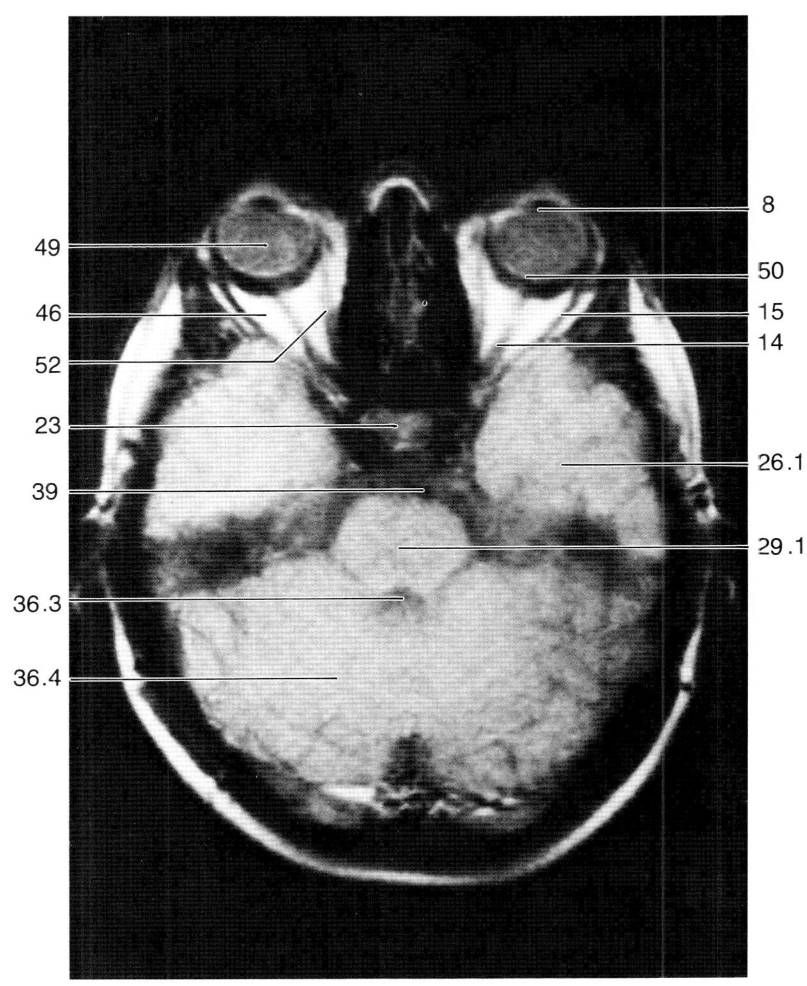

MRI, SE 1050/75

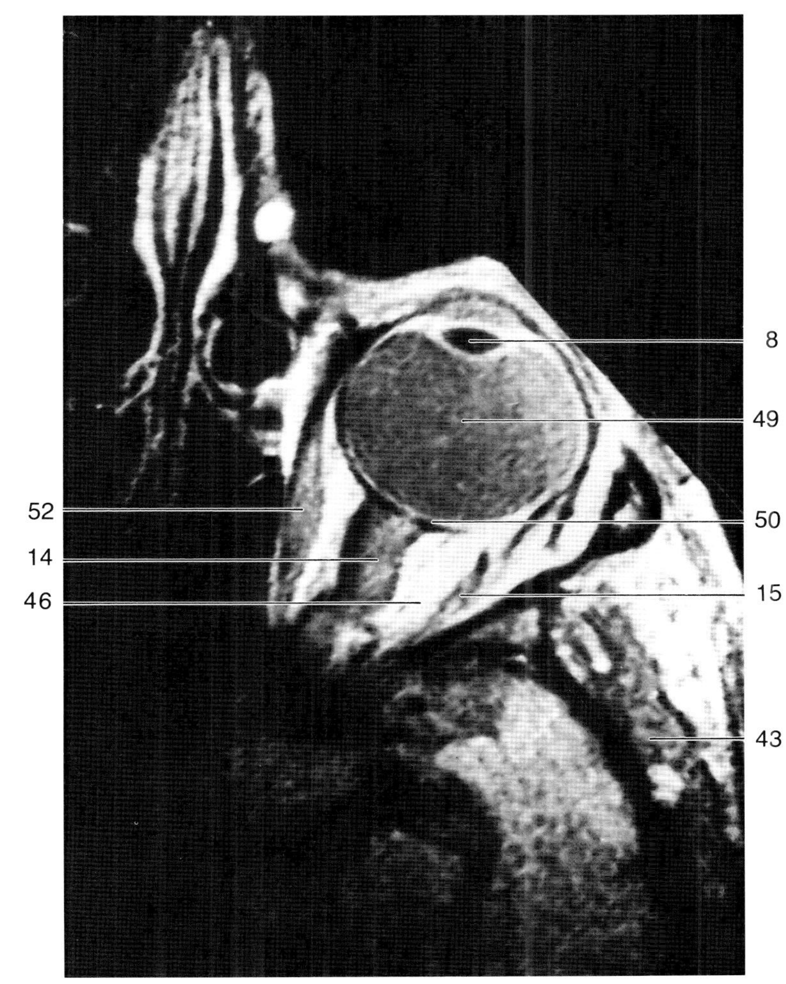

MRI, SE 1000/30

1 Nasal cavity
3 Anterior ethmoidal air cells
4 Posterior ethmoidal air cells
5 Sphenoid sinus
8 Cornea
14 Optic nerve
15 Lateral rectus muscle
21 Optic canal
22 Internal carotid artery
22.1 Middle cerebral artery
22.2 Posterior communicating artery
22.3 Posterior cerebral artery
23 Optic chiasma
26.1 Temporal lobe
28 Tentorial incisure
28.1 Choroid plexus
28.2 Rectal sinus
29 Cerebral falx
29.1 Pons
31 Superior sagittal sinus
36.1 Suprasellar cistern
36.2 Supracerebellar cistern
36.3 Fourth ventricle
36.4 Cerebellar hemisphere
39 Basilar artery
43 Temporal muscle
45 Zygomatic bone
45.1 Sphenoid bone, lesser wing
46 Orbital fat pad
49 Vitreous chamber of the bulb
50 Sclera
52 Medial rectus muscle

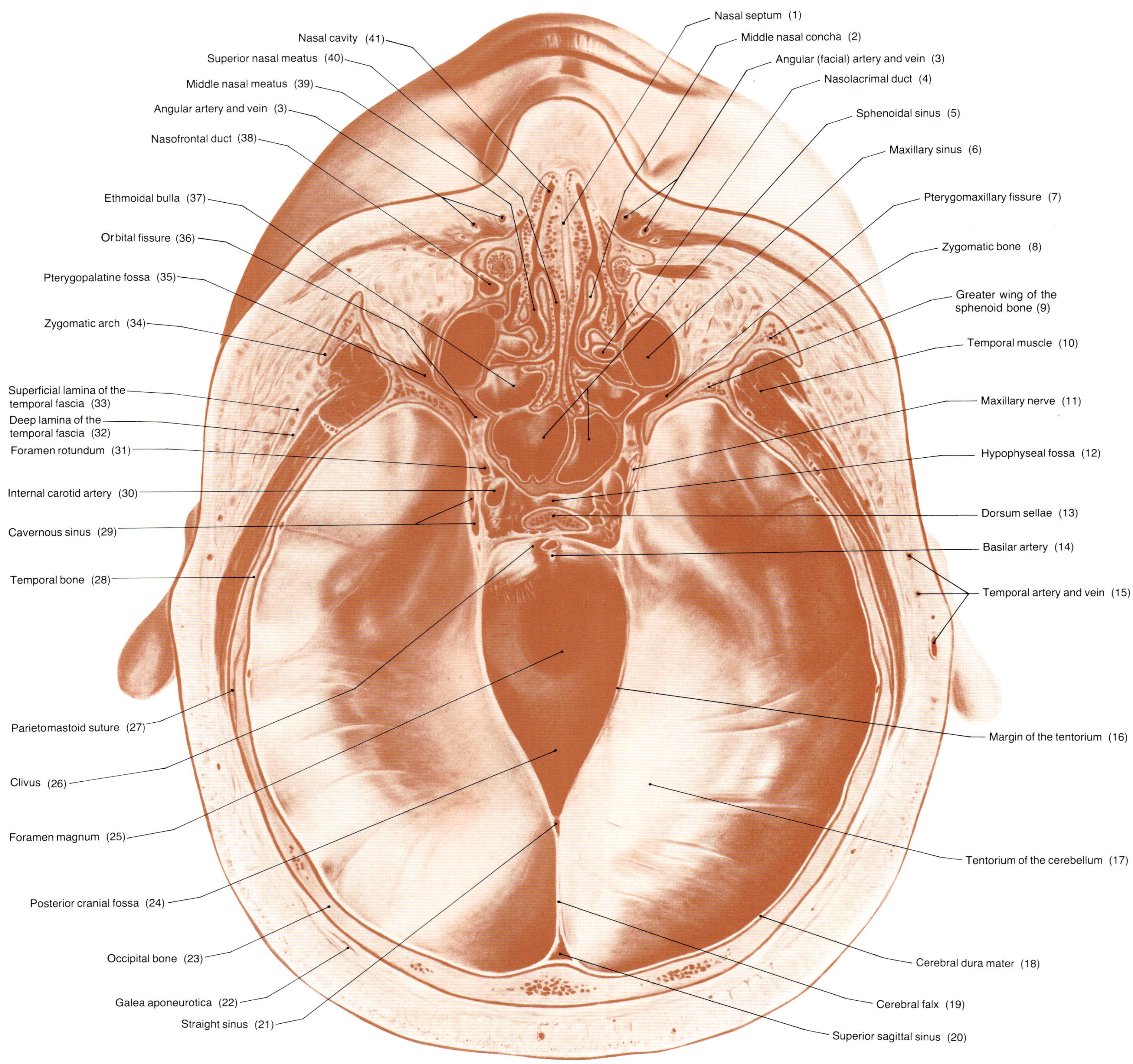

1 Septum nasi
2 Concha nasalis media
3 A. et V. angularis (facialis)
4 Ductus nasolacrimalis
5 Sinus sphenoidalis
6 Sinus maxillaris
7 Fissura orbitalis inferior
8 Os zygomaticum
9 Ala major (oss. sphen.)
10 M. temporalis
11 N. maxillaris
12 Fossa hypophysialis
13 Dorsum sellae
14 A. basilaris
15 A. et V. temporalis
16 Margo tentorii
17 Tentorium cerebelli
18 Dura mater encephali
19 Falx cerebri
20 Sinus sagittalis superior
21 Sinus rectus
22 Galea aponeurotica
23 Os occipitale
24 Fossa cranii posterior
25 Foramen magnum
25.1 Ventriculus IV
25.2 Cerebellum
25.3 Pons
26 Clivus
26.1 M. masseter
26.2 Medulla oblongata
26.3 M. pterygoideus lateralis
27 Sutura parietomastoidea
28 Os temporale
28.1 Lobus temporalis
28.2 Pars petrosa ossis temporalis
28.3 Cellulae mastoideae
28.4 Cisterna pontis
29 Sinus cavernosus
30 A. carotis interna
31 Foramen rotundum
32 Lamina profunda (Fascia temporalis)
33 Lamina superficialis (Fascia temporalis)
34 Arcus zygomaticus
35 Fossa pterygopalatina
36 Fissura orbitalis
37 Bulla ethmoidalis
38 Ductus nasofrontalis
39 Meatus nasi medius
40 Meatus nasi superior
41 Cavum nasi proprium

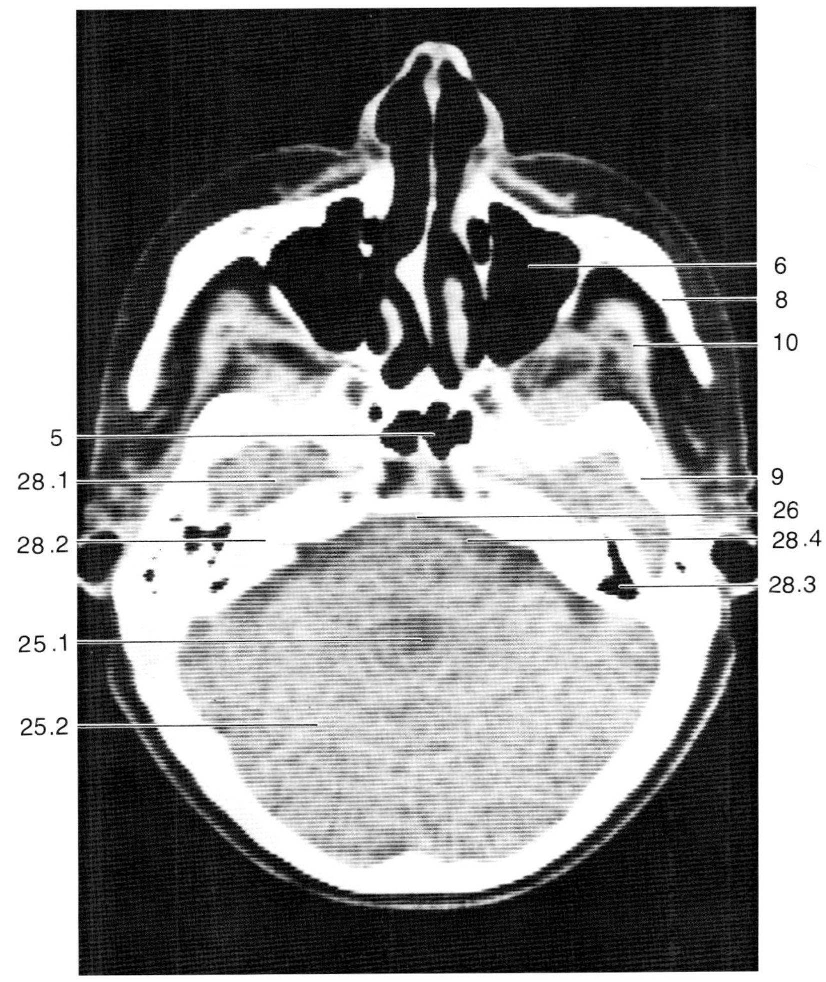

CT scan

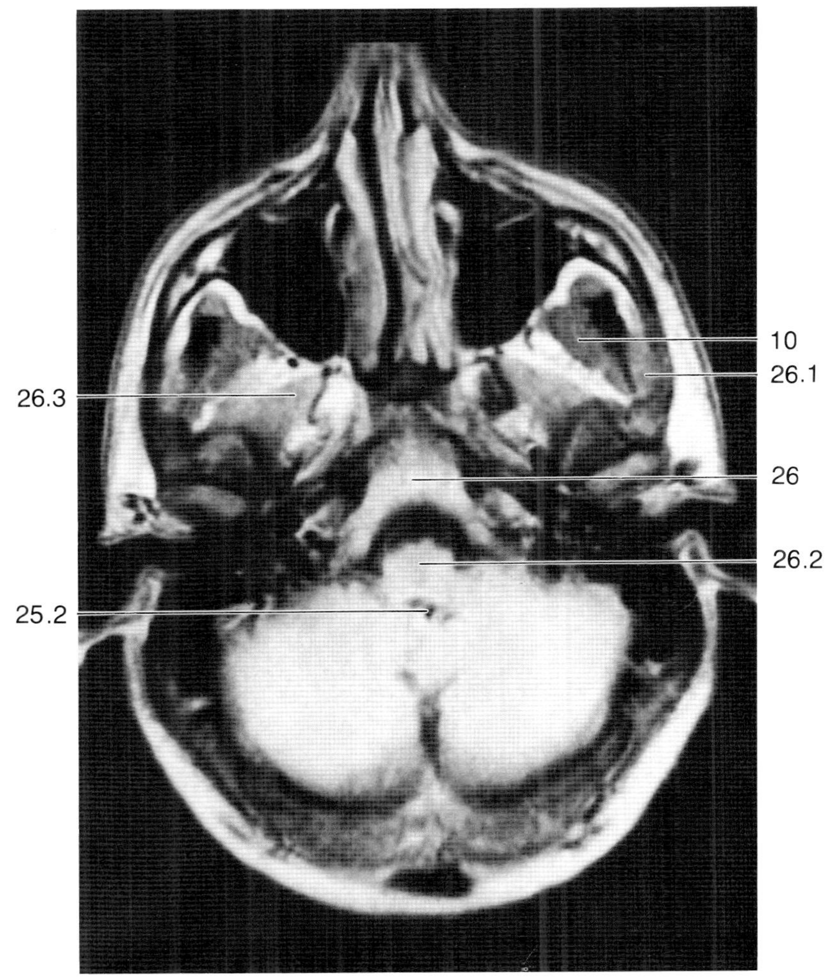

MRI, SE 700/30

5 Sphenoidal sinus
6 Maxillary sinus
8 Zygomatic bone
9 Greater wing of the sphenoid
10 Temporal muscle
25.1 Fourth ventricle
25.2 Cerebellar hemisphere
26 Clivus
26.1 Masseter muscle
26.2 Medulla oblongata
26.3 Lateral pterygoid muscle
28.1 Temporal bone
28.2 Petrous bone
28.3 Mastoid cells
28.4 Pontine cistern

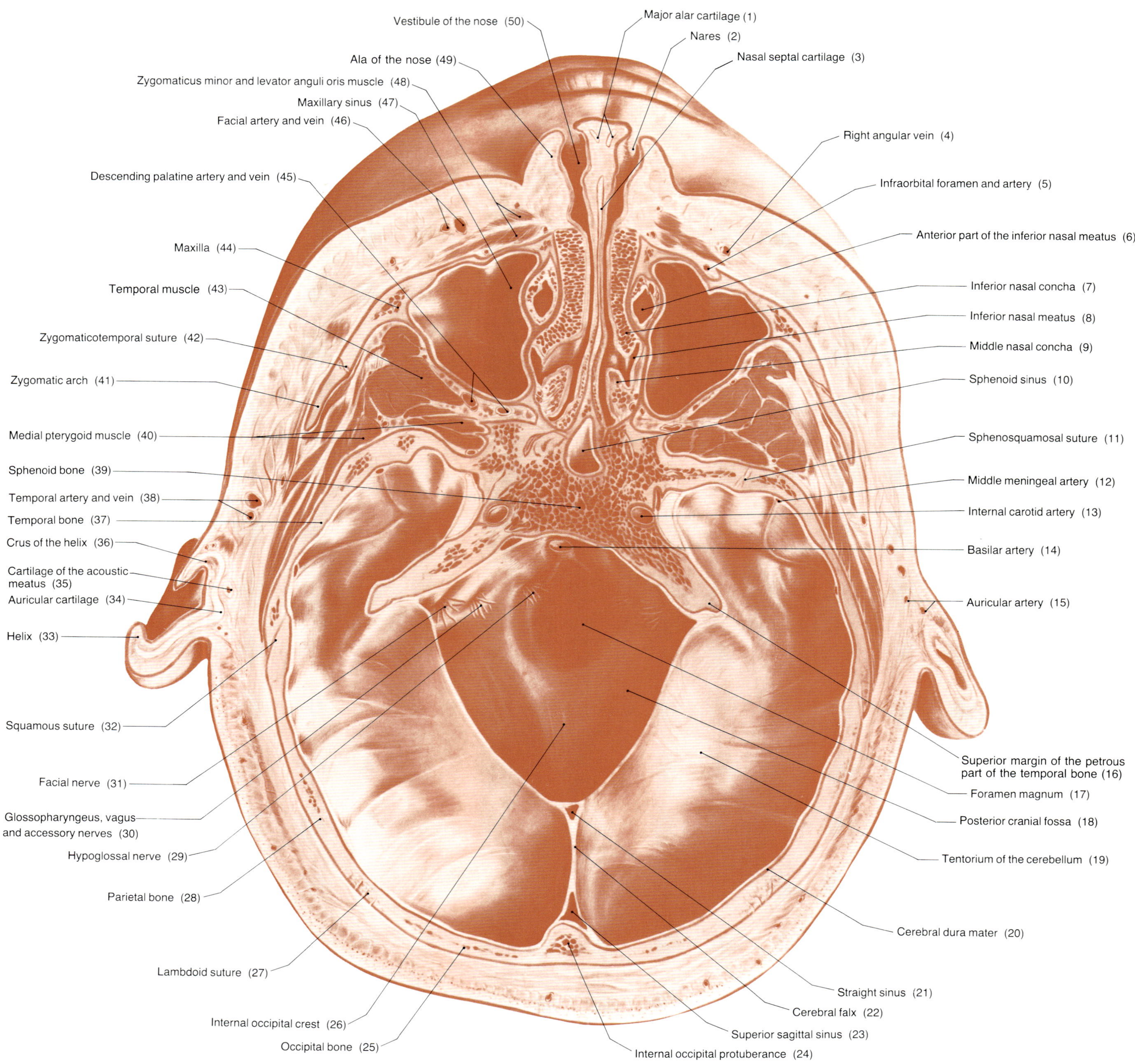

1 Cartilago alaris major
1.1 Sinus frontalis
1.2 Vena supraorbitalis
2 Nares
3 Cartilago septi nasi
4 V. angularis dextra
5 Foramen infraorbitale et A. infraorbitalis
6 Meatus nasi inferior, Pars anterior
7 Concha nasalis inferior
8 Meatus nasi inferior
9 Concha nasalis media
10 Sinus sphenoidalis
11 Sutura sphenosquamosa
11.1 Cavum tympani
11.2 Canalis semicircularis
11.3 Antrum mastoideum
11.4 Cellulae mastoideae
12 A. meningea media
13 A. carotis interna
14 A. basilaris
15 A. auricularis
16 Margo superior partis petrosae ossis temporalis
17 Foramen magnum
18 Fossa cranii posterior
19 Tentorium cerebelli
19.1 Fossa cranii posterior
19.2 Foramen magnum
20 Dura mater encephali
21 Sinus rectus
22 Falx cerebri
23 Sinus sagittalis superior
24 Protuberantia occipitalis interna
25 Os occipitale
25.1 M. rectus capitis posterior
25.2 M. semispinalis capitis
25.3 Cerebellum
26 Crista occipitalis interna
27 Sutura lambdoidea
28 Os parietale
29 N. hypoglossus
30 N. glossopharyngeus, N. vagus et N. accessorius
30.1 Pons
30.2 Ventriculus IV
31 N. facialis
32 Sutura squamosa
33 Helix
34 Cartilago auriculae
35 Cartilago meatus acustici
36 Crus helicis
37 Os temporale
37.1 Pars petrosa ossis temporalis
37.2 Meatus acusticus internus
37.3 Condylus mandibularis
37.4 Meatus acusticus externus
38 A. et V. temporalis
39 Os sphenoidale
39.1 Clivus
40 M. pterygoideus medialis
41 Arcus zygomaticus
42 Sutura temporozygomatica
43 M. temporalis
43.1 Crista galli
43.2 Fossa cranii anterior
43.3 Fossa cranii media
43.4 M. pterygoideus lateralis
44 Maxilla
45 A. et V. palatina descendens
46 A. et V. facialis
47 Sinus maxillaris
48 M. zygomaticus minor et M. levator anguli oris
49 Ala nasi
50 Vestibulum nasi

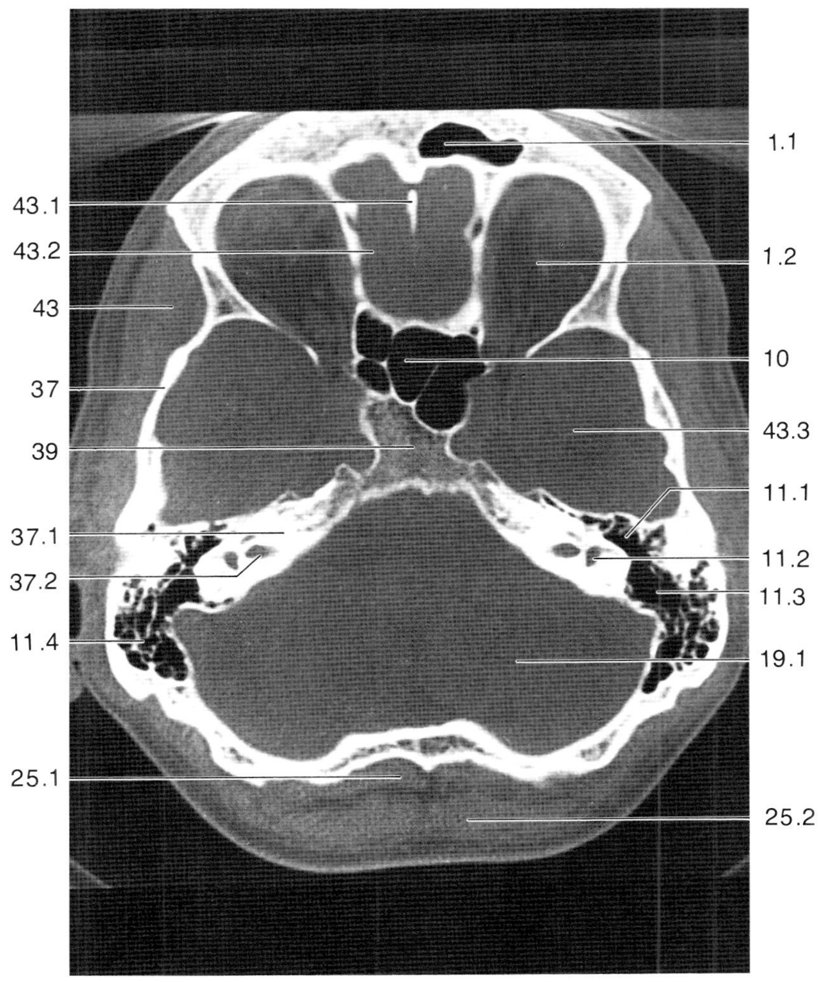

CT scan

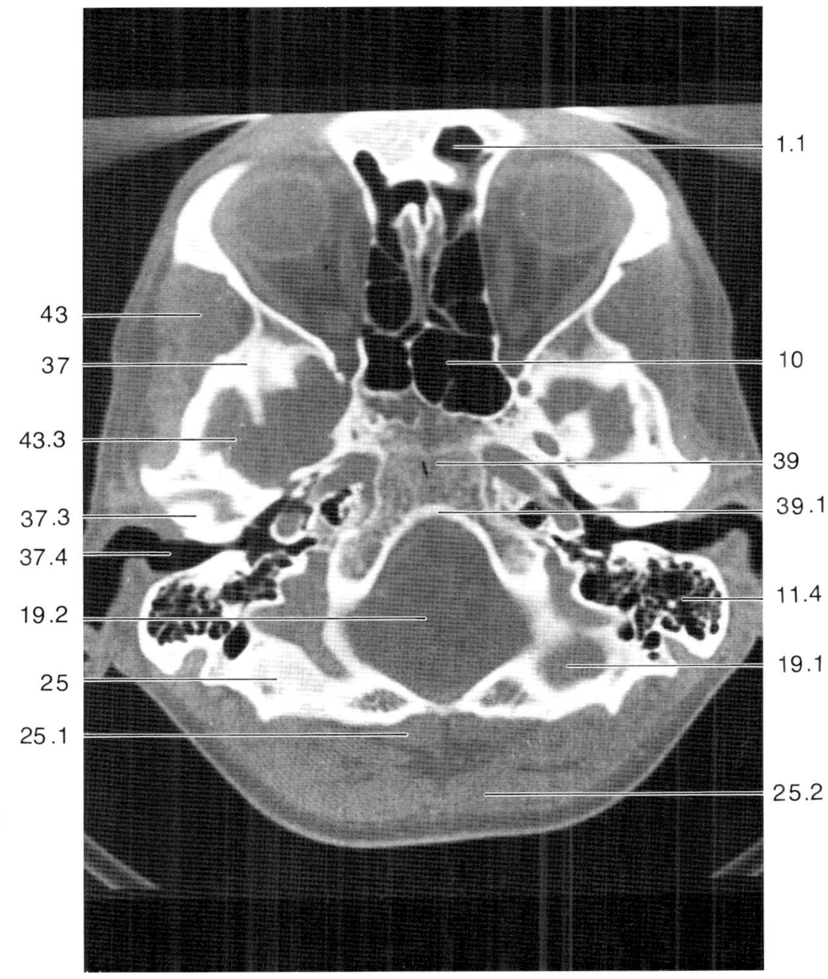

CT scan

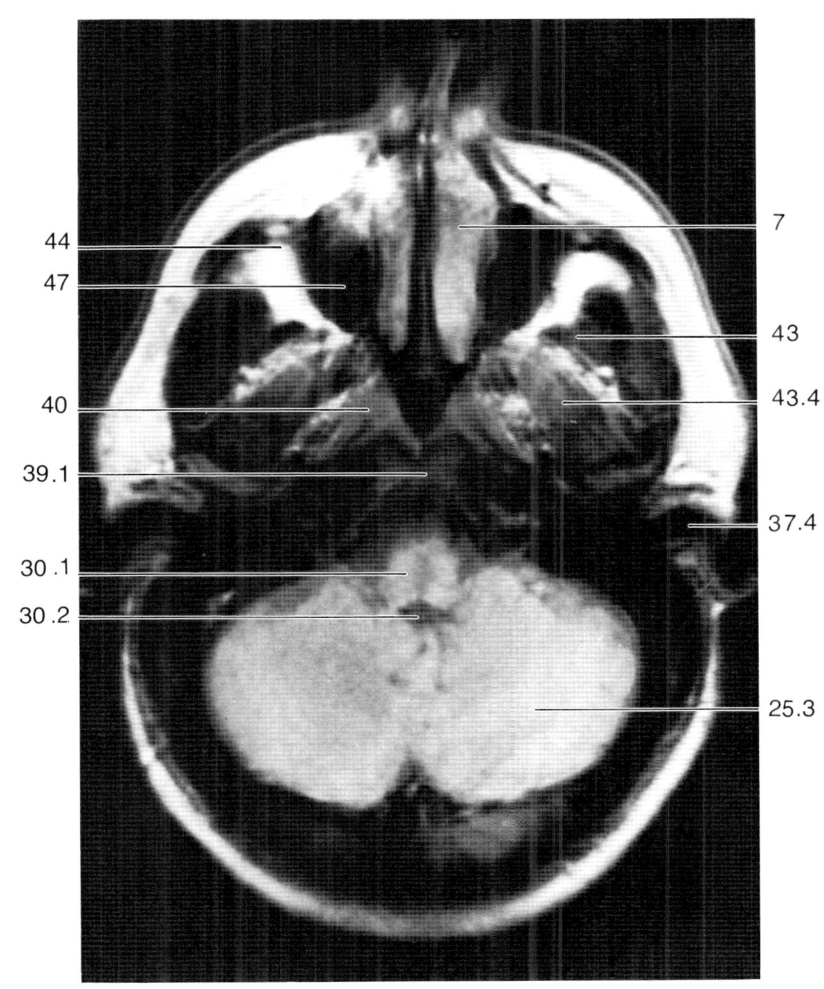

MRI, SE 500/50

1.1 Frontal sinus
1.2 Supraorbital vein
7 Inferior nasal concha
10 Sphenoid sinus
11.1 Tympanic cavity
11.2 Semicircular canal
11.3 Mastoid antrum
11.4 Mastoid air cells
19.1 Posterior cranial fossa
19.2 Foramen magnum
25 Occipital bone
25.1 Rectus capitis posterior muscle
25.2 Semispinalis capitis muscle
25.3 Cerebellar hemisphere
30.1 Pons
30.2 Fourth ventricle
37 Temporal bone
37.1 Petrous bone
37.2 Internal auditory meatus
37.3 Mandibular condyle
37.4 External auditory meatus
39 Sphenoid bone
39.1 Clivus
40 Medial pterygoid muscle
43 Temporal muscle
43.1 Crista galli
43.2 Anterior cranial fossa
43.3 Middle cranial fossa
43.4 Lateral pterygoid muscle
44 Maxilla
47 Maxillary sinus

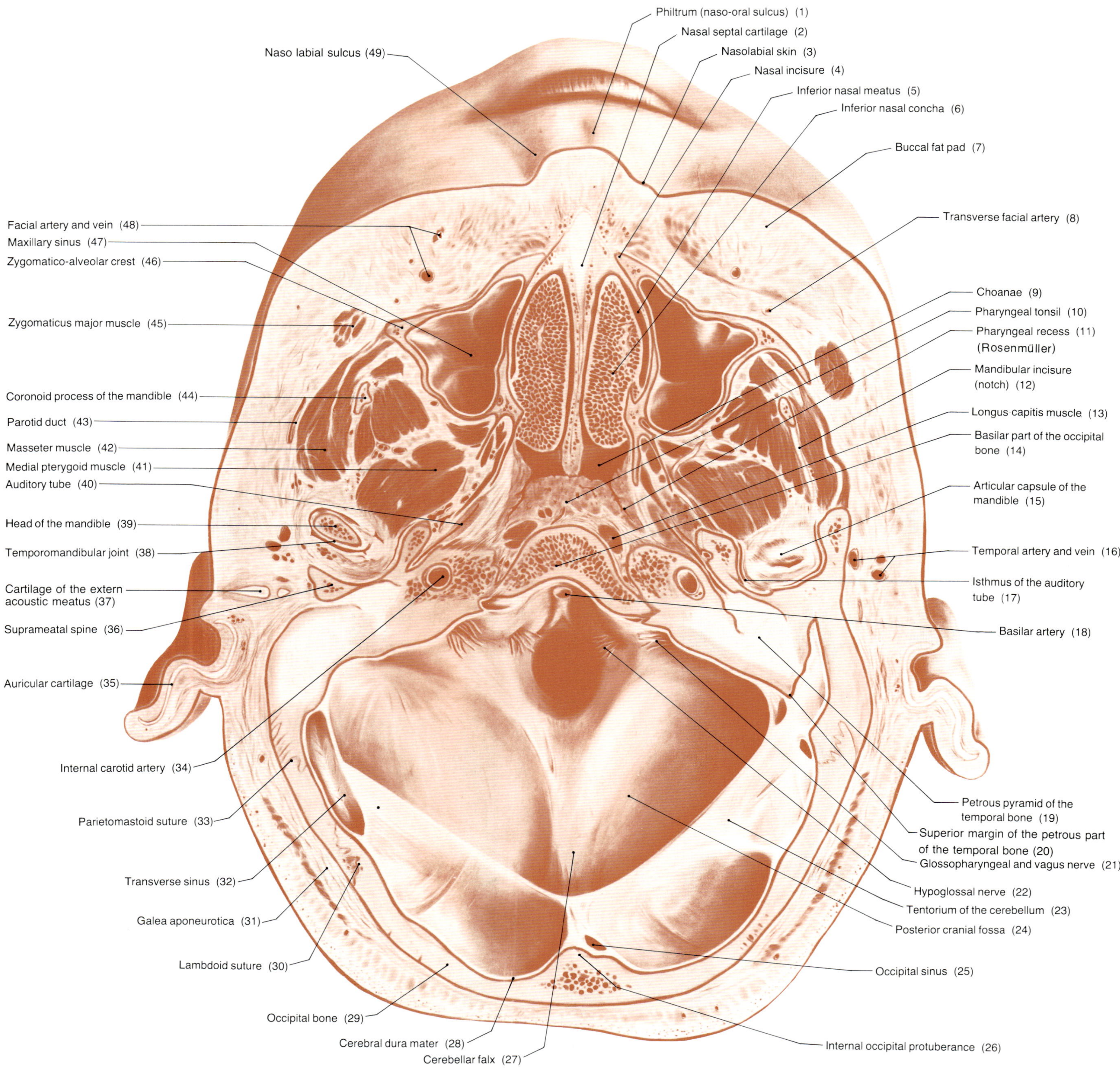

1 Philtrum (Sulcus nasooralis)
2 Cartilago septi nasi
3 Integumentum nasolabiale
4 Incisura nasalis
5 Meatus nasi inferior
6 Concha nasalis inferior
7 Corpus adiposum buccae
8 A. transversa faciei
9 Choanae
10 Tonsilla pharyngea
11 Recessus pharyngeus (Rosenmüller)
12 Incisura mandibulae
13 M. longus capitis
14 Pars basilaris ossis occipitalis
15 Capsula articularis mandibulae
16 A. et V. temporalis
17 Isthmus tubae auditivae
18 A. basilaris
18.1 Medulla oblongata
19 Pyramis, Pars petrosa, Os temporale
20 Margo superior partis petrosae ossis temporalis
21 Nn. glossopharyngeus et vagus
22 N. hypoglossus
23 Tentorium cerebelli
24 Fossa cranii posterior
24.1 Fossa cranii posterior
25 Sinus occipitalis
26 Protuberantia occipitalis interna
27 Falx cerebelli
28 Dura mater encephali
29 Os occipitale
30 Sutura lambdoidea
31 Galea aponeurotica
32 Sinus transversus
33 Sutura parietomastoidea
33.1 Cellulae mastoideae
34 A. carotis interna
35 Cartilago auriculae
36 Spina suprameatalis
37 Cartilago meatus acustici
37.1 Cavum tympani
37.2 Cochlea
37.3 Meatus acusticus internus
37.4 Vestibulum labyrinthi
37.5 Canales semicirculares
37.6 Malleus
37.7 Incus
37.8 Synchondrosis petrooccipitalis
38 Articulatio temporomandibularis
39 Caput mandibulae
40 Tuba auditiva
41 M. pterygoideus medialis
42 M. masseter
43 Ductus parotideus
44 Processus coronoideus (mandib.)
45 M. zygomaticus major
46 Crista zygomatico-alveolaris
47 Sinus maxillaris
48 A. et V. facialis
49 Sulcus nasolabialis

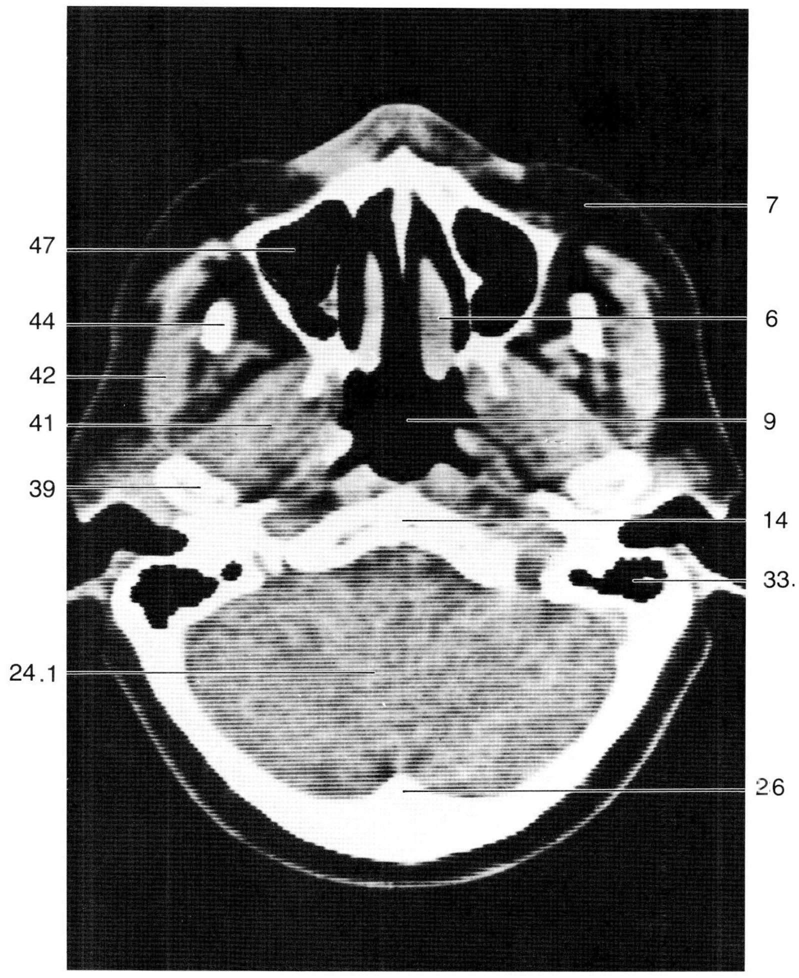

CT scan

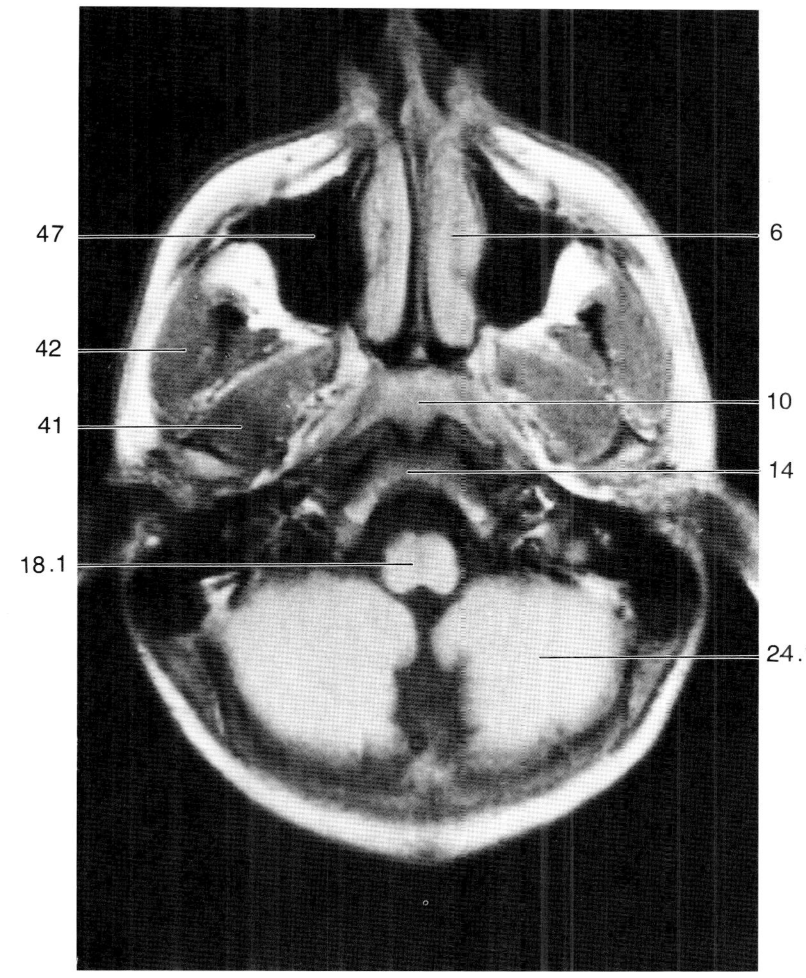

MRI, SE 1000/50

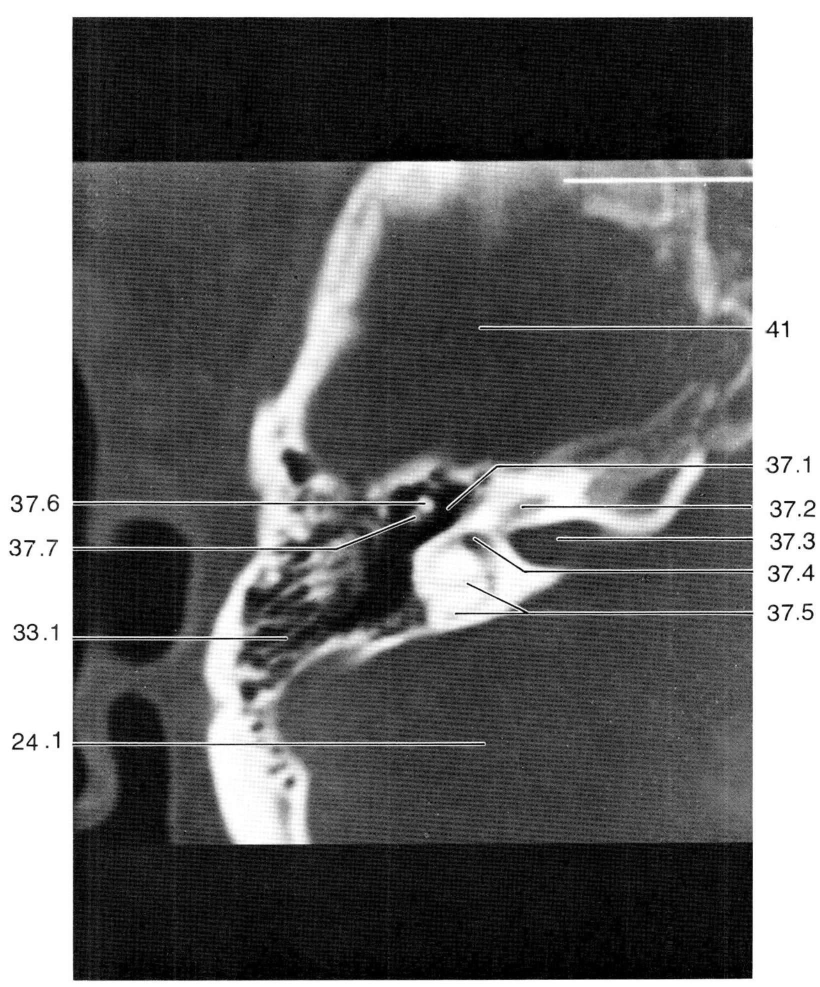

CT scan

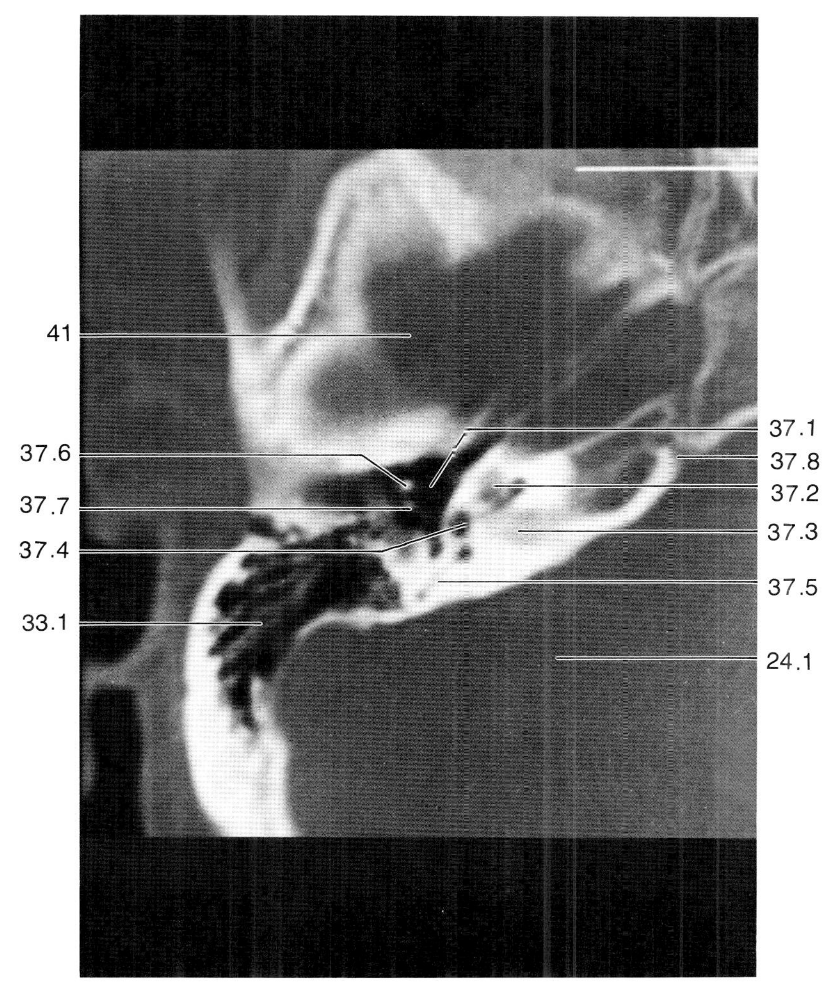

CT scan

6	Inferior nasal concha
7	Buccal fat pad
9	Choanae
10	Pharyngeal tonsil
14	Basilar part of the occipital bone
18.1	Medulla
24.1	Posterior cranial fossa
26	Internal occipital protuberance
33.1	Mastoid air cells
37.1	Tympanic cavity
37.2	Cochlea
37.3	Internal auditory meatus
37.4	Vestibule
37.5	Semicircular canals
37.6	Malleus
37.7	Incus
37.8	Petrooccipital synchondrosis
39	Head of the mandible
41	Middle cranial fossa
42	Masseter muscle
44	Coronoid process of the mandible
47	Maxillary sinus

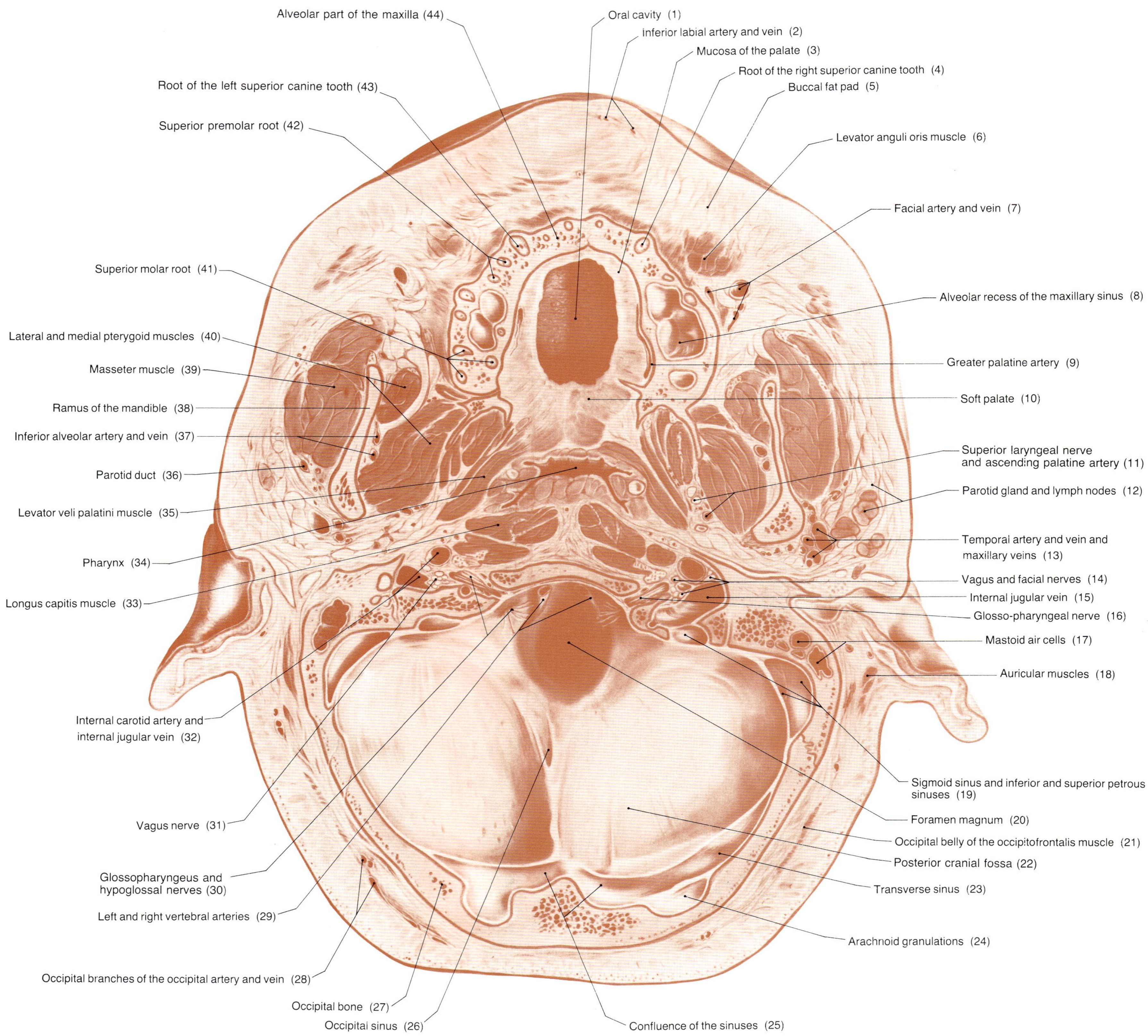

1 Cavum oris proprium
2 A. et V. labialis inferior
3 Tunica mucosa palati
4 Radix dentis canini superioris dextri
5 Corpus adiposum buccae
6 M. levator anguli oris
7 A. et V. facialis
8 Recessus alveolaris sinus maxillaris
9 A. palatina major
10 Palatum molle
11 Nn. vagus et laryngeus superior et A. palatina ascendens
12 Nodi lymphatici parotidei
13 A. et V. temporalis et Vv. maxillares
14 Nn. vagus et facialis
15 V. jugularis interna
16 N. glossopharyngeus
17 Cellulae mastoideae
17.1 Medulla oblongata
17.2 Cerebellum
17.3 Vermis
17.4 Tonsilla cerebelli
18 Mm. auriculares
19 Sinus sigmoideus et sinus petrosus inferior et superior
20 Foramen magnum
20.1 Corpus vitreum
20.2 Cellulae ethmoidales
20.3 Foramen ovale
20.4 Os sphenoidale
20.5 Meatus acusticus externus
20.6 Os zygomaticum
20.7 Os temporale
20.8 Foramen lacerum
20.9 Canalis hypoglossalis
21 Venter occipitalis m. occipitofrontalis
22 Fossa posterior cranii
23 Sinus transversus
24 Granulationes arachnoideales
25 Confluens sinuum
26 Sinus occipitalis
27 Os occipitale
27.1 Processus odontoideus
27.2 Foramen jugulare
27.3 Tuberculum jugulare
28 Rr. occipitales a. et v. occipitalis
29 A. vertebralis sinistra et dextra
30 Nn. glossopharyngeus et hypoglossus
31 N. vagus
32 A. carotis interna et V. jugularis interna
33 M. longus capitis
34 Pharynx
35 M. levator veli palatini
36 Ductus parotideus
37 A. et V. alveolaris inferior
38 R. mandibulae
39 M. masseter
40 M. pterygoideus lateralis et medialis
40.1 Processus styloideus ossis temporalis
40.2 Condylus occipitalis
41 Radix dentis molaris superioris
42 Radix dentis praemolaris superioris
43 Radix dentis canini superioris sinistri
44 Processus alveolaris maxillaris
44.1 Maxilla

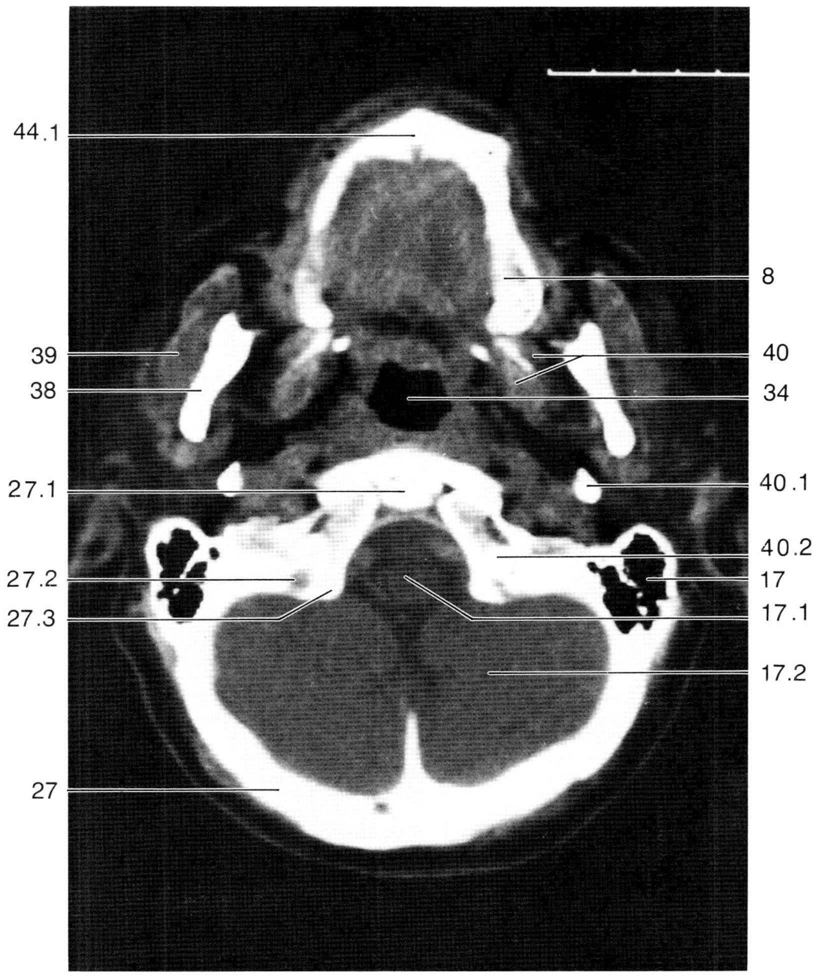

CT scan

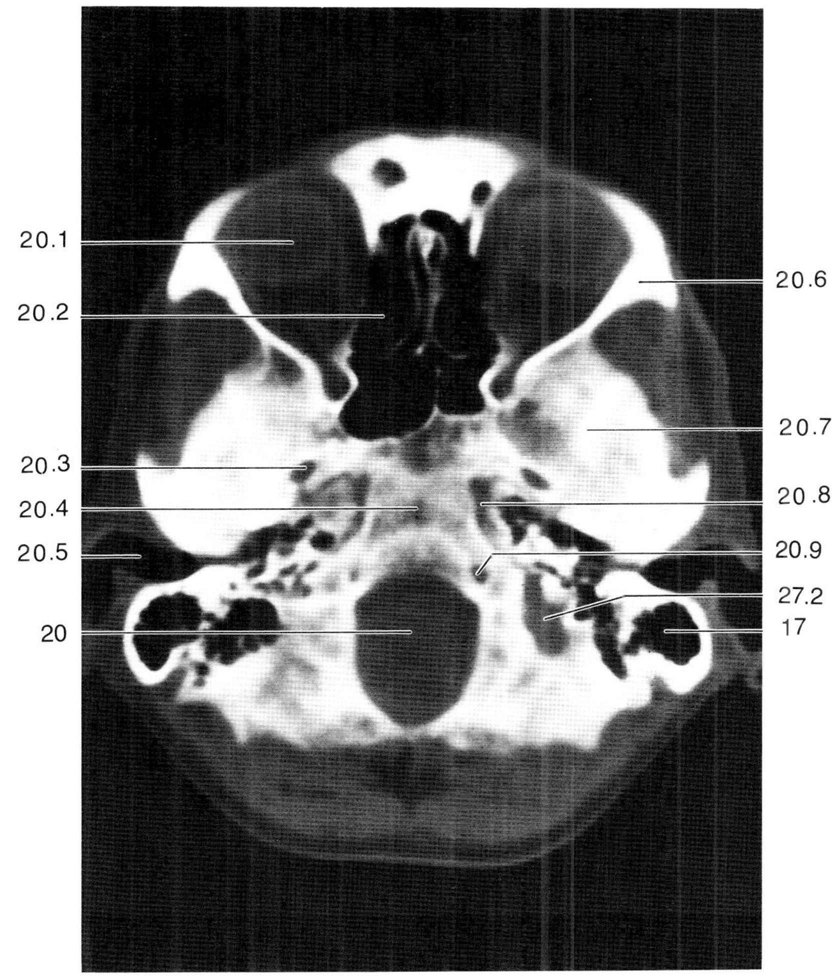

CT scan

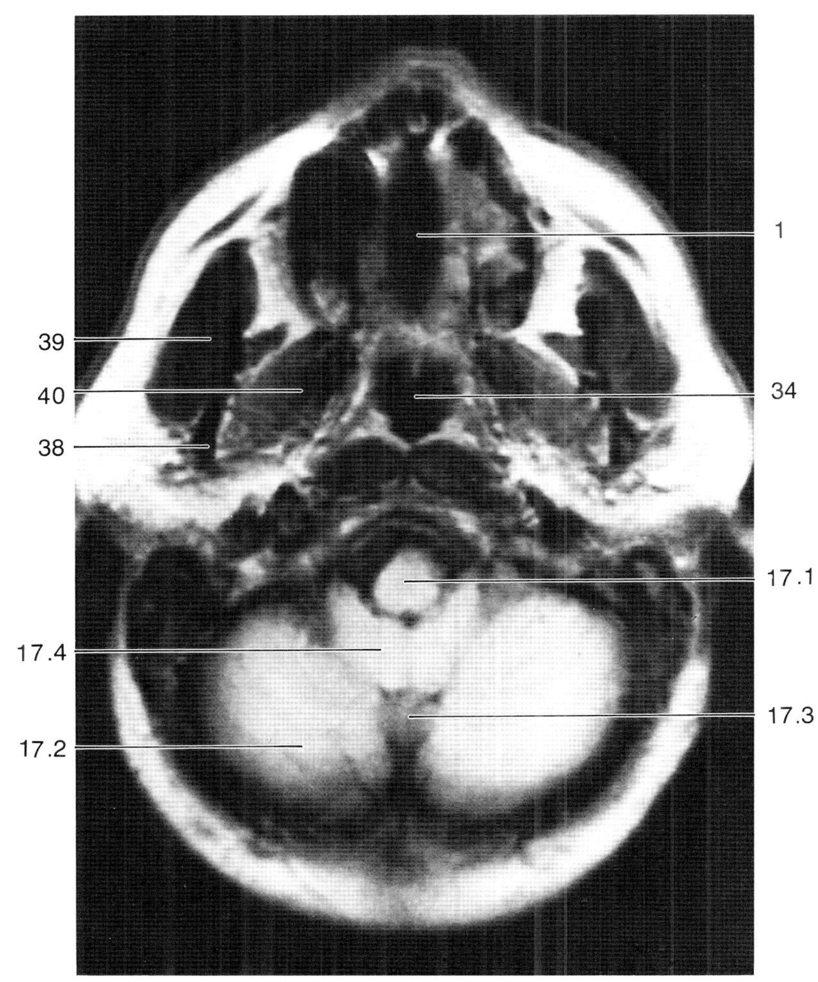

MRI, SE 500/50

1 Oral cavity
8 Alveolar recess of the maxillary sinus
17 Mastoid air cells
17.1 Medulla
17.2 Cerebellum
17.3 Vermis
17.4 Cerebellar tonsil
20 Foramen magnum
20.1 Vitreous body
20.2 Ethmoidal cells
20.3 Foramen ovale
20.4 Sphenoid body
20.5 External auditory meatus
20.6 Zygomatic bone
20.7 Temporal bone
20.8 Foramen lacerum
20.9 Hypoglossal canal
27 Occipital bone
27.1 Odontoid process
27.2 Jugular foramen
27.3 Jugular tuberculum
34 Pharynx
38 Ramus of the mandible
39 Masseter muscle
40 Medial pterygoid muscles
40.1 Styloid process
40.2 Occipital condyle
44.1 Maxilla

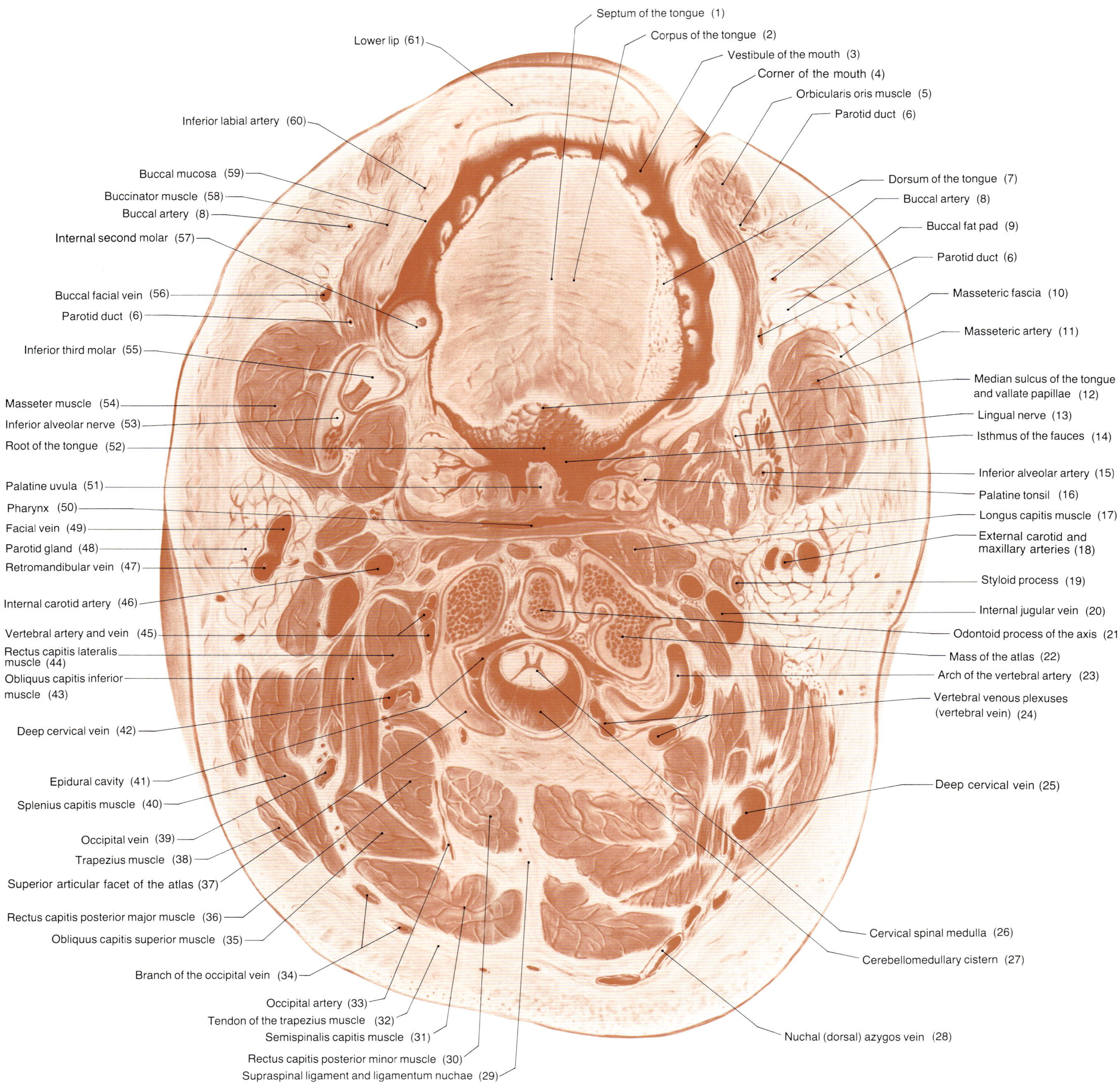

1 Septum linguae
2 Corpus linguae
2.1 Maxilla
2.2 R. mandibularis
2.3 Processus styloideus
3 Vestibulum oris
4 Angulus oris
5 M. orbicularis oris
6 Ductus parotideus
7 Dorsum linguae
8 A. buccalis
9 Corpus adiposum buccae
10 Fascia masseterica
11 A. masseterica
12 Sulcus medianus linguae et Papillae vallatae
13 N. lingualis
14 Isthmus faucium
15 A. alveolaris inferior
16 Tonsilla palatina
17 M. longus capitis
18 Aa. carotis externa et maxillaris
19 Processus styloideus
20 V. jugularis interna
20.1 M. sternocleidomastoideus
21 Dens (axis)
21.1 Processus articularis atlantis
21.1 Arcus vertebrae atlantis
22 Massa atlantis
23 Arcus a. vertebralis
24 Plexus venosi vertebrales (V. vertebralis)
25 V. cervicalis profunda
26 Medulla spinalis cervicalis
26.1 Tuberculum anterius atlantis
26.2 Foramen transversum
27 Cisterna cerebellomedullaris
28 V. azygos nuchae (dorsi)
29 Ligg. supraspinale et nuchae
30 M. rectus capitis posterior minor
31 M. semispinalis capitis
32 Tendo m. trapezii
33 A. occipitalis
34 R. v. occipitalis
35 M. obliquus capitis superior
36 M. rectus capitis posterior major
37 Fovea articularis superior atlantis
38 M. trapezius
39 V. occipitalis
40 M. splenius capitis
40.1 Processus transversus
41 Cavum epidurale
42 V. cervicalis profunda
43 M. obliquus capitis inferior
44 M. rectus capitis lateralis
45 A. et V. vertebralis
45.1 Axis
46 A. carotis interna
47 V. retromandibularis
48 Glandula parotis
49 V. facialis
50 Pharynx
50.1 Lamina lateralis processus pterygoidis
50.2 Lamina medialis processus pterygoidis
50.3 Vomer
50.4 Processus frontalis maxillae
50.5 Sinus maxillaris
50.6 R. mandibularis
50.7 M. pterygoideus medialis
51 Uvula palatina
52 Radix linguae
53 N. alveolaris inferior
54 M. masseter
55 Dens molaris III inferior
56 V. facialis buccalis
57 Dens molaris II superior
57.1 Dentes mandibulae
58 M. buccinator
59 Tunica mucosa buccae
60 A. labialis inferior
61 Labium inferius

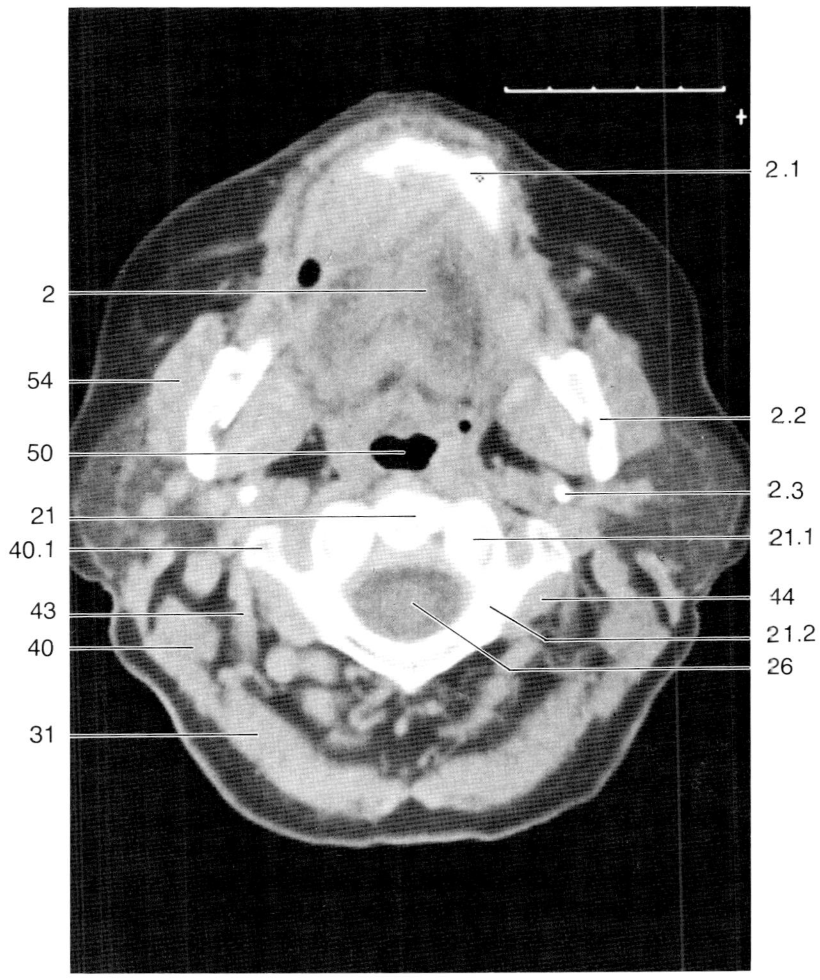

CT scan

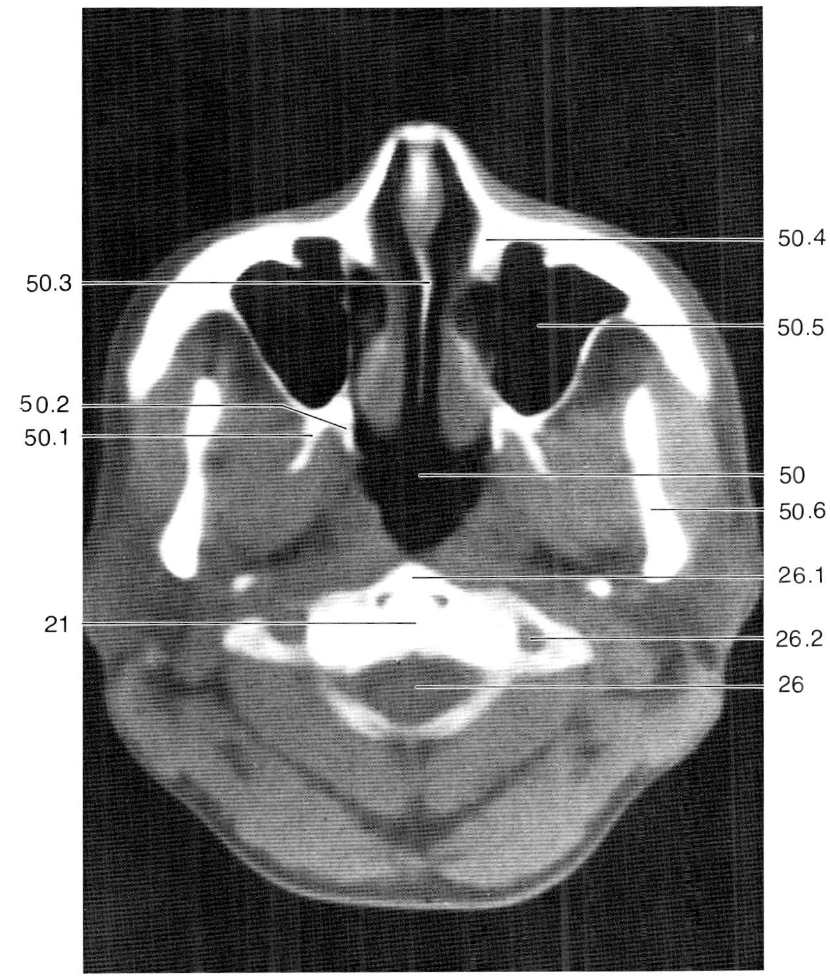

CT scan

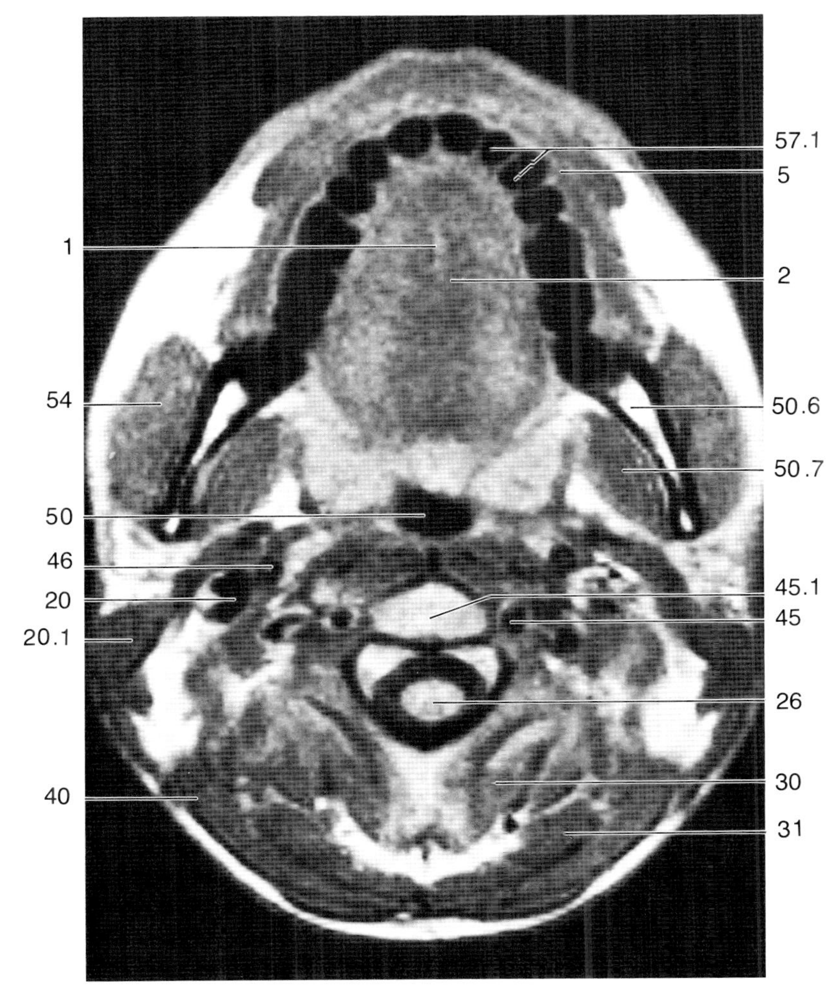

MRI, SE 600/30

1 Septum of the tongue
2 Corpus of the tongue
2.1 Maxilla
2.2 Mandibular ramus
2.3 Styloid process
5 Orbicularis oris muscle
20 Internal jugular vein
20.1 Sternocleidomastoid muscle
21 Odontoid process of the axis
21.1 Articular process of the atlas
21.2 Posterior arch of the atlas
26 Cervical spinal medulla
26.1 Anterior tubercle of the atlas
26.2 Transverse foramen
30 Rectus capitis posterior minor muscle
31 Semispinalis capitis muscle
40 Splenius capitis muscle
40.1 Transverse process of the atlas
43 Obliquus capitis inferior muscle
44 Rectus capitis lateralis muscle
45 Vertebral artery
45.1 Body of the axis
46 Internal carotid artery
50 Pharynx
50.1 Lateral pterygoid plate of the sphenoid bone
50.2 Medial pterygoid plate of the sphenoid bone
50.3 Vomer bone
50.4 Frontal process of the maxilla
50.5 Maxillary sinus
50.6 Mandibular ramus
50.7 Pterygoideus medialis muscle
54 Masseter muscle
57.1 Mandibular tooth

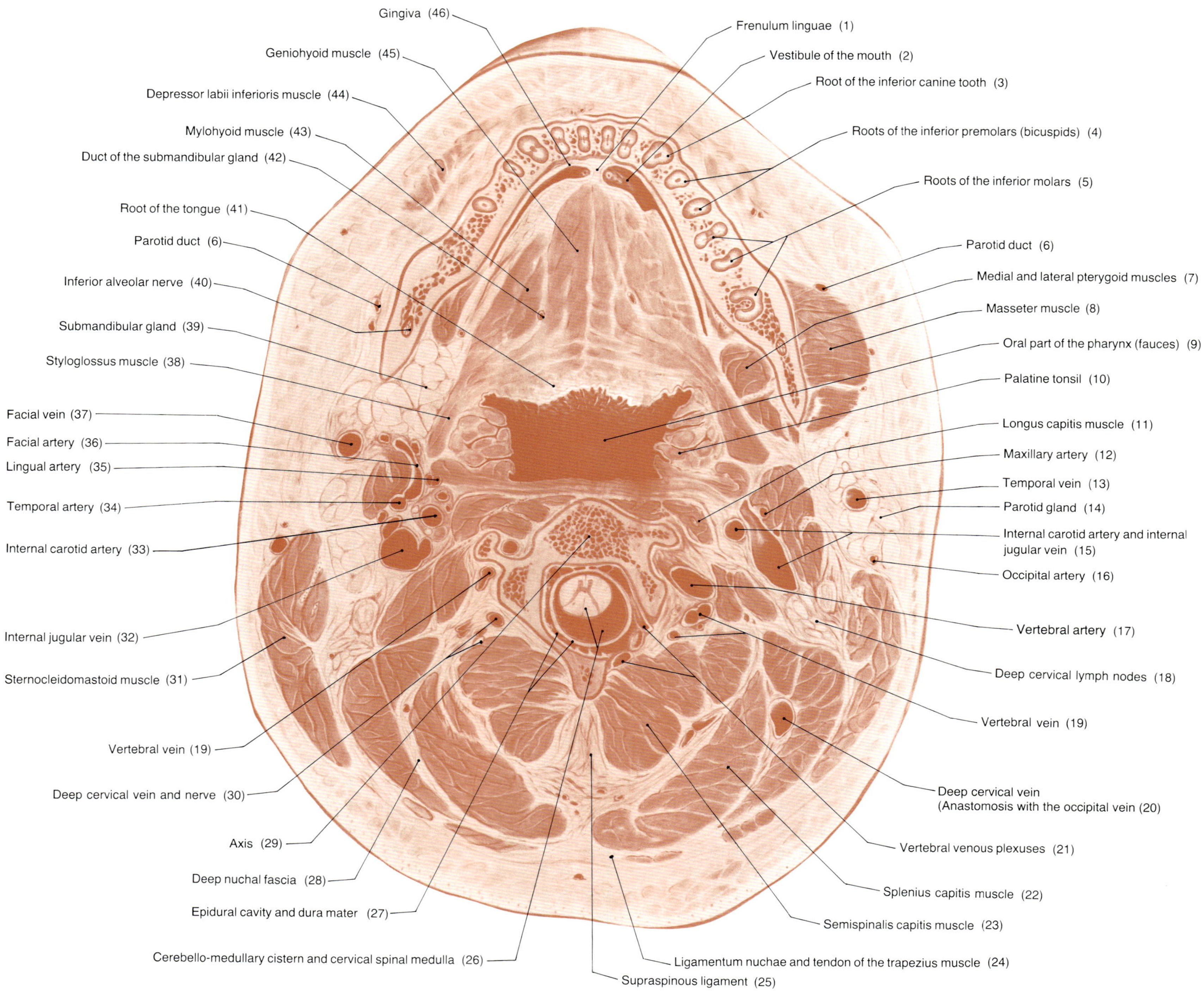

1 Frenulum linguae
2 Vestibulum oris
3 Radix dentis canini inferioris
4 Radices dentium praemolarium inferiorum
5 Radices dentium molarium inferiorum
6 Ductus parotideus
7 M. pterygoideus medialis et lateralis
8 M. masseter
9 Pars oralis pharyngis
9.1 Mandibula
9.2 R. mandibulae
9.3 Processus styloideus
9.4 Processus transversus
9.5 Processus articularis
9.6 Medulla spinalis
9.7 A. carotis externa
10 Tonsilla palatina
11 M. longus capitis
12 A. maxillaris
13 V. temporalis
14 Glandula parotis
15 A. carotis interna et V. jugularis interna
16 A. occipitalis
17 A. vertebralis
17.1 M. obliquus capitis
18 Nodi lymphatici cervicales profundi
19 V. vertebralis
20 V. cervicalis profunda (Anastomosis v. occipitalis)
21 Plexus venosi vertebrales
22 M. splenius capitis
23 M. semispinalis capitis
23.1 M. trapezius
24 Lig. nuchae et Tendo m. trapezii
25 Lig. supraspinale
26 Cisterna cerebellomedullaris et Medulla spinalis cervicalis
27 Cavum epidurale et Dura mater
28 Fascia nuchae profunda
29 Axis
30 V. cervicalis profunda et N. cervicalis
31 M. sternocleidomastoideus
32 V. jugularis interna
33 A. carotis interna
34 A. temporalis
35 A. lingualis
36 A. facialis
37 V. facialis
38 M. styloglossus
39 Glandula submandibularis
40 N. alveolaris inferior
41 Radix linguae
42 Ductus glandulae submandibularis
43 M. mylohyoideus
44 M. depressor labii inferioris
45 M. geniohyoideus
46 Gingiva

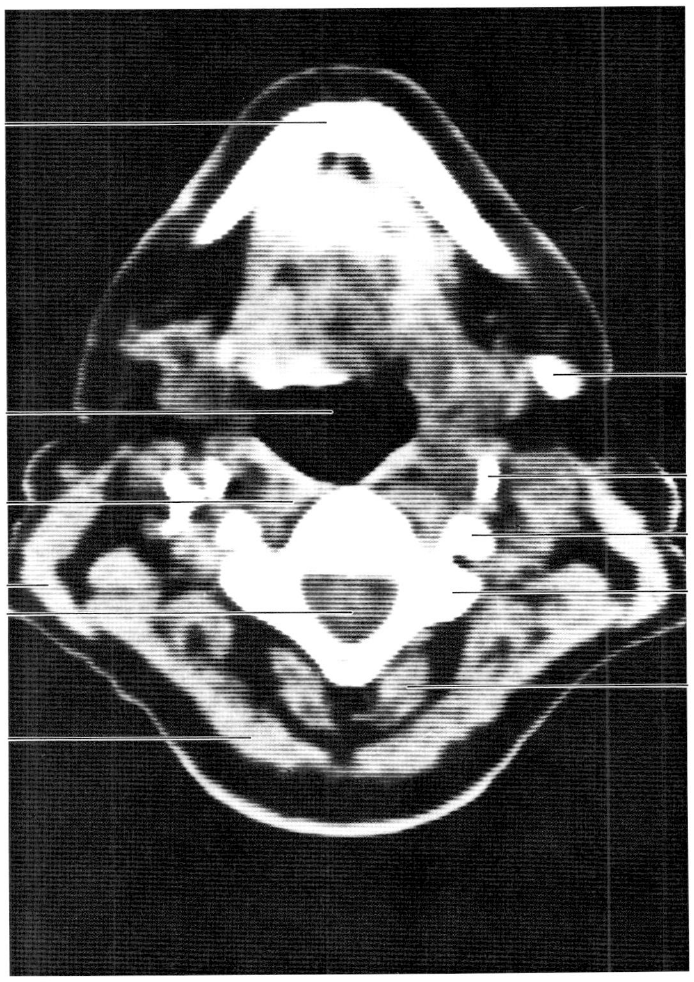

CT scan

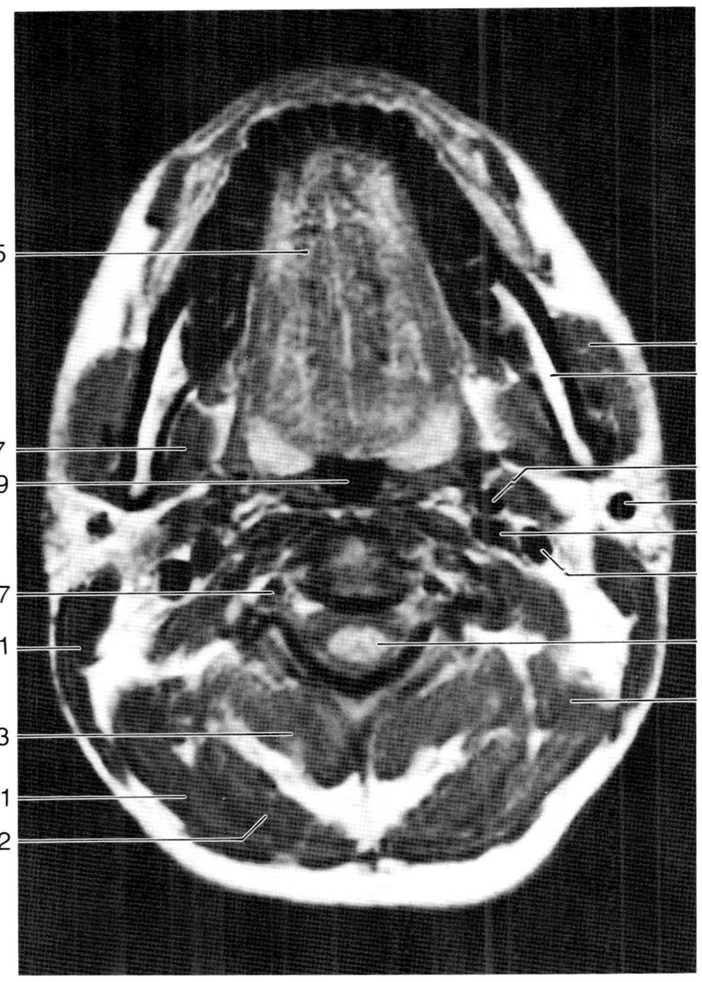

MRI, SE 700/30

7 Medial and lateral pterygoid muscles
8 Masseter muscle
9 Oral part of the pharynx (fauces)
9.1 Mandibula
9.2 Mandibular ramus
9.3 Styloid process
9.4 Transverse process of the axis
9.5 Articular process of the axis
9.6 Spinal cord
9.7 External carotid artery
11 Longus capitis muscle
13 Temporal vein
17 Vertebral artery
17.1 Obliquus capitis muscle
22 Splenius capitis muscle
23 Semispinalis capitis muscle
23.1 Trapezius muscle
31 Sternocleidomastoid muscle
32 Internal jugular vein
33 Internal carotid artery
45 Geniohyoid muscle

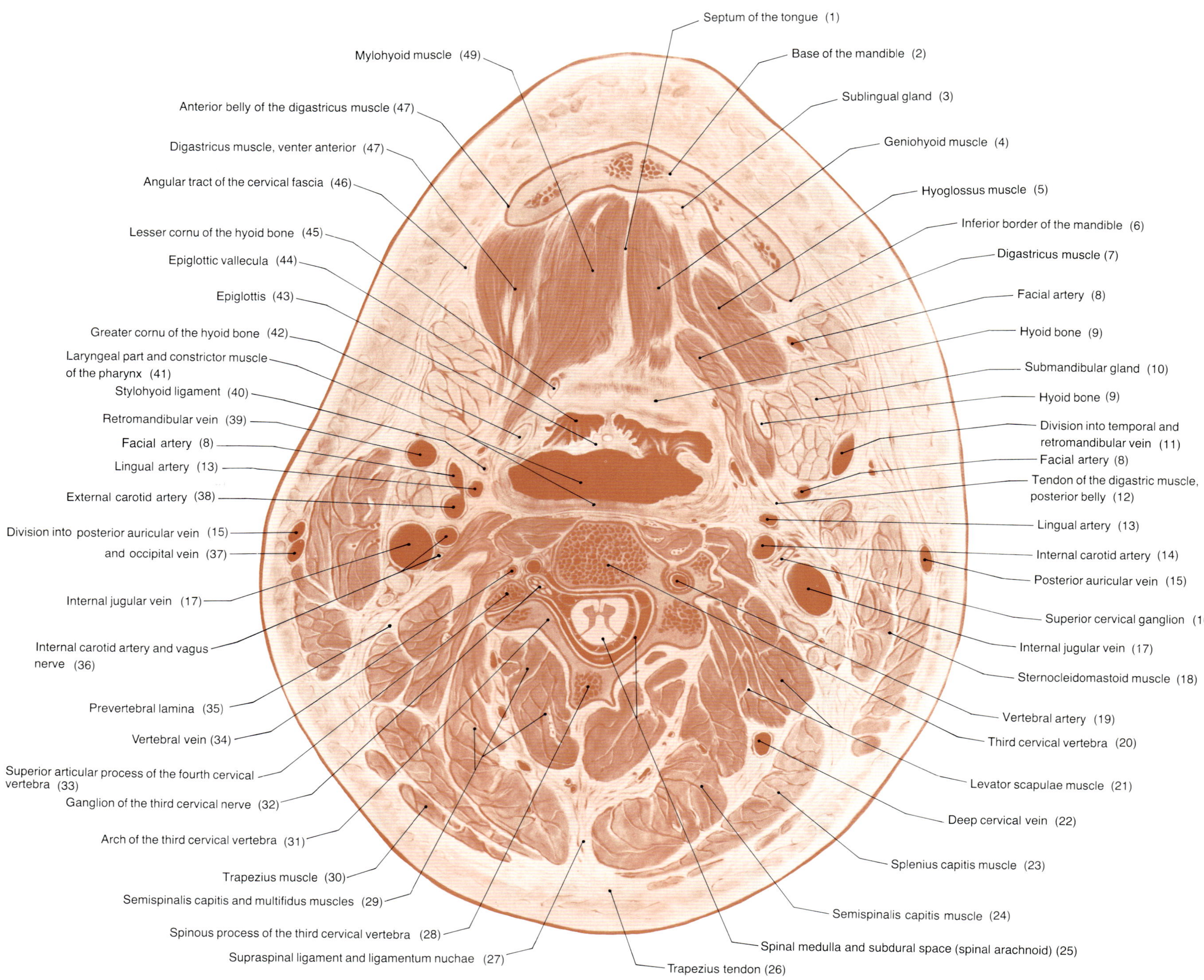

1 Septum linguae
2 Basis mandibulae
2.1 Pharynx
3 Glandula sublingualis
4 M. geniohyoideus
5 M. hyoglossus
6 Margo inferior mandibularis
7 M. digastricus
8 A. facialis
9 Os hyoideum
10 Glandula submandibularis
11 Bifurcatio V. temporalis et V. retromandibularis
12 Tendo m. digastrici Venter posterior
13 A. lingualis
14 A. carotis interna
15 V. auricularis posterior
16 Ganglion cervicale superior
17 V. jugularis interna
18 M. sternocleidomastoideus
19 A. vertebralis
19.1 M. longus capitis
20 Vertebra cervicalis III
21 N. levator scapulae
22 V. cervicalis profunda
23 M. splenius capitis
24 M. semispinalis capitis
25 Medulla spinalis et Spatium subdurale (Arachnoidea spinalis)
26 Tendo m. trapezii
27 Lig. supraspinale et Lig. nuchae
28 Processus spinosus cervicalis III
29 M. semispinalis capitis et M. multifidus
30 M. trapezius
31 Arcus vertebrae cervicalis III
32 Ganglion n. cervicalis III
33 Processus articularis superior vertebr. cervic. IV
34 V. vertebralis
35 Lamina praevertebralis
36 A. carotis interna et N. vagus
37 Bifurcatio V. auricularis posterioris (15) et V. occipitalis
38 A. carotis externa
39 V. retromandibularis
40 Lig. stylohyoideum
41 Pars laryngea pharyngis et M. constrictor pharyngis
42 Cornu majus ossis hyoideus
43 Epiglottis
44 Vallecula epiglottica
45 Cornu minus ossis hyoideus
46 Tractus angularis fasciae cervicis
47 M. digastricus, Venter anterior
48 Fascia cervicalis submandibularis
49 M. mylohyoideus

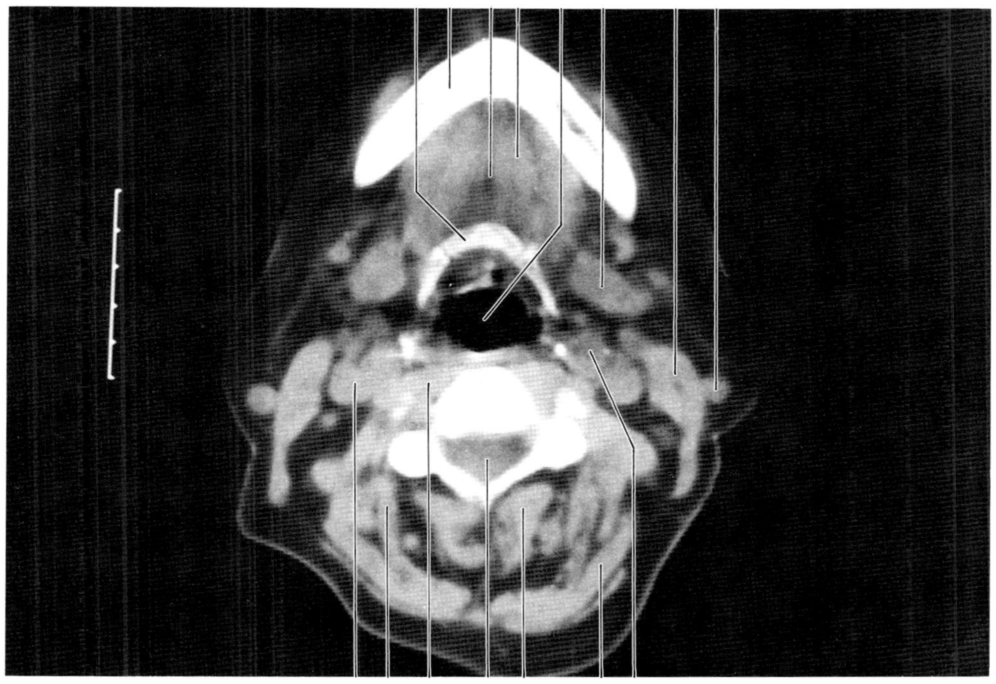

CT scan

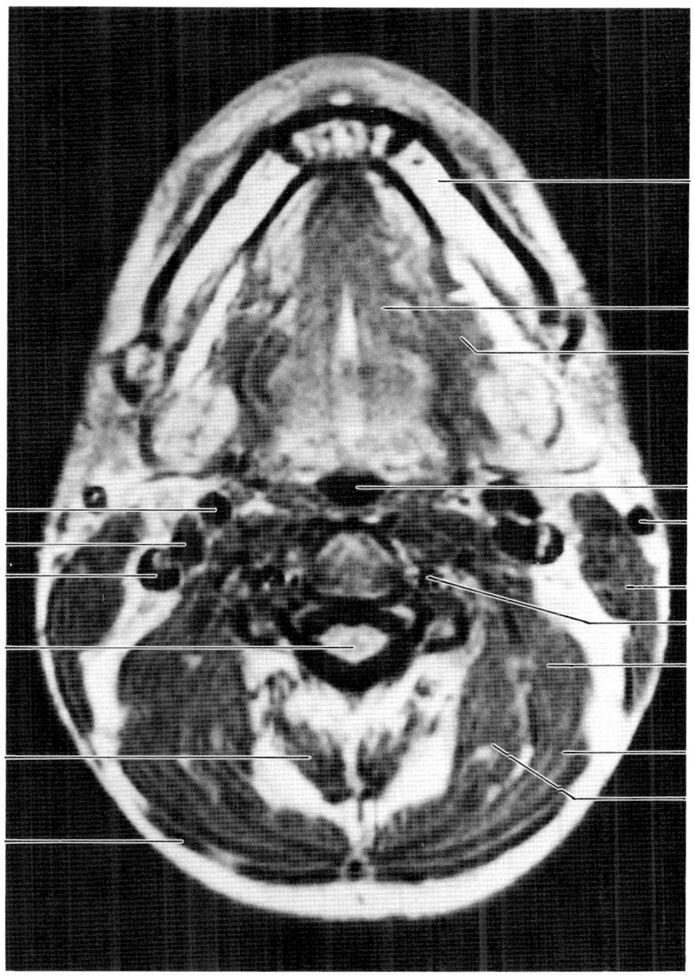

MRI, SE 700/30

1 Septum of the tongue
2 Basis of the mandible
2.1 Pharynx
4 Geniohyoid muscle
5 Hyoglossus muscle
9 Hyoid bone
14 Internal carotid artery
15 Posterior auricular vein
17 Internal jugular vein
18 Sternocleidomastoid muscle
19 Vertebral artery
19.1 Longus capitis muscle
21 Levator scapulae muscle
23 Splenius capitis muscle
24 Semispinalis capitis muscle
25 Spinal medulla and subdural space (spinal arachnoid)
29 Semispinalis capitis and multifidus muscles
30 Trapezius muscle
38 External carotid artery

Axial Sections of the Neck and Thorax

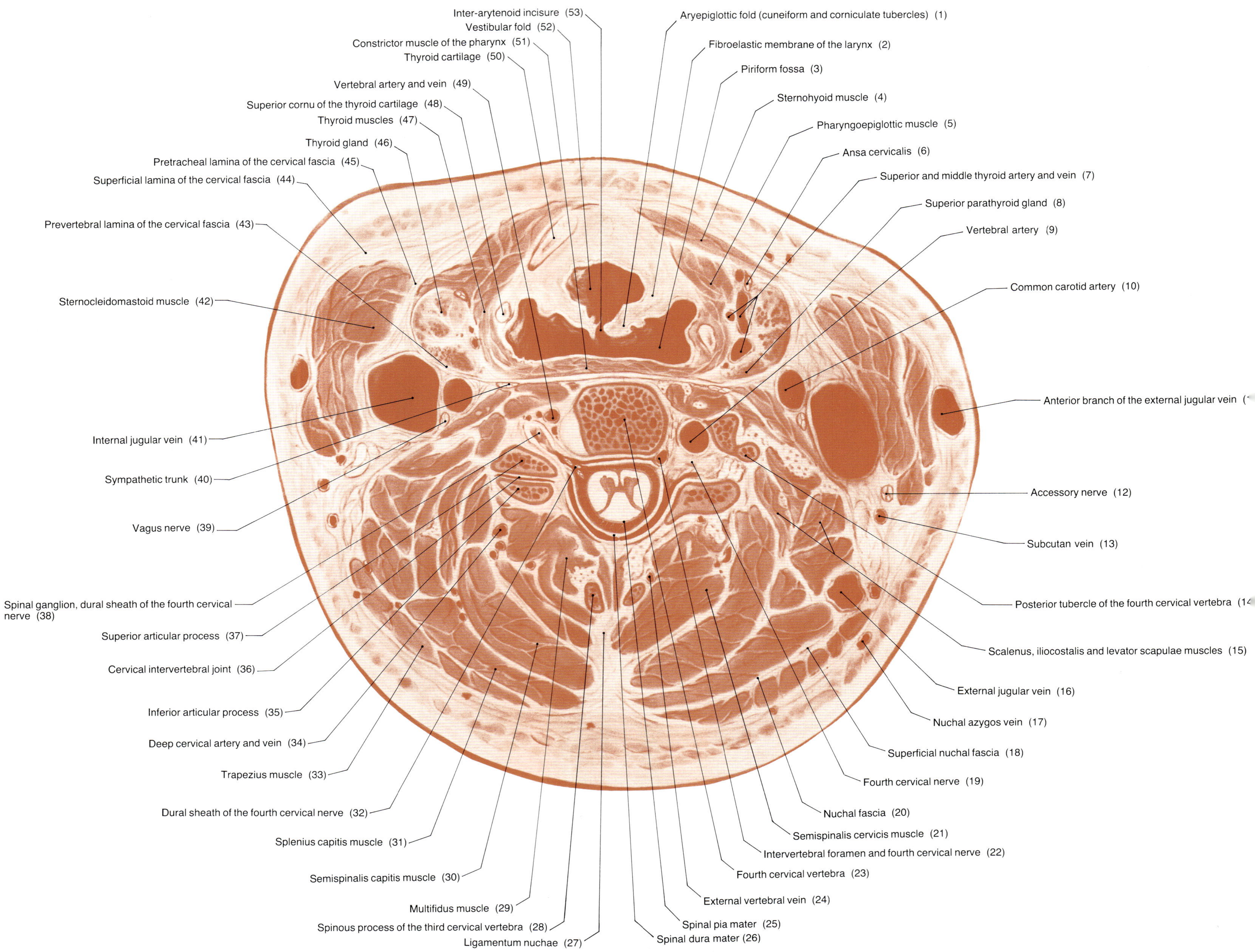

1 Plica aryepiglottica (Tuberculum cuneiforme et corniculatum)
2 Membrana fibroelastica laryngis
3 Recessus piriformis
4 M. sternohyoideus
5 M. pharyngoepiglotticus
6 Ansa cervicalis
7 A. et V. thyroidea superior et media
8 Glandula parathyroidea superior
9 A. vertebralis
10 A. carotis communis
11 V. jugularis externa (R. anterior)
12 N. accessorius
13 V. subcutanea
14 Tuberculum posterius vertebrae
15 Mm. scalenus, iliocostalis et levator scapulae
16 V. jugularis externa
17 V. azygos nuchae
18 Fascia nuchae superficialis
19 N. cervicalis IV
19.1 N. cervicalis VII, Vagina durae matris
20 Fascia nuchae
21 M. semispinalis cervicis
22 Foramen intervertebrale, N. cervicalis IV
23 Vertebra cervicalis IV
23.1 Vertebra cervicalis VII
24 V. vertebralis externa
25 Pia mater spinalis
26 Dura mater spinalis
26.1 Cavum epidurale
26.2 Processus spinosus
26.3 Medulla spinalis
27 Lig. nuchae
28 Processus spinosus cervicalis III
29 M. multifidus
30 M. semispinalis capitis
31 M. splenius capitis
32 N. cervicalis IV, Vagina durae matris
33 M. trapezius
34 A. et V. cervicalis profunda
35 Processus articularis inferior
35.1 Lamina arcus vertebrae
36 Articulus intervertebralis cervicis
37 Processus articularis superior
37.1 Processus transversus, tuberculum anterius
37.2 Processus transversus, tuberculum posterius
37.3 Foramen transversarium
38 Ganglion spinale, N. cervicalis IV (Vagina durae matris)
39 N. vagus
40 Truncus n. sympathici
41 V. jugularis interna
41.1 A. carotis interna
41.2 A. carotis externa
41.3 V. retromandibularis
42 M. sternocleidomastoideus
43 Lamina praevertebralis, Fascia cervicalis
44 Lamina superficialis, Fascia cervicalis
45 Lamina praetrachealis, Fascia cervicalis
46 Glandula thyroidea
47 M. thyrohyoideus
48 Cornu superius (cart. thyroid.)
49 A. et V. vertebralis
50 Cartilago thyroidea
51 M. constrictor pharyngis
52 Plica vestibularis
53 Incisura interarytaenoidea

3 Piriform fossa
4 Sternohyoid muscle
9 Vertebral artery
10 Common carotid artery
15 Scalenus, iliocostalis and levator scapulae muscles
19.1 Dural sheath of the seventh cervical nerve
21 Semispinalis cervicis muscle
23.1 Seventh cervical vertebra
26.1 Dural sac
26.2 Spinous process
26.3 Spinal medulla
29 Multifidus muscle
30 Semispinalis capitis muscle
31 Splenius capitis muscle
33 Trapezius muscle
35 Inferior articular process
35.1 Vertebral lamina
37 Superior articular process
37.1 Transverse process, anterior tubercle
37.2 Transverse process, posterior tubercle
37.3 Transverse foramen
41 Internal jugular vein
41.1 Internal carotid artery
41.2 External carotid artery
41.3 Retromandibular vein
42 Sternocleidomastoid muscle
46 Thyroid gland
48 Superior cornu of the thyroid cartilage
48.1 Fifth cervical vertebra
48.2 Sixth cervical vertebra
50 Thyroid cartilage
52 Vestibular fold

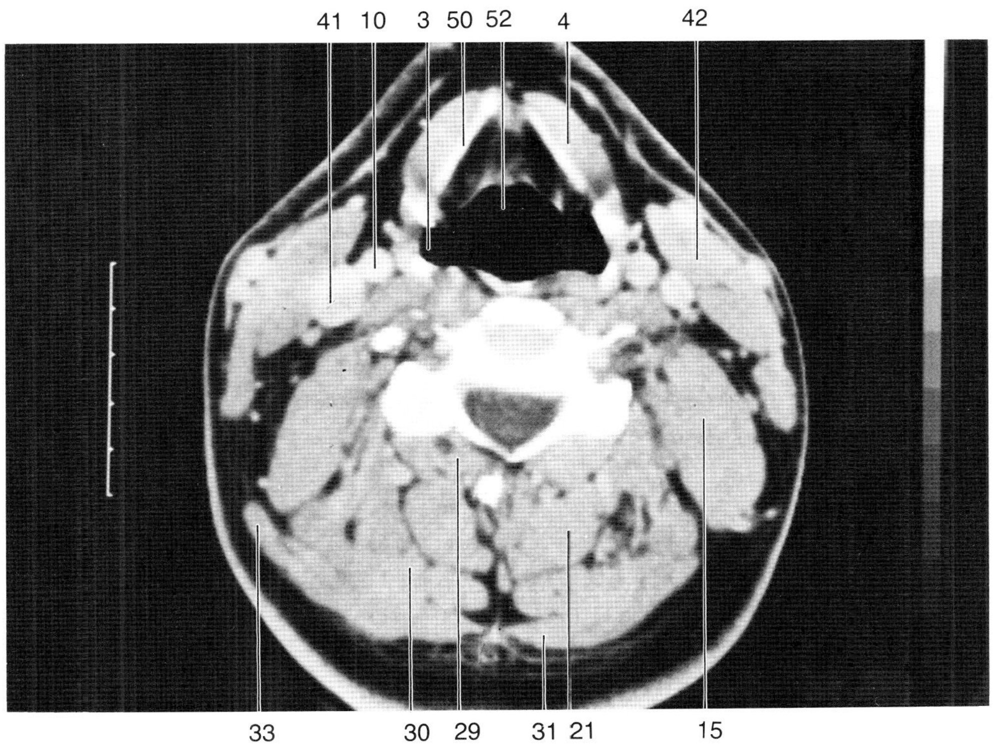

CT scan, unenhanced

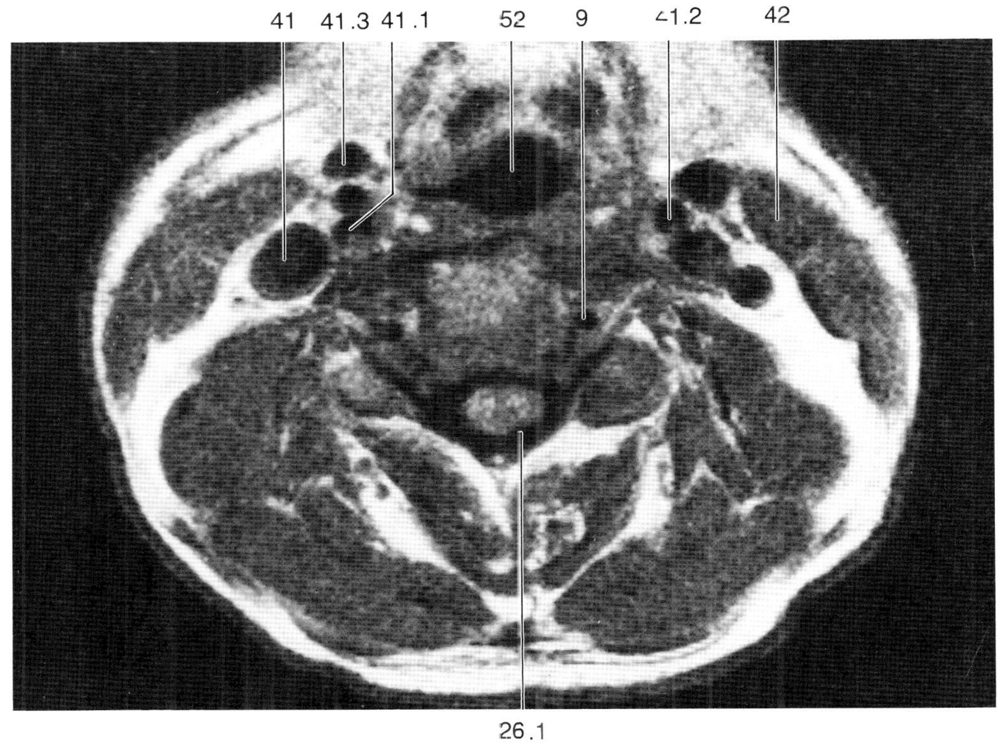

MRI, SE 1000/50

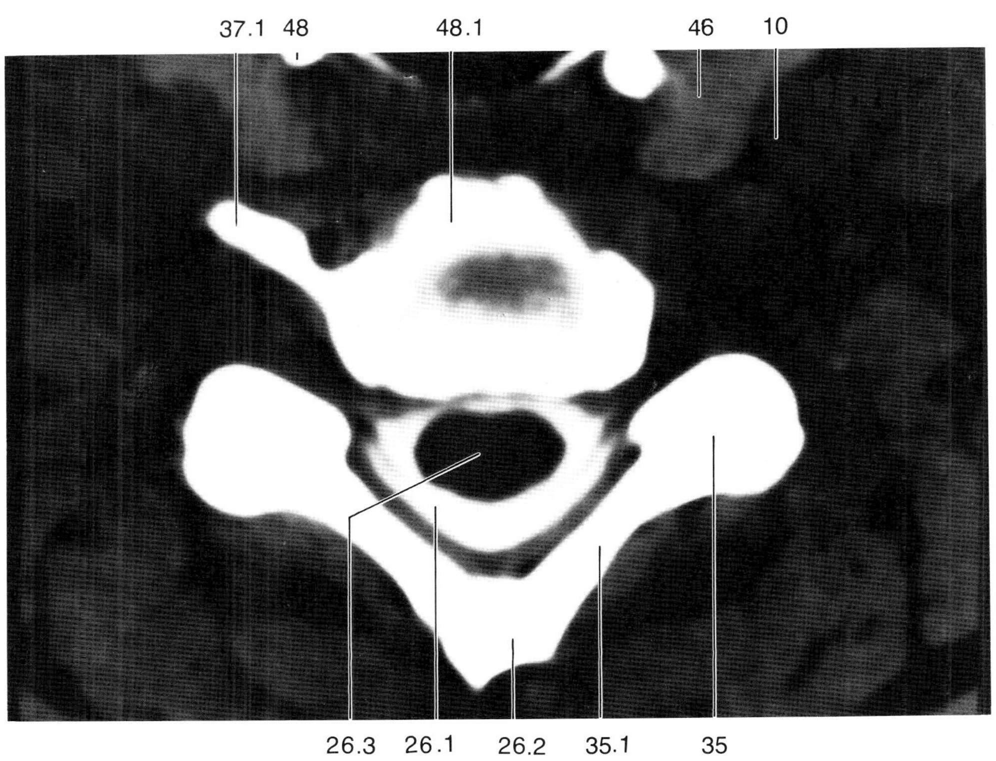

CT with contrast enhancement of the dural sac at CV level

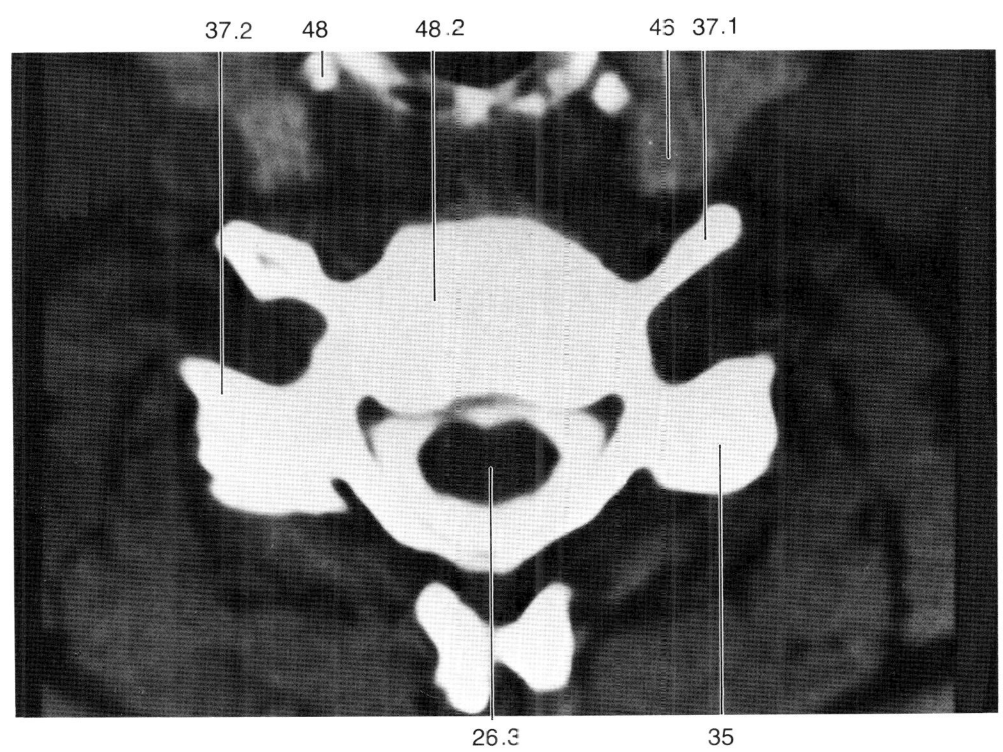

CT with contrast enhancement of the dural sac at CVI level

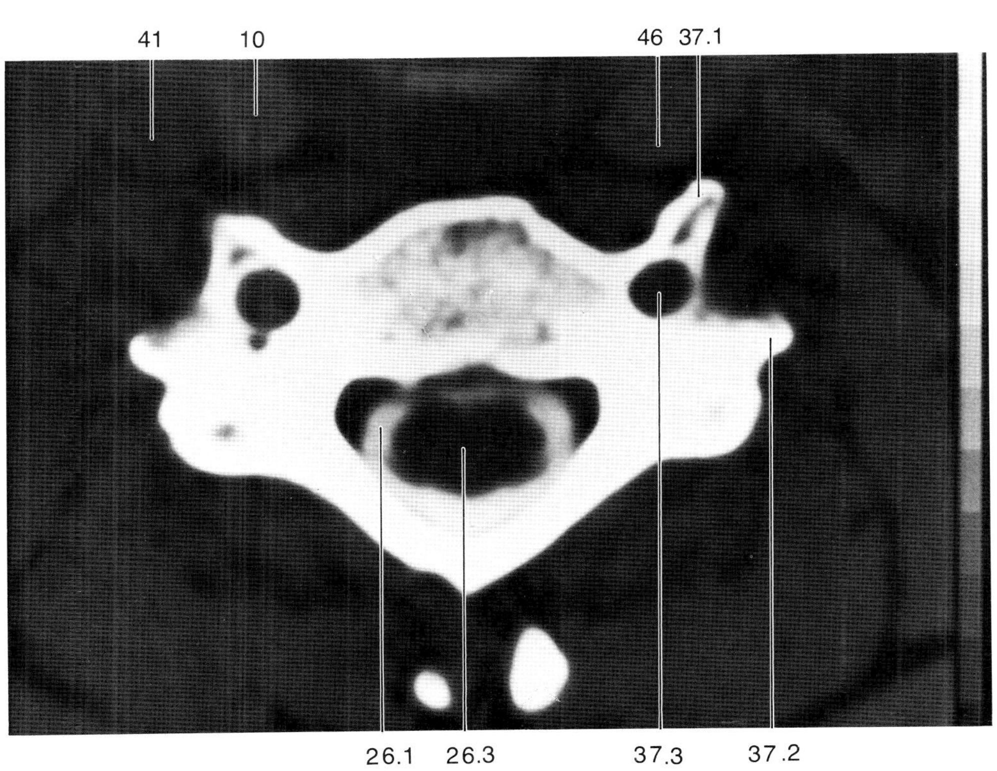

CT with contrast enhancement of the dural sac at CVI level

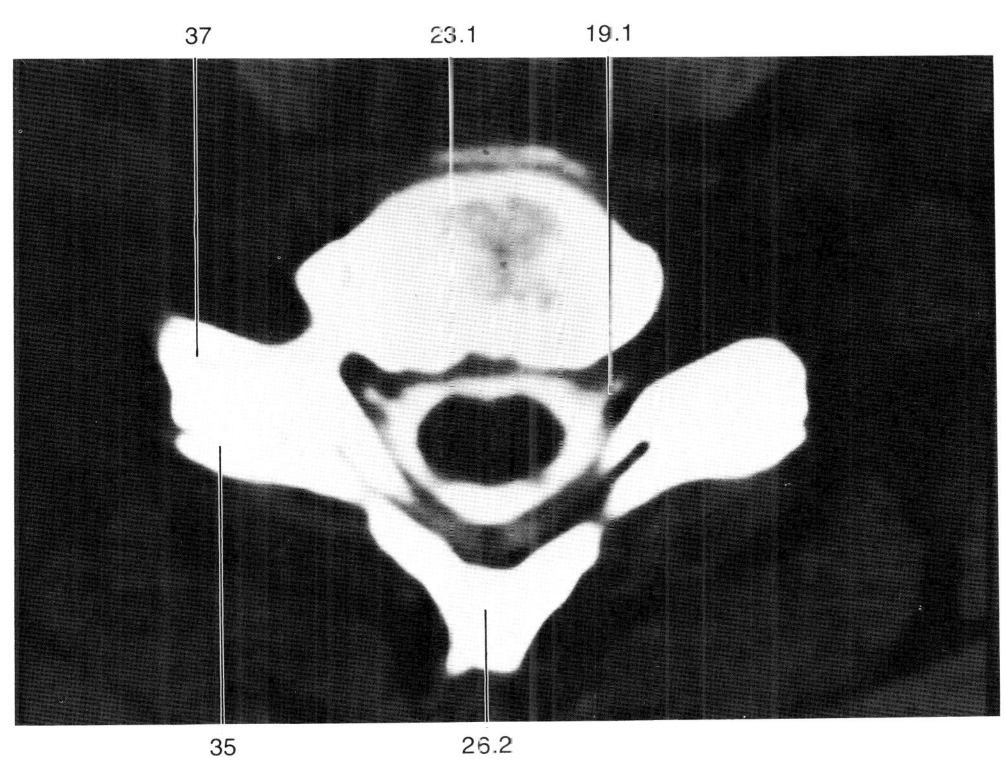

CT with contrast enhancement of the dural sac at CVII level

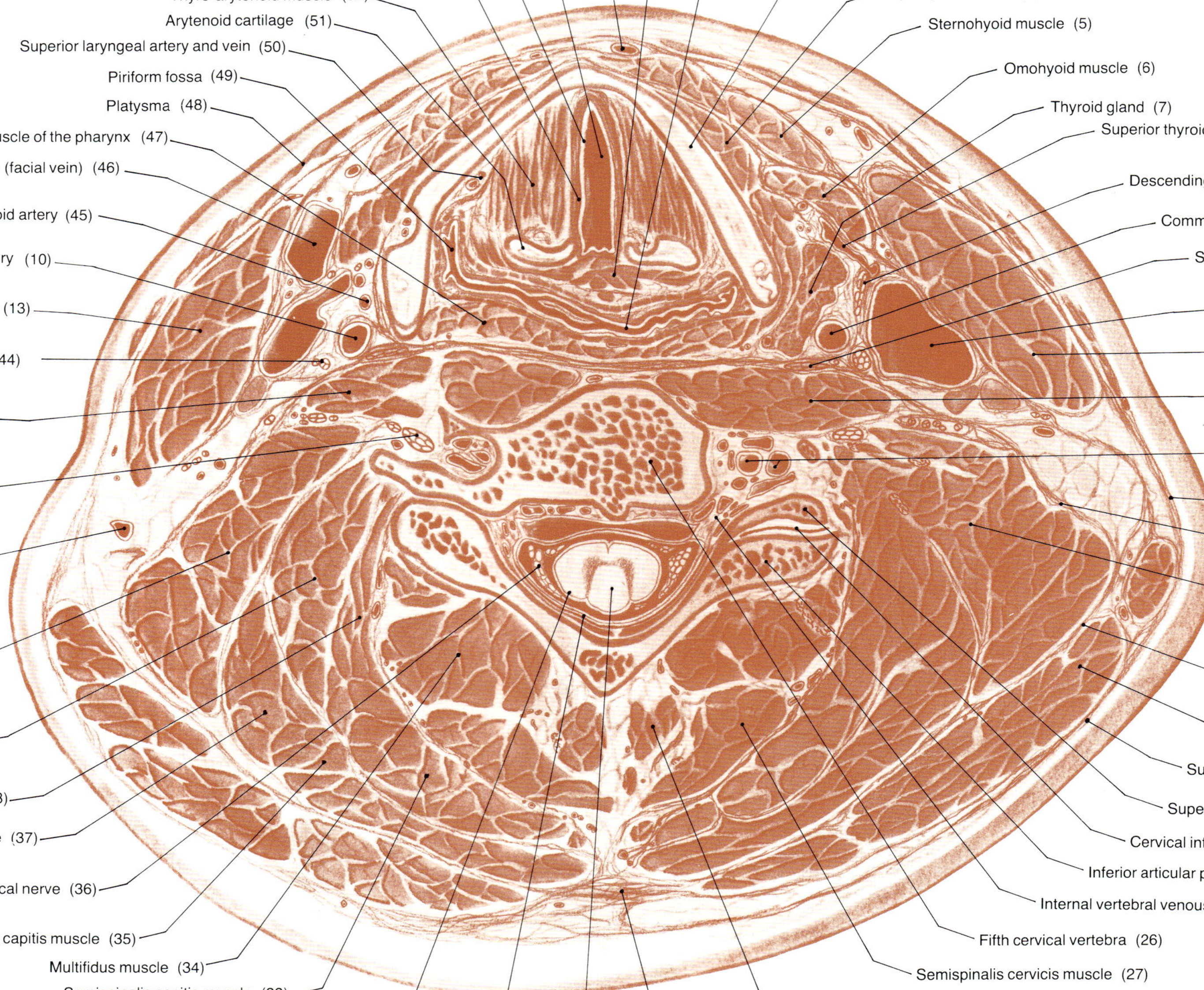

1 M. arytaenoideus
2 Pharynx
3 Cartilago thyroidea
4 M. thyrohyoideus
5 M. sternohyoideus
6 M. omohyoideus
7 Glandula thyroidea
8 V. thyroidea superior
9 R. descendens n. hypoglossi
10 A. carotis communis
11 Truncus sympathicus
12 Bifurcatio V. jugularis internae et V. jugularis externae
13 M. sternocleidomastoideus
14 M. longus colli
15 A. et V. vertebralis
16 Lamina superficialis fasciae cervicalis
17 Lamina praevertebralis fasciae cervicalis
18 M. scalenus medius
19 Fascia nuchae profunda
20 M. trapezius
21 Fascia nuchae superficialis
22 Processus articularis superior
23 Articulus intervertebralis cervicis
24 Processus articularis inferior
25 Plexus venosus vertebralis internus
26 Vertebra cervicalis V
27 M. semispinalis cervicis
28 M. interspinalis cervicis
29 Lig. nuchae
30 Medulla spinalis cervicalis
31 Dura mater spinalis
32 Pia mater spinalis
33 M. semispinalis capitis
34 M. multifidus
35 M. splenius capitis
36 Radix dorsalis n. cervicis IV
37 M. splenius cervicis
38 M. longissimus capitis
39 M. longissimus cervicis
40 M. levator scapulae
41 V. jugularis externa
42 N. cervicalis VI
43 M. scalenus cervicalis
44 N. vagus
45 A. thyroidea superior
46 V. jugularis externa
47 M. constrictor pharyngis
48 Platysma
49 Recessus piriformis
50 A. et V. laryngea superior
51 Cartilago arytaenoidea
52 M. thyroarytaenoideus
53 M. vocalis
54 Lig. vocale
55 Rima glottidis
56 V. colli mediana

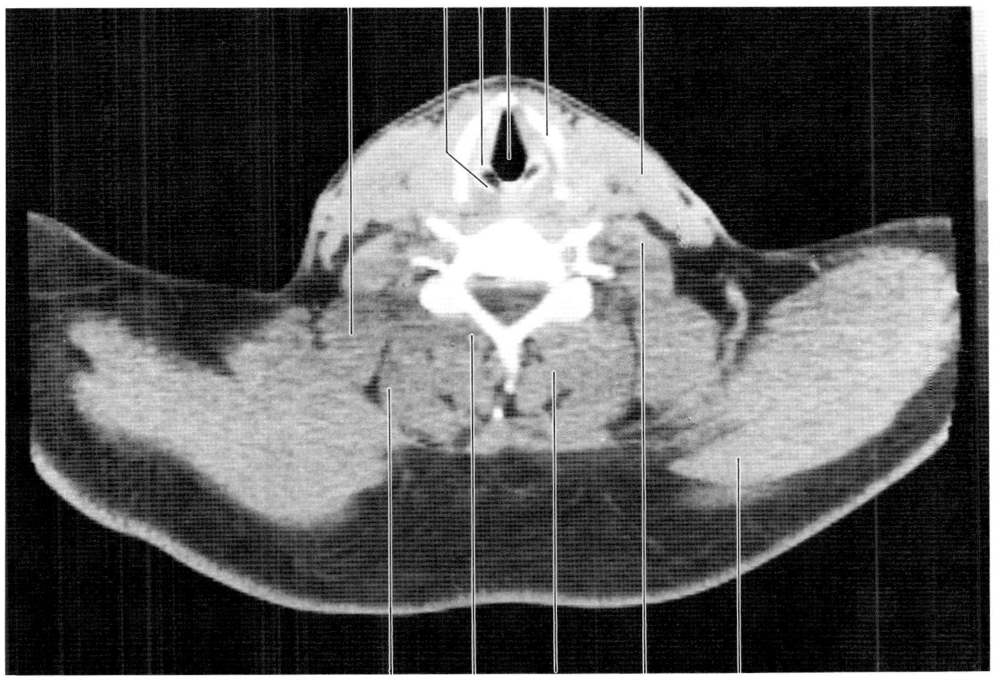

CT scan

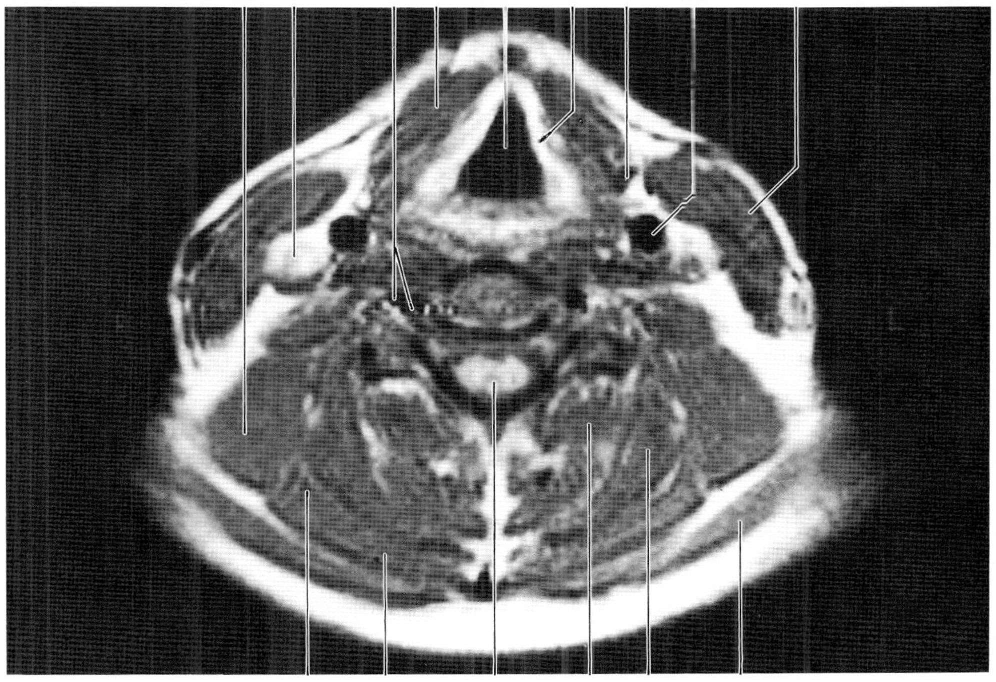

MRI, SE 700/30

2 Pharynx
3 Thyroid cartilage
5 Sternohyoid muscle
10 Common carotid artery
12 Division of internal and external jugular veins
13 Sternocleidomastoid muscle
15 Vertebral artery and vein
18 Scalenus medius muscle
20 Trapezius muscle
27 Semispinalis cervicis muscle
30 Cervical spinal medulla
34 Multifidus muscle
35 Splenius capitis muscle
37 Splenius cervicis muscle
39 Longissimus cervicis muscle
40 Levator scapulae muscle
45 Superior thyroid artery
51 Arytenoid cartilage
52 Thyro-arytenoid muscle
55 Rima glottidis

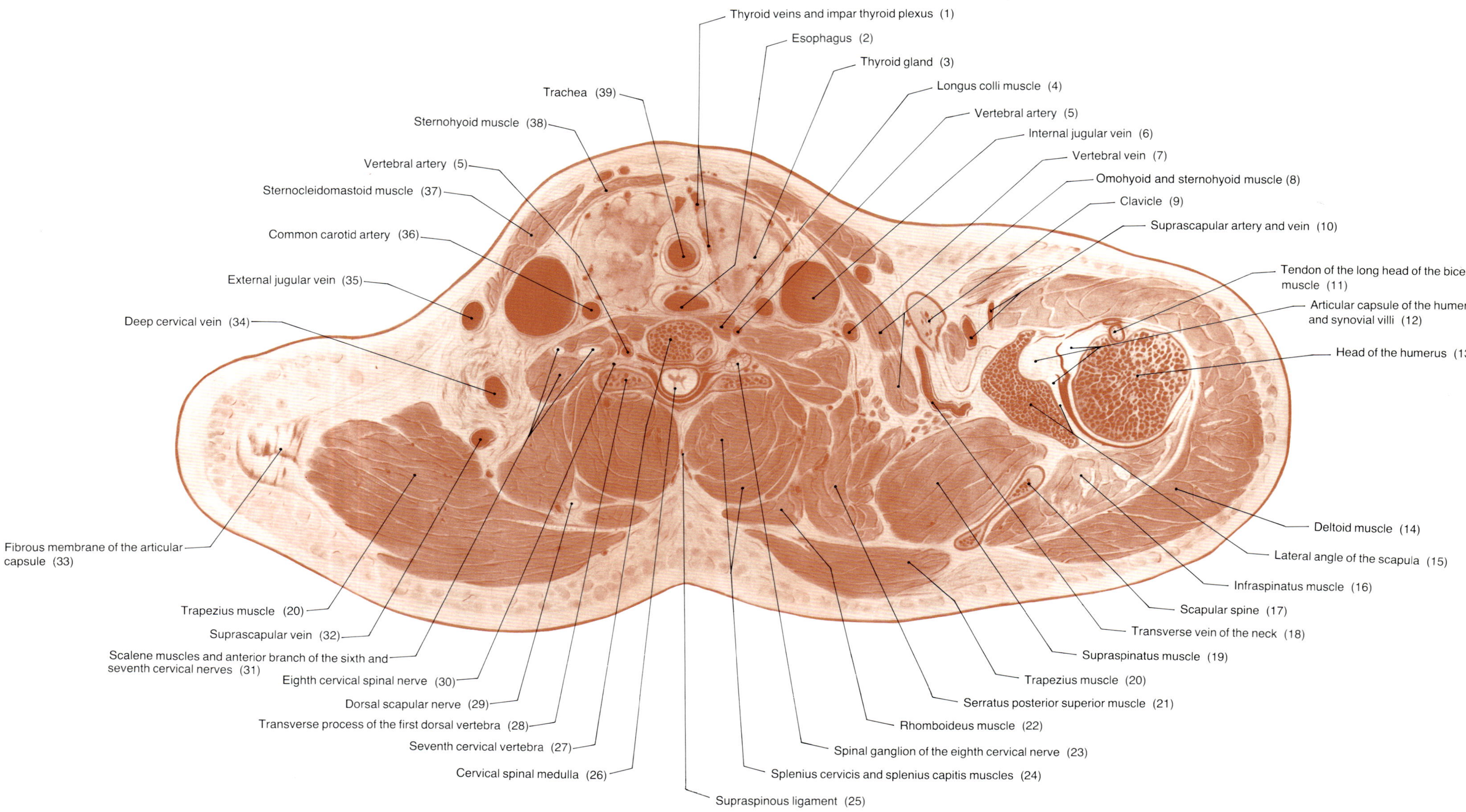

1 Vv. thyroideae imae et plexus thyroideus impar
2 Oesophagus
3 Glandula thyroidea
4 M. longus colli
5 A. vertebralis
6 V. jugularis interna
7 V. vertebralis
8 M. omohyoideus et sternohyoideus
9 Clavicula
10 A. et V. suprascapularis
11 Tendo capitis longi m. bicepitis brachii
12 Capsula articularis humeri et Villi synoviales
13 Caput humeri
14 M. deltoideus
15 Angulus lateralis scapulae
16 M. infraspinatus
17 Spina scapulae
18 V. transversae colli
19 M. supraspinatus
20 M. trapezius
21 M. serratus posterior superior
22 M. rhomboideus
23 Ganglion spinale (N. cervic. VIII)
24 M. splenius cervicis et M. splenius capitis
25 Lig. supraspinale
26 Medulla spinalis cervicalis
27 Vertebra cervicalis VII
28 Processus transversus (Vert. thor. I)
29 N. dorsalis scapulae
30 N. spinalis cervicalis VIII
31 Mm. scaleni et R. ventralis (N. cerv. VI + VII)
32 V. suprascapularis
33 Membrana fibrosa capsulae articularis
34 V. cervicalis profunda
35 V. jugularis externa
36 A. carotis communis
37 M. sternocleidomastoideus
38 M. sternohyoideus
39 Trachea
39.1 Cartilago thyroidea

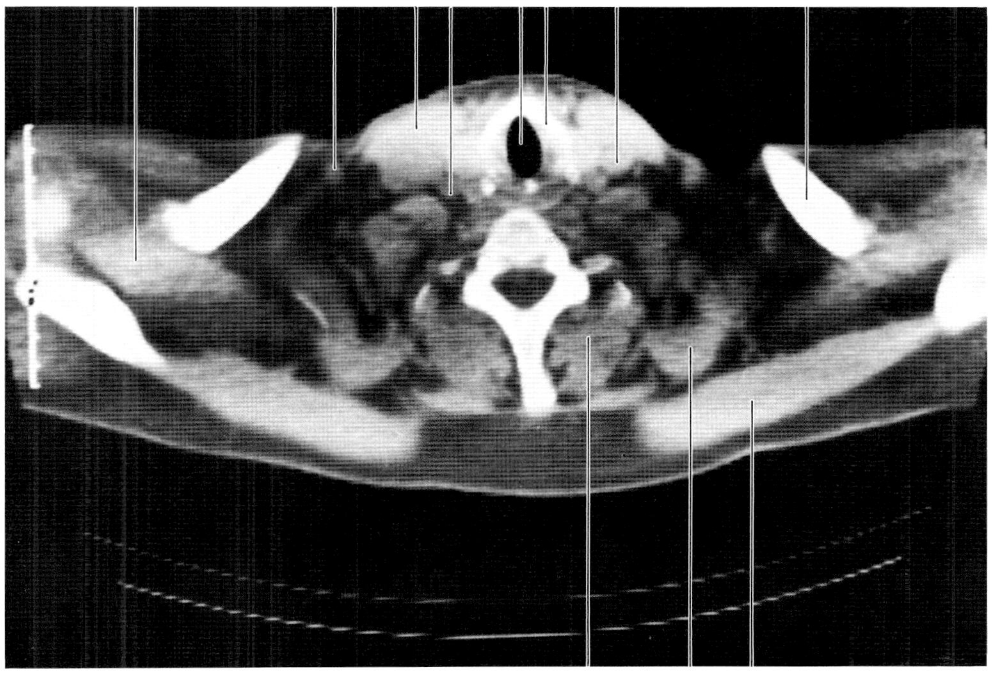

CT, enhanced after bolus injection of contrast medium

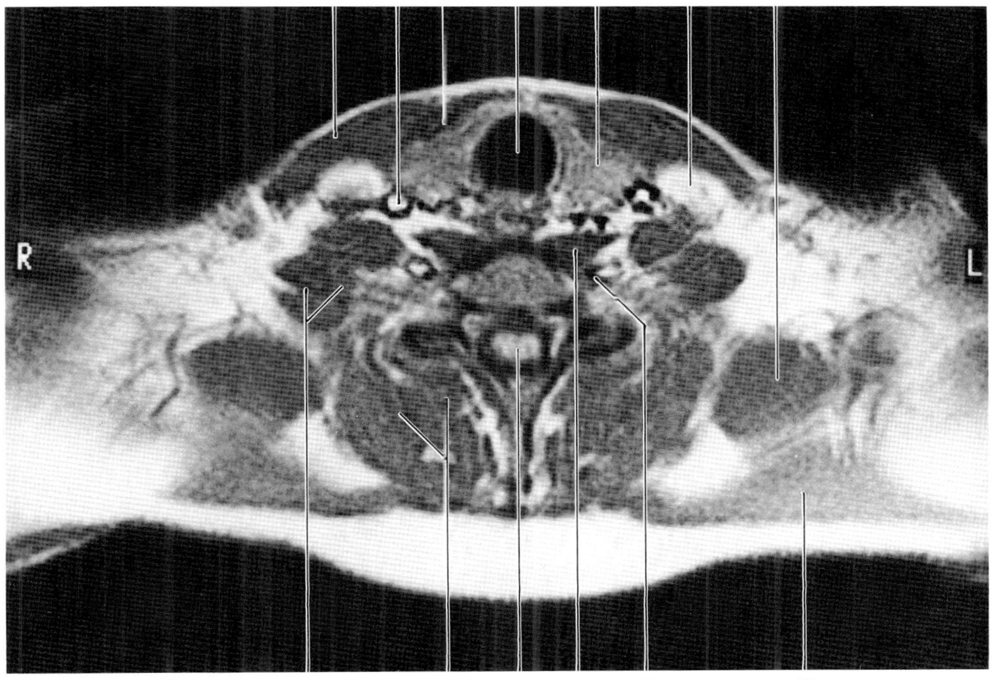

MRI, SE 700/30

3	Thyroid gland
4	Longus colli muscle
5	Vertebral artery
6	Internal jugular vein
9	Clavicle
19	Supraspinatus muscle
20	Trapezius muscle
21	Serratus posterior superior muscle
24	Splenius cervicis and splenius capitis muscles
26	Cervical spinal medulla
31	Scalene muscles and anterior branch of the sixth and seventh cervical nerve
35	External jugular vein
36	Common carotid artery
37	Sternocleidomastoid muscle
38	Sternohyoid muscle
39	Trachea
39.1	Thyroid cartilage

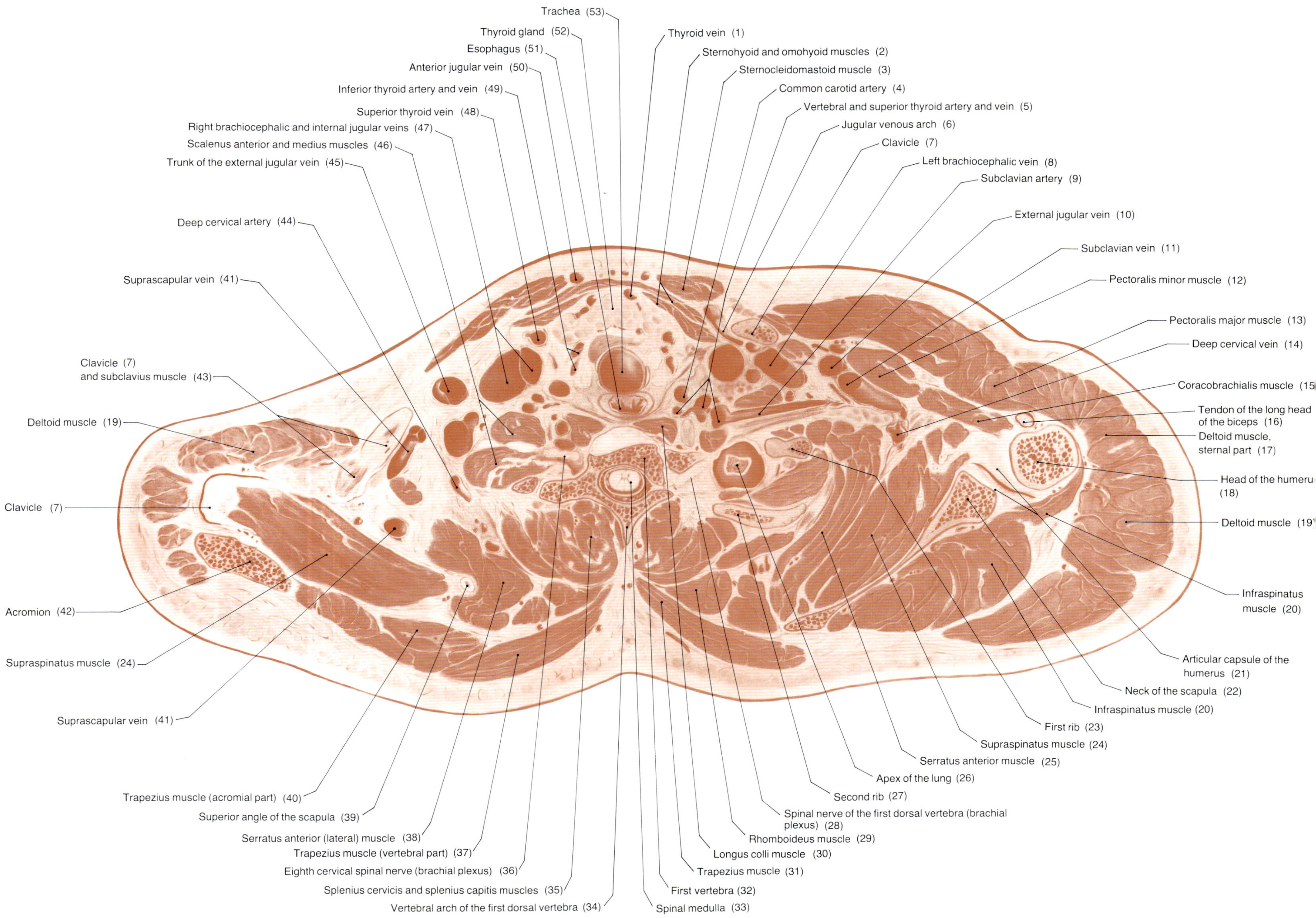

1 V. thyroidea ima
2 M. sternohyoideus et omohyoideus
3 M. sternocleidomastoideus
4 A. carotis communis
5 A. et V. vertebralis et thyroidea superior
6 Arcus venosus juguli
7 Clavicula
8 V. brachiocephalica sinistra
9 A. subclavia
10 V. jugularis externa
11 V. subclavia
12 M. pectoralis minor
13 M. pectoralis major
14 V. cervicalis profunda
15 M. coracobrachialis
16 Tendo capitis longi m. bicepitis brachii
17 M. deltoideus (Pars sternalis)
18 Caput humeri
19 M. deltoideus
20 M. infraspinatus
21 Capsula articularis humeri
22 Collum scapulae
23 Costa I
24 M. supraspinatus
25 M. serratus anterior
26 Apex pulmonis
27 Costa II
28 N. spinalis plexus brachialis
29 M. rhomboideus
30 M. longus colli
31 M. trapezius
32 Vertebra dorsalis I
33 Medulla spinalis
34 Arcus vertebrae (Thor. I)
35 M. splenius cervicis et M. splenius capitis
36 N. spinalis cervicalis VIII (Plexus brachialis)
37 M. trapezius (Pars vertebralis)
38 M. serratus anterior (lateralis)
38.1 Spina scapulae
39 Angulus superior scapulae
40 M. trapezius (Pars acromialis)
41 V. suprascapularis
42 Acromion
43 M. subclavius
44 A. cervicalis profunda
45 V. jugularis externa (Truncus)
46 M. scalenus anterior et medius
47 V. brachiocephalica dextra et V. jugularis interna
48 V. thyroidea superior
49 A. et V. thyroidea inferior
50 V. jugularis anterior
51 Oesophagus
52 Glandula thyroidea
53 Trachea

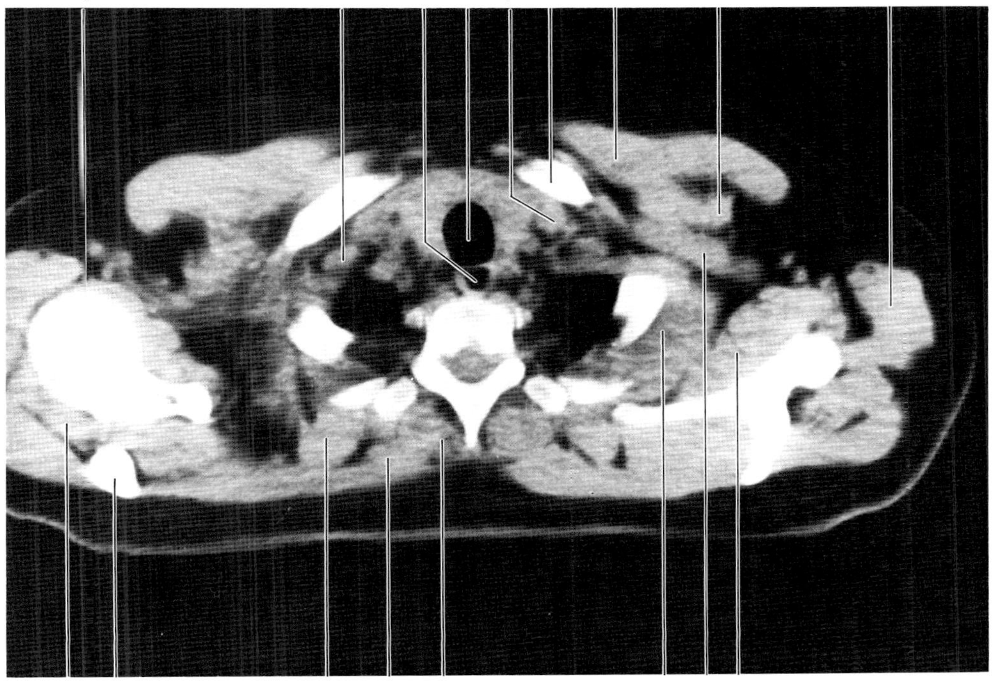

CT scan

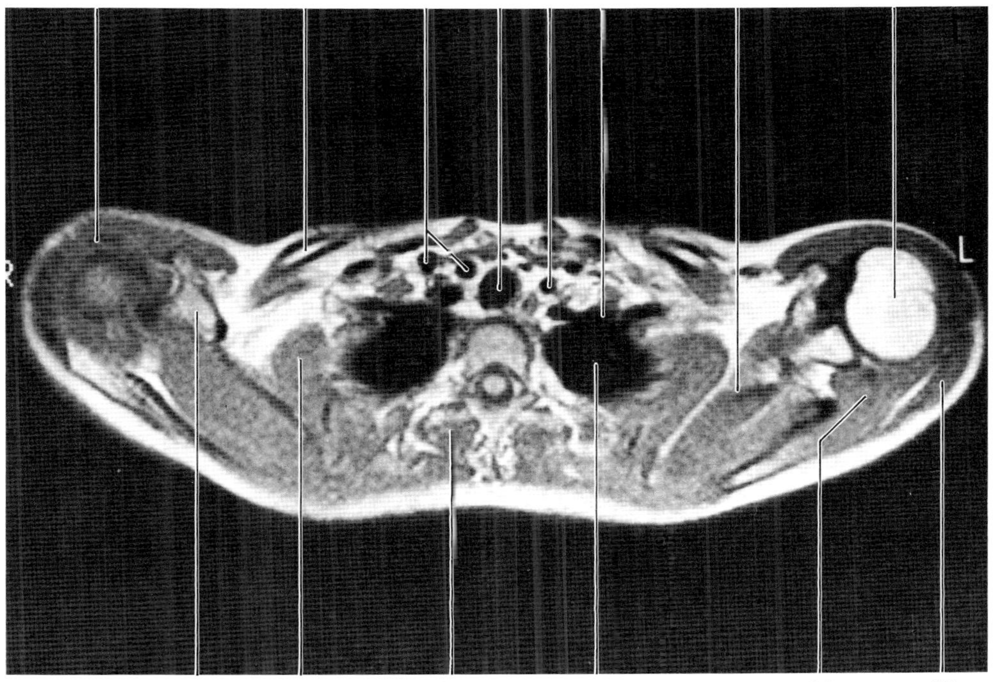

MRI, SE 700/30

4 Common carotid artery
7 Clavicle
8 Left brachiocephalic vein
9 Subclavian artery
12 Pectoralis minor muscle
13 Pectoralis major muscle
15 Coracobrachialis muscle
18 Head of the humerus
19 Deltoid muscle
20 Infraspinatus muscle
22 Neck of the scapula
24 Supraspinatus muscle
25 Serratus anterior muscle
26 Apex of the lung
35 Splenius cervicis and splenius capitis muscles
37 Trapezius muscle (vertebral part)
38 Serratus anterior (lateral) muscle
38.1 Spine of scapula
47 Right brachiocephalic and internal jugular veins
51 Esophagus
53 Trachea

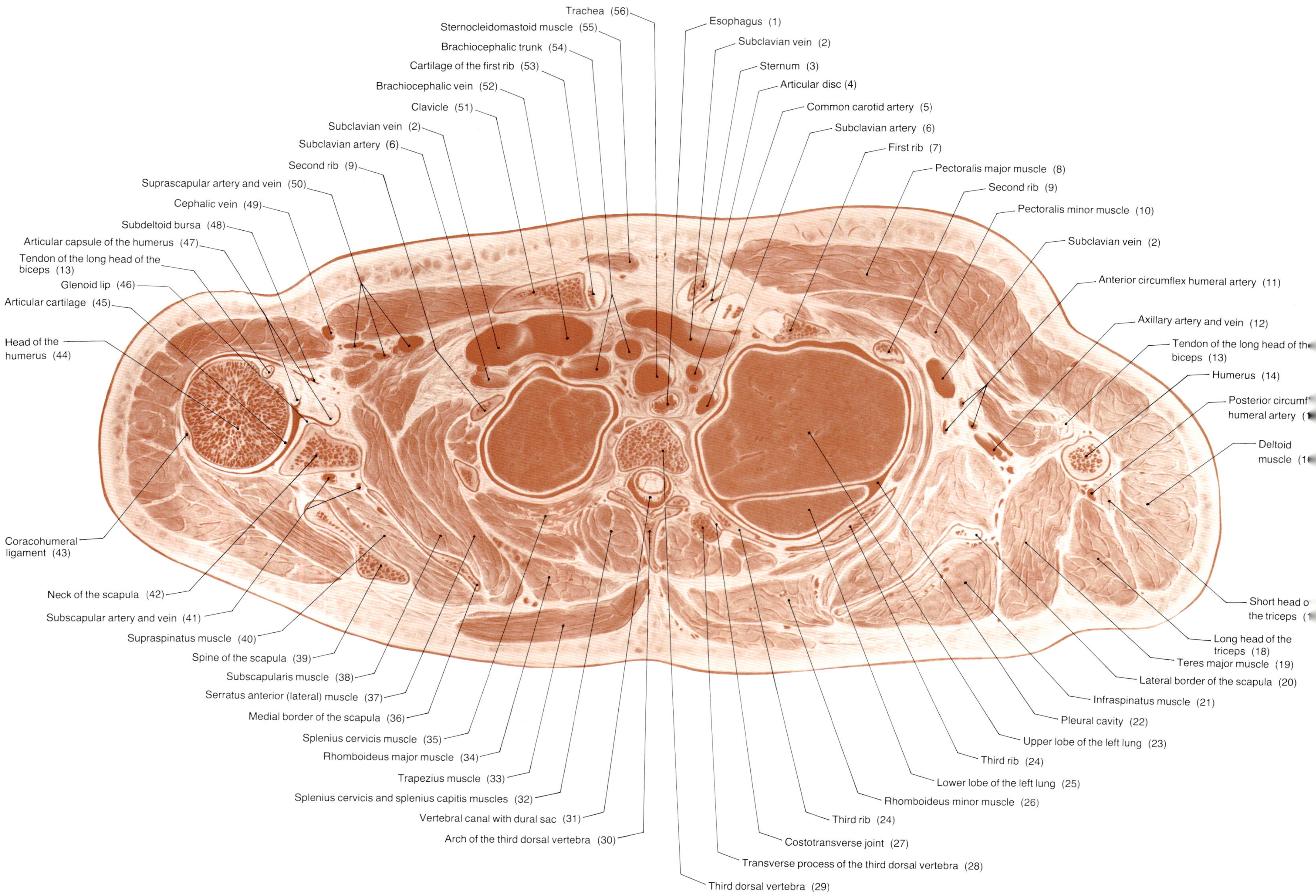

1 Oesophagus
2 V. subclavia
3 Sternum
4 Discus articularis
5 A. carotis communis
6 A. subclavia
7 Costa I
8 M. pectoralis major
9 Costa II
10 M. pectoralis minor
11 A. circumflexa humeri anterior
12 A. et V. axillaris
13 Tendo capitis longi m. bicipitis brachii
14 Humerus
15 A. circumflexa humeri posterior
16 M. deltoideus
17 Caput breve m. tricipitis brachii
18 Caput longum m. tricipitis brachii
19 M. teres major
20 Margo lateralis scapulae
21 M. infraspinatus
22 Cavitas pleuralis
23 Lobus superior pulmonis sinistri
24 Costa III
25 Lobus inferior pulmonis sinistri
26 M. rhomboideus minor
27 Articulatio costatransversaria
28 Processus transversus (Vert. thor. III)
29 Vertebra thoracica III
30 Arcus vertebrae thoracicae III
31 Canalis vertebralis et spatium subdurale
32 M. splenius cervicis et M. splenius capitis
33 M. trapezius
34 M. rhomboideus major
35 M. splenius cervicis
36 Margo medialis scapulae
37 M. serratus anterior (lateralis)
38 M. subscapularis
39 Spina scapulae
40 M. supraspinatus
41 A. et V. subscapularis
42 Collum scapulae
43 Lig. coracohumerale
44 Caput humeri
45 Cartilago articularis
46 Labrum glenoidale
47 Capsula articularis humeri
48 Bursa subdeltoidea
49 V. cephalica
50 A. et V. suprascapularis
51 Clavicula
52 V. brachiocephalica
53 Cartilago costae I
54 Truncus brachiocephalicus
55 M. sternocleidomastoideus
56 Trachea

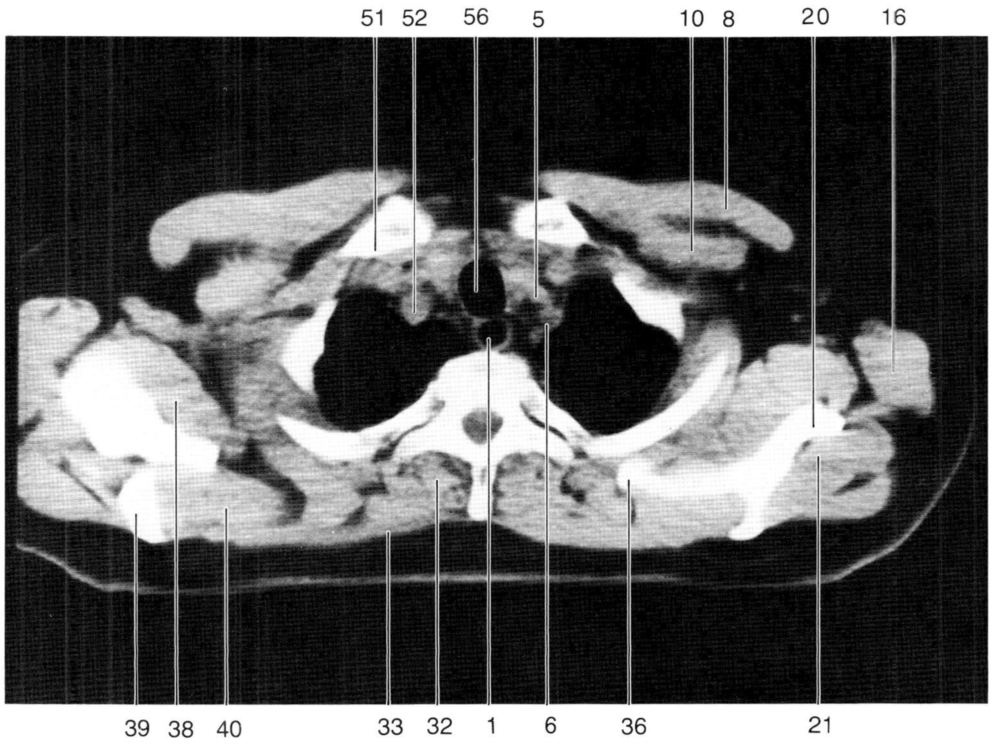

CT scan

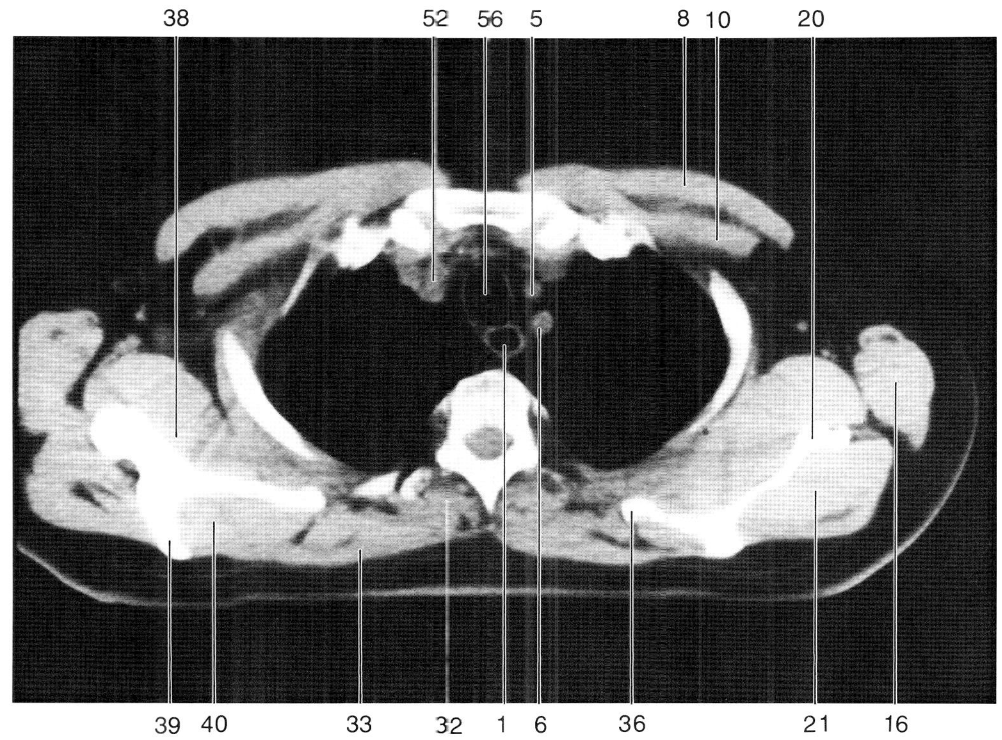

CT scan

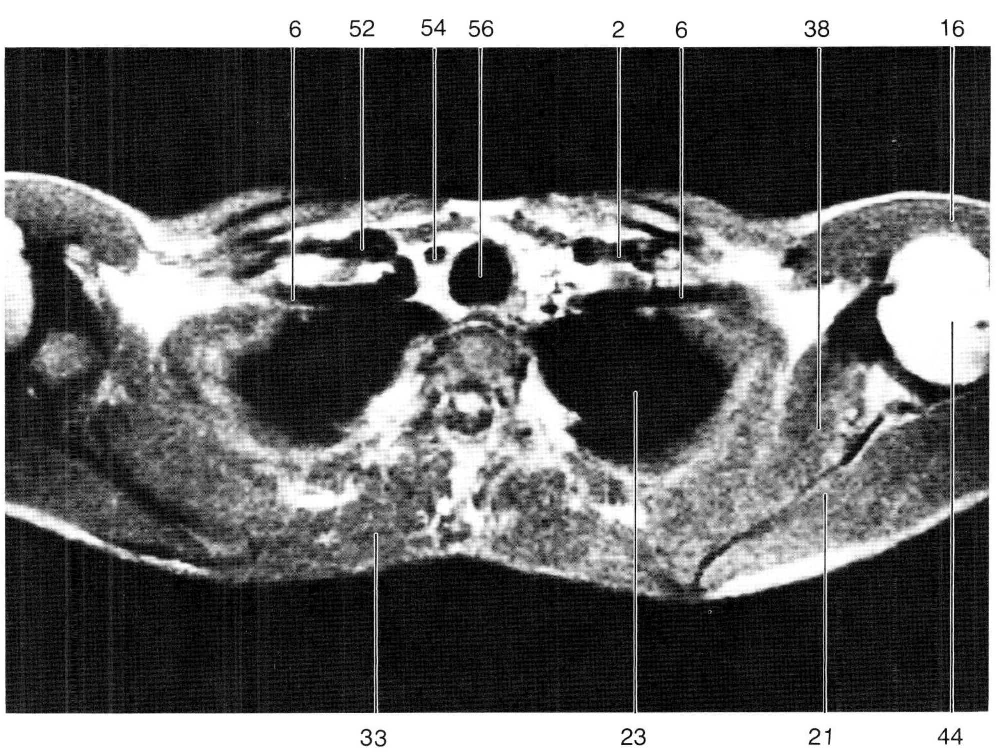

MRI, SE 600/30

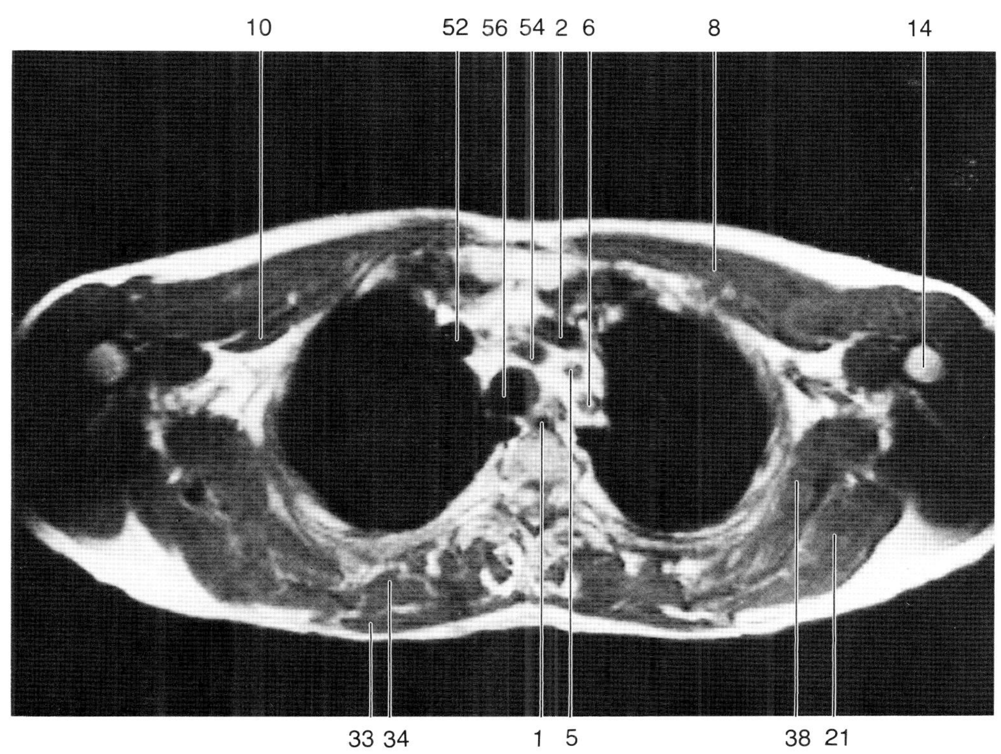

MRI, SE 600/30

1 Esophagus
2 Subclavian vein
5 Common carotid artery
6 Subclavian artery
8 Pectoralis major muscle
10 Pectoralis minor muscle
14 Humerus
16 Deltoid muscle
20 Lateral border of the scapula
21 Infraspinatus muscle
23 Upper lobe of the left lung
32 Splenius cervicis and splenius capitis muscles
33 Trapezius muscle
34 Rhomboideus major muscle
36 Medial border of the scapula
38 Subscapularis muscle
39 Spina of the scapula
40 Supraspinatus muscle
44 Head of the humerus
51 Clavicle
52 Brachiocephalic vein
54 Brachiocephalic trunk
56 Trachea

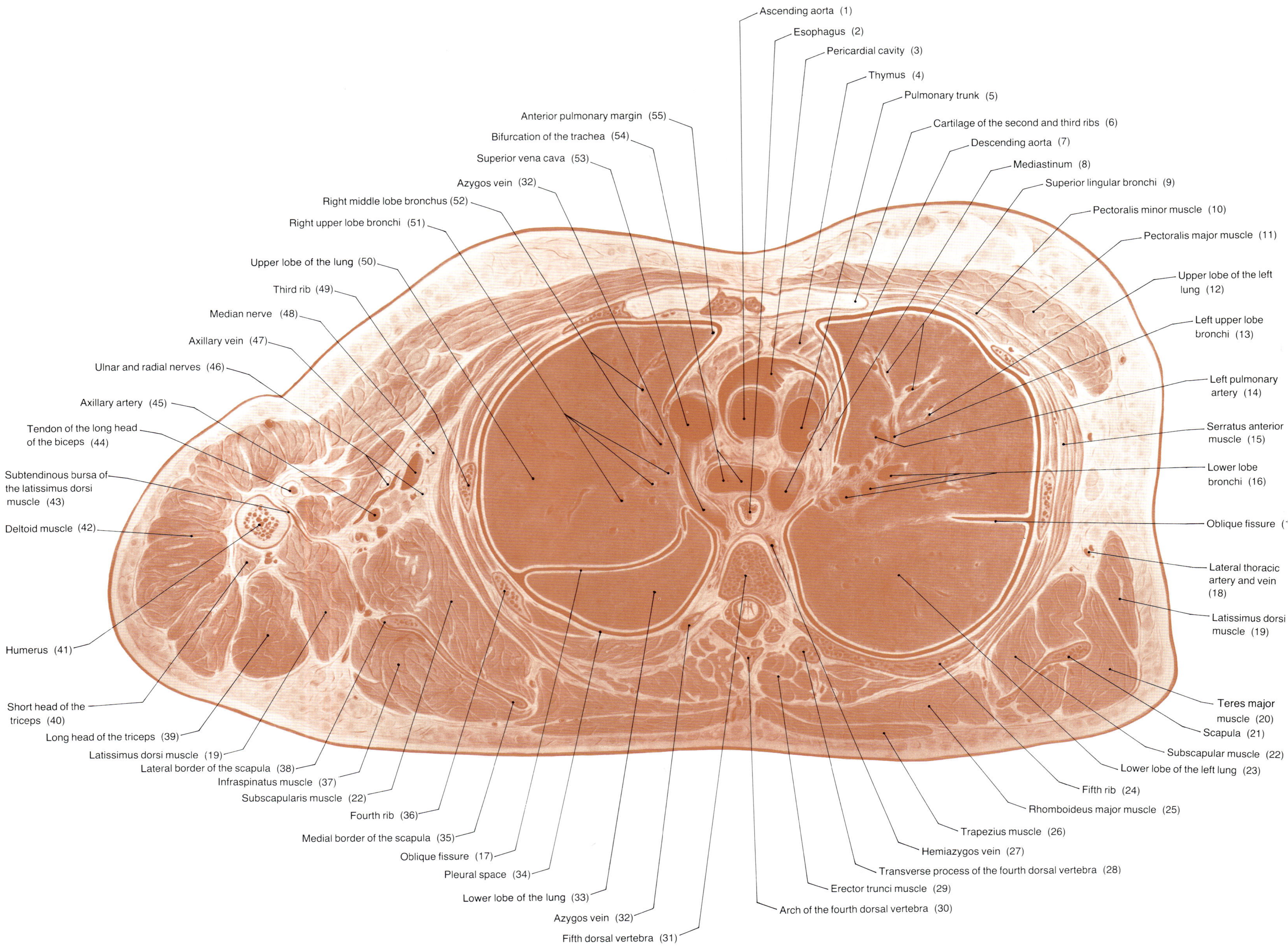

1 Aorta ascendens
1.1 Arcus aortae
2 Oesophagus
3 Cavum pericardii
4 Thymus
5 Truncus pulmonalis
6 Cartilago costae III et II
7 Aorta descendens
8 Mediastinum
9 Bronchi lingulares superiores
10 M. pectoralis minor
11 M. pectoralis major
12 Lobus superior pulmonis sinistri
13 Bronchi lobares superiores sinistri
14 A. pulmonalis sinistra
15 M. serratus anterior
16 Bronchi lobares inferiores
17 Fissura obliqua
18 A. et V. thoracica lateralis
19 M. latissimus dorsi
20 M. teres major
21 Scapula
22 M. subscapularis
23 Lobus inferior pulmonis sinistri
24 Costa V
25 M. rhomboideus major
26 M. trapezius
27 V. hemiazygos
28 Processus transversus (Vert. thor. IV)
29 M. erector trunci
30 Arcus vertebrae thoracicae IV
31 Vertebra thoracica V
32 V. azygos
33 Lobus inferior pulmonis
34 Spatium pleurae
35 Margo medialis scapulae
36 Costa IV
37 M. infraspinatus
38 Margo lateralis scapulae
39 Caput longum m. tricipitis brachii
40 Caput breve m. tricipitis brachii
41 Humerus
42 M. deltoideus
43 Bursa subtendinea m. latissimi dorsi
44 Tendo capitis longi m. bicipitis brachii
45 A. axillaris
46 N. ulnaris et radialis
47 V. axillaris
48 N. medianus
49 Costa III
50 Lobus superior pulmonis
51 Bronchi lobares superiores dextri
52 Bronchus lobaris medius dexter
53 V. cava superior
54 Bifurcatio trachea
54.1 Trachea
55 Margo pulmonalis anterior

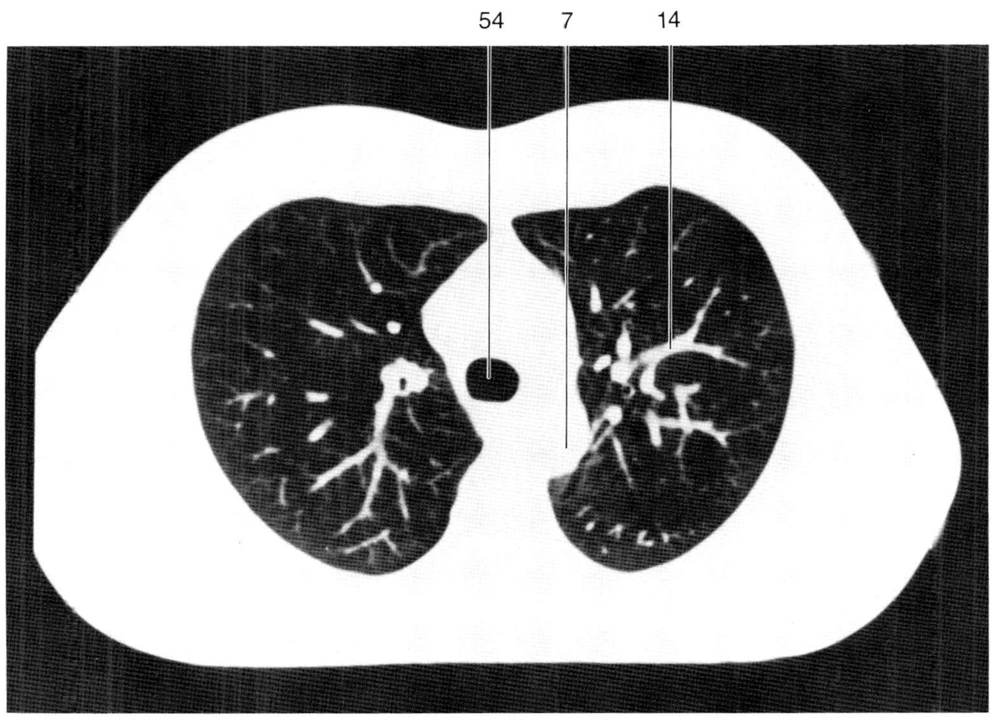

CT scan

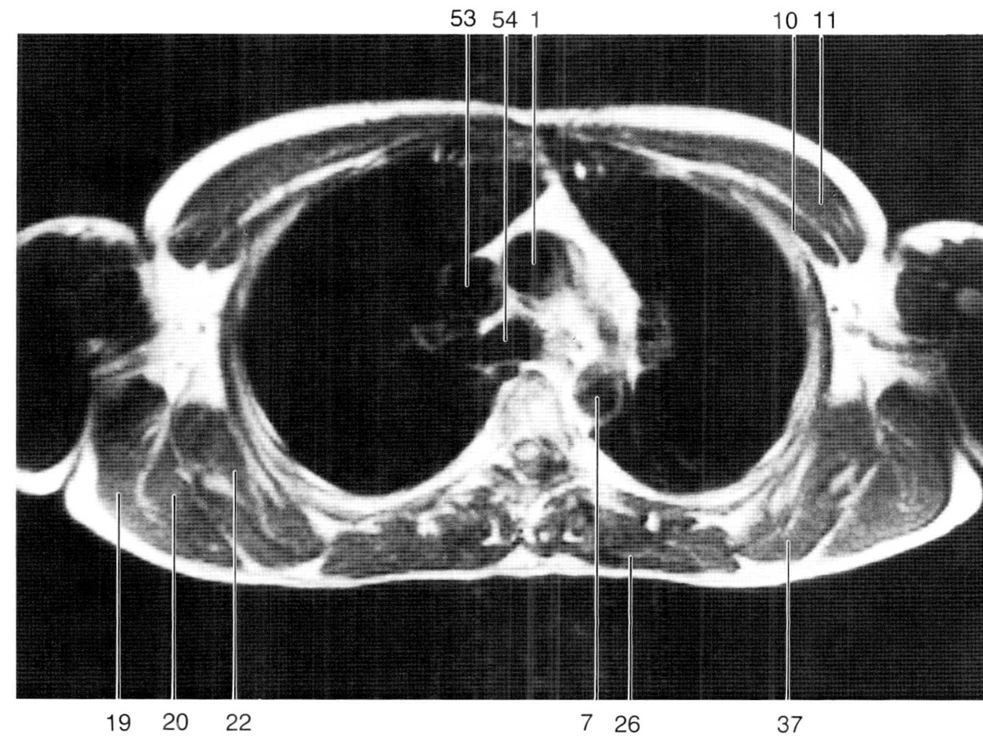

CT scan

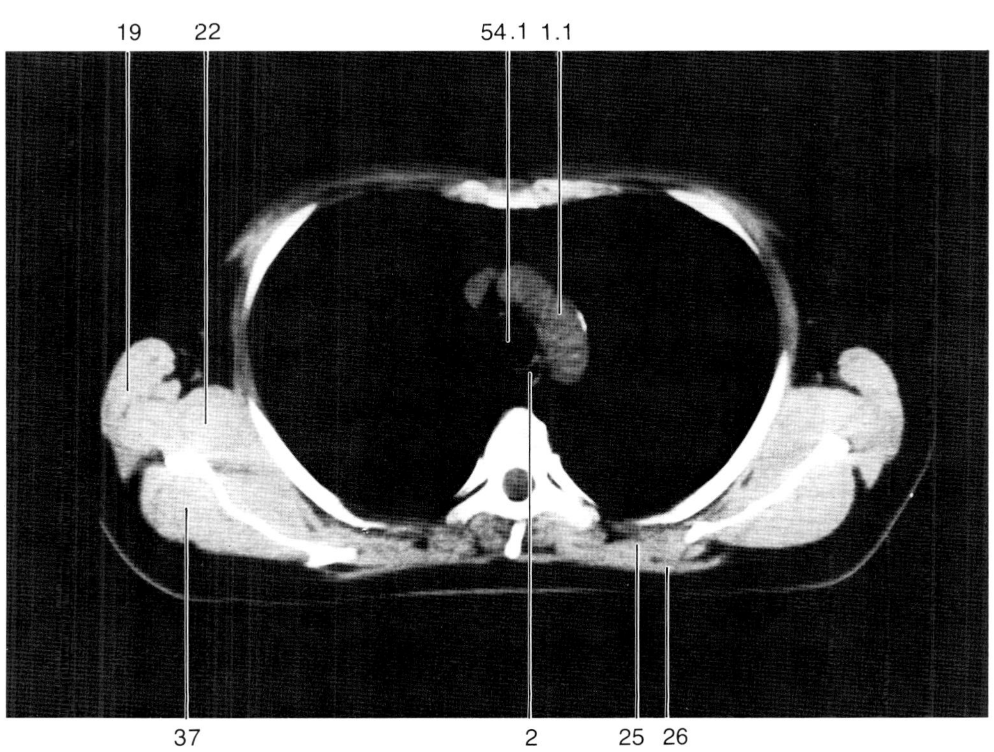

CT scan

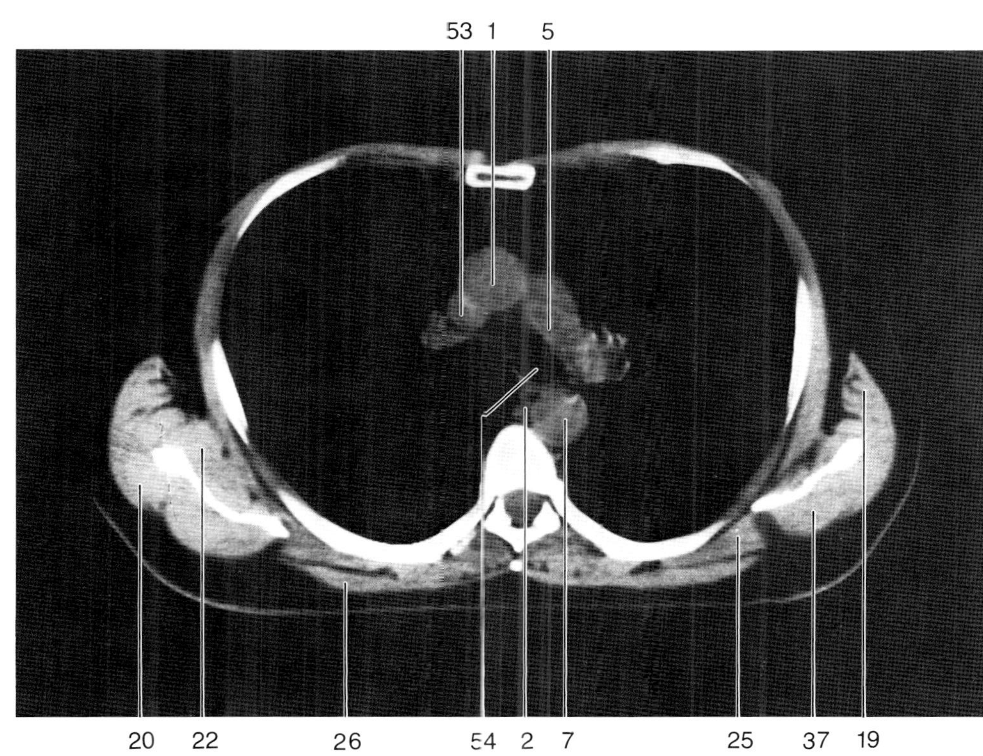

MRI, SE 600/30

1 Ascending aorta
1.1 Aortic arch
2 Esophagus
5 Pulmonary trunk
7 Descending aorta
10 Pectoralis minor muscle
11 Pectoralis major muscle
14 Left pulmonary artery
19 Latissimus dorsi muscle
20 Teres major muscle
22 Subscapularis muscle
25 Rhomboideus major muscle
26 Trapezius muscle
37 Infraspinatus muscle
53 Superior vena cava
54 Bifurcation of the trachea
54.1 Trachea

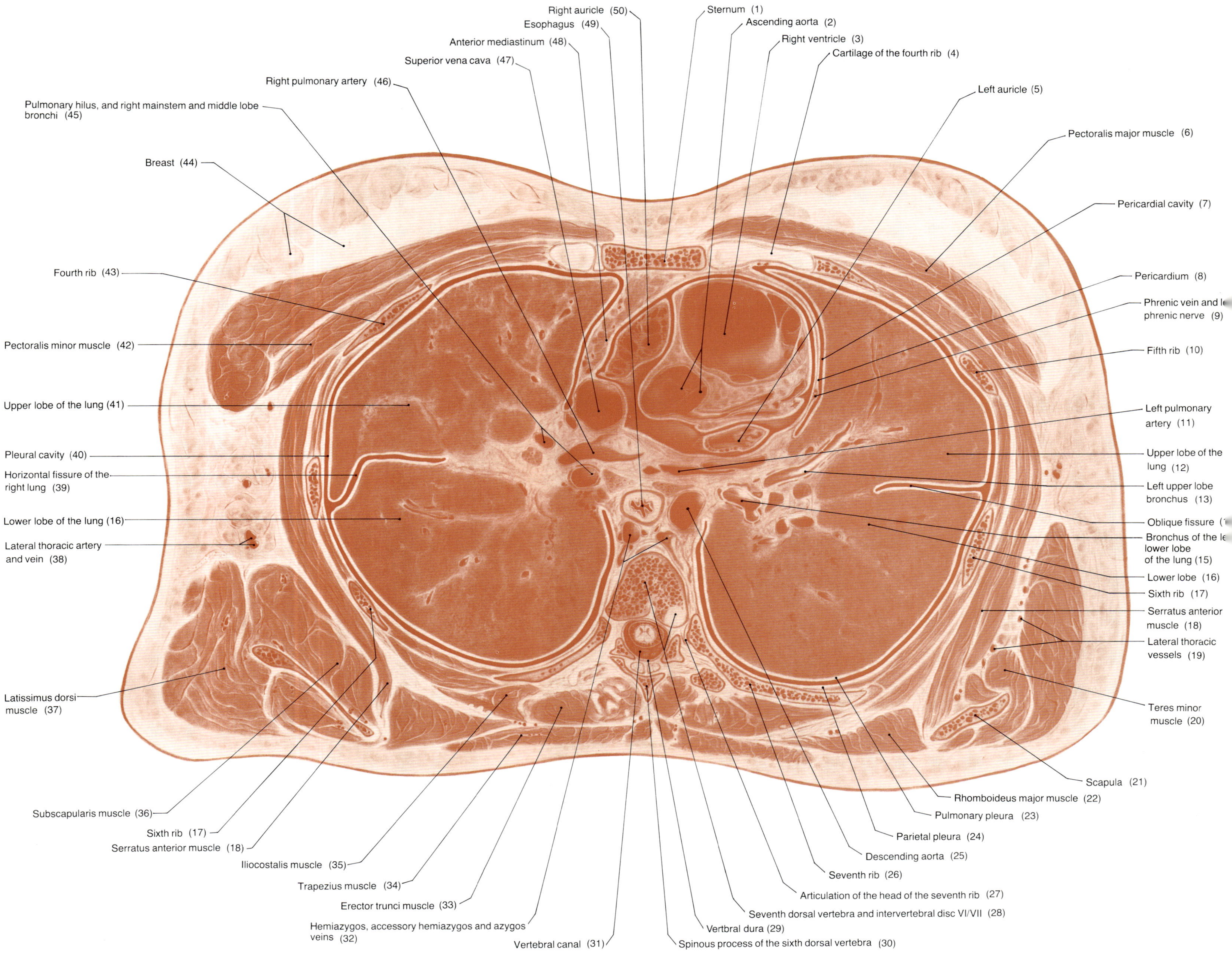

1 Sternum
2 Aorta ascendens
2.1 Atrium sinistrum
3 Ventriculus dexter
3.1 Ventriculus sinister
4 Cartilago costa IV
5 Auricula sinistra
6 M. pectoralis major
7 Cavum pericardii
8 Pericardium
9 V. phrenica et N. phrenicus sinister
10 Costa V
11 A. pulmonalis sinistra
12 Lobus superior pulmonis sinistri
13 Bronchus lobaris superior sinister
14 Fissura obliqua
15 Bronchus lobaris inferior sinister
16 Lobus inferior pulmoniis
17 Costa VI
18 M. serratus anterior
19 Vasa thoraco-lateralia
20 M. teres minor
21 Scapula
22 M. rhomboideus major
23 Pleura pulmonalis
24 Pleura parietalis
25 Aorta descendens
26 Costa VII
27 Articulatio capitis costae VII
28 Vertebra thoracica VII et Discus intervertebralis VI/VII
29 Dura mater spinalis
30 Processus spinosus (Vert. thor. VI)
31 Canalis vertebralis
32 V. hemiazygos/V. hemiazygos accessoria
33 M. erector trunci
34 M. trapezius
35 M. iliocostalis
36 M. subscapularis
37 M. latissimus dorsi
38 A. et V. thoracica lateralis
39 Fissura obliqua (pulm. dext.)
40 Cavum pleurae
41 Lobus superior pulmonis
42 M. pectoralis minor
43 Costa IV
44 Corpus mammae
45 Hilus pulmonis et Bronchus principalis dexter et Bronchus lobarius medius dexter
46 A. pulmonalis dextra
47 V. cava superior
47.1 Atrium dextrum
48 Mediastinum anterius
49 Oesophagus
50 Auricula dextra

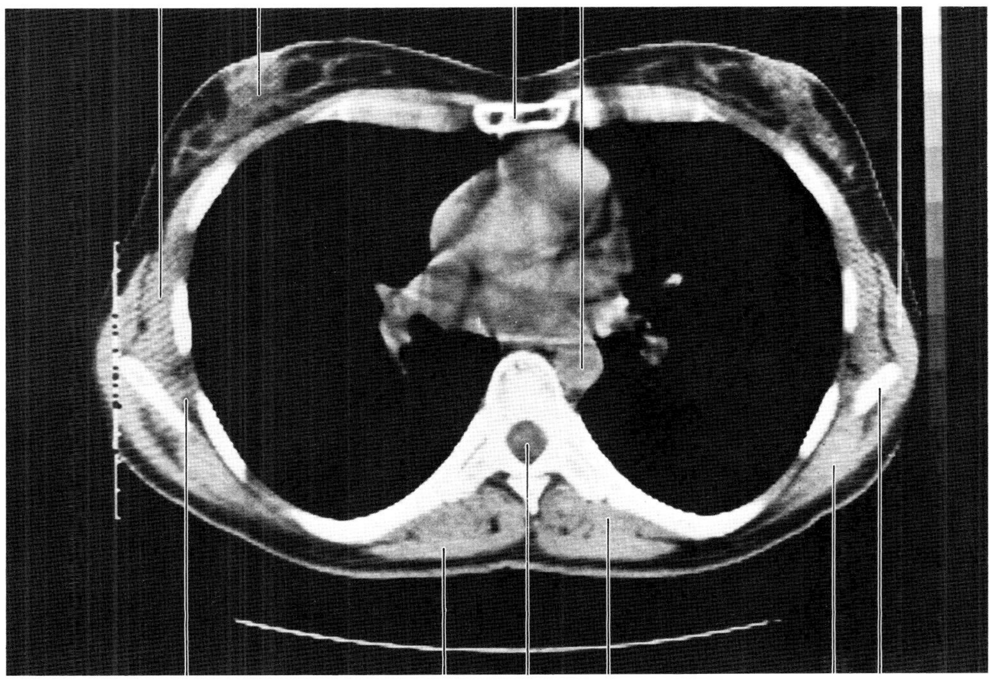

CT scan

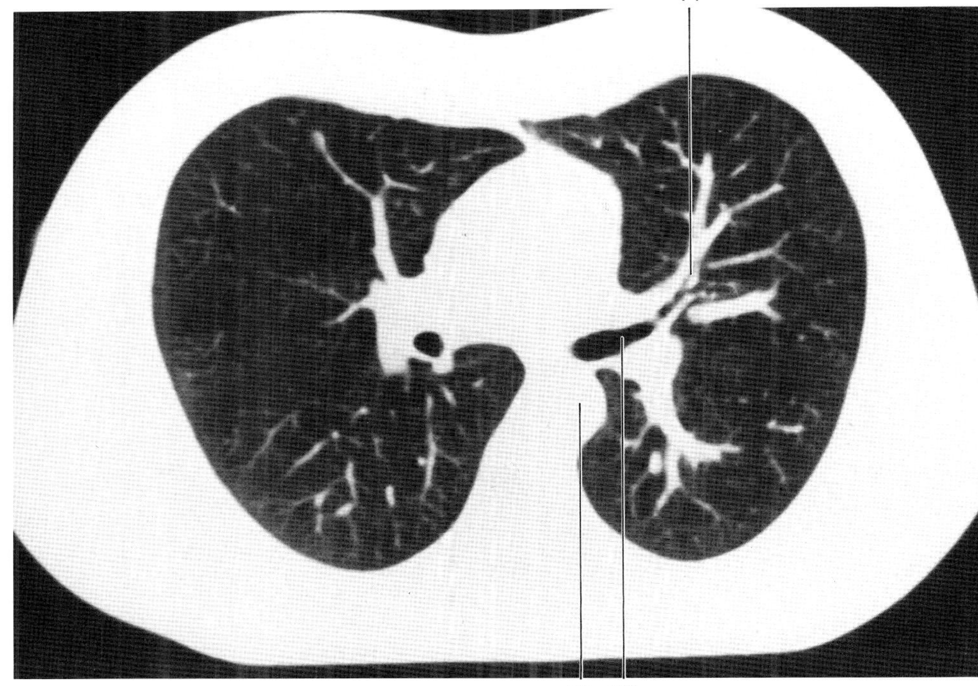

CT scan

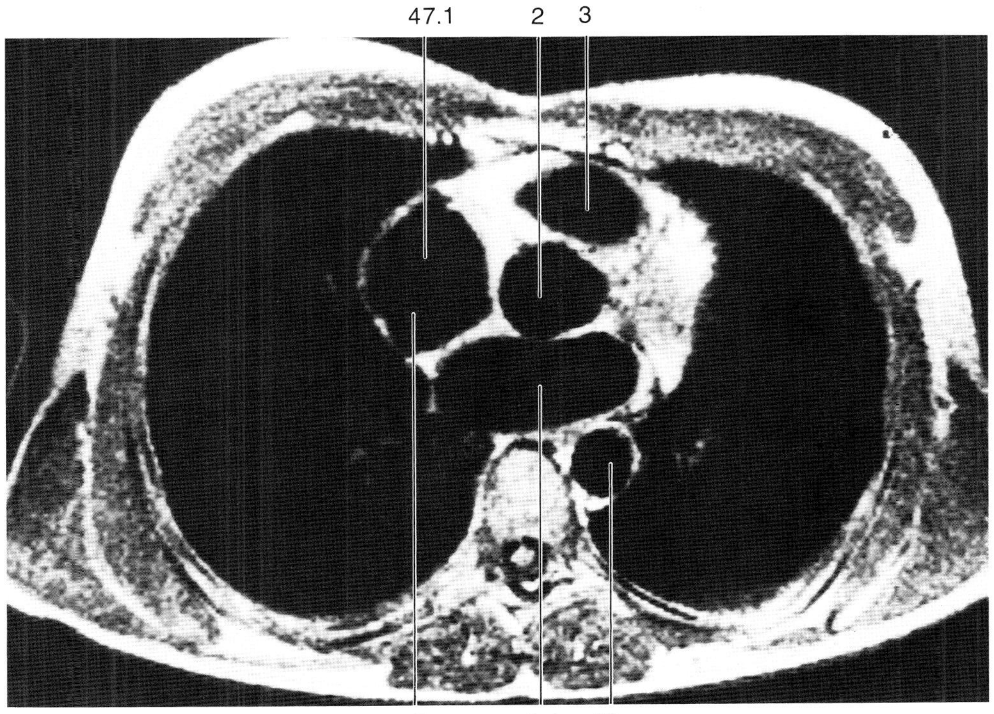

MRI, ECG-triggered, $T_E = 50$

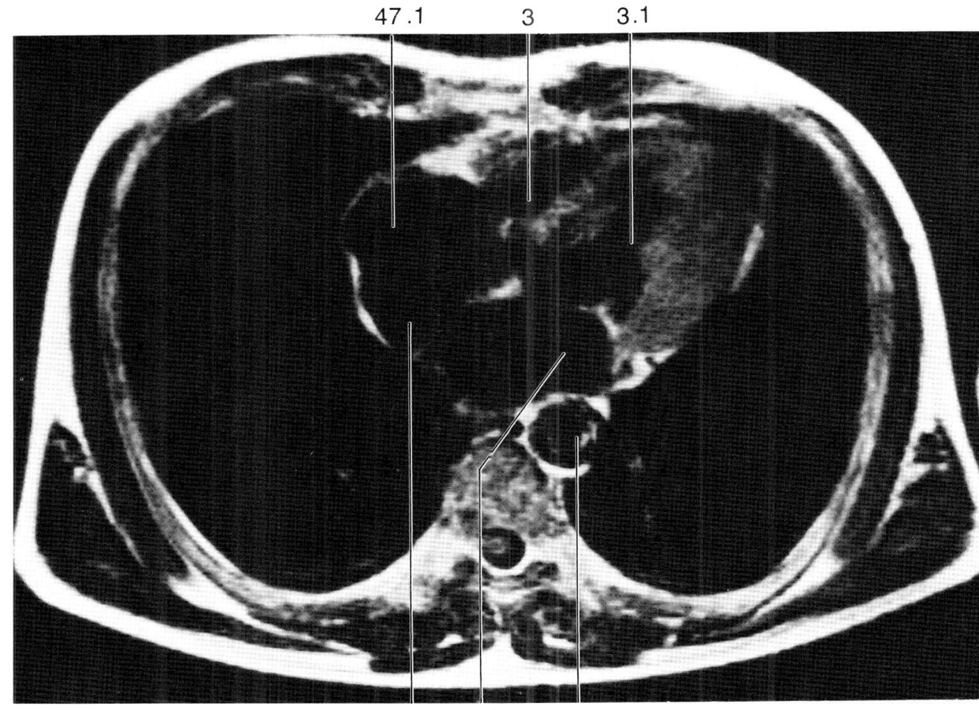

MRI, ECG-triggered, $T_E = 50$

1 Sternum
2 Ascending aorta
2.1 Left atrium
3 Right ventricle
3.1 Left ventricle
11 Left pulmonary artery
13 Left upper lobe bronchus
18 Serratus anterior muscle
21 Scapula
22 Rhomboideus major muscle
25 Descending aorta
31 Vertebral canal
33 Erector trunci muscle
34 Trapezius muscle
36 Subscapularis muscle
37 Latissimus dorsi muscle
44 Breast
47 Superior vena cava
47.1 Right atrium

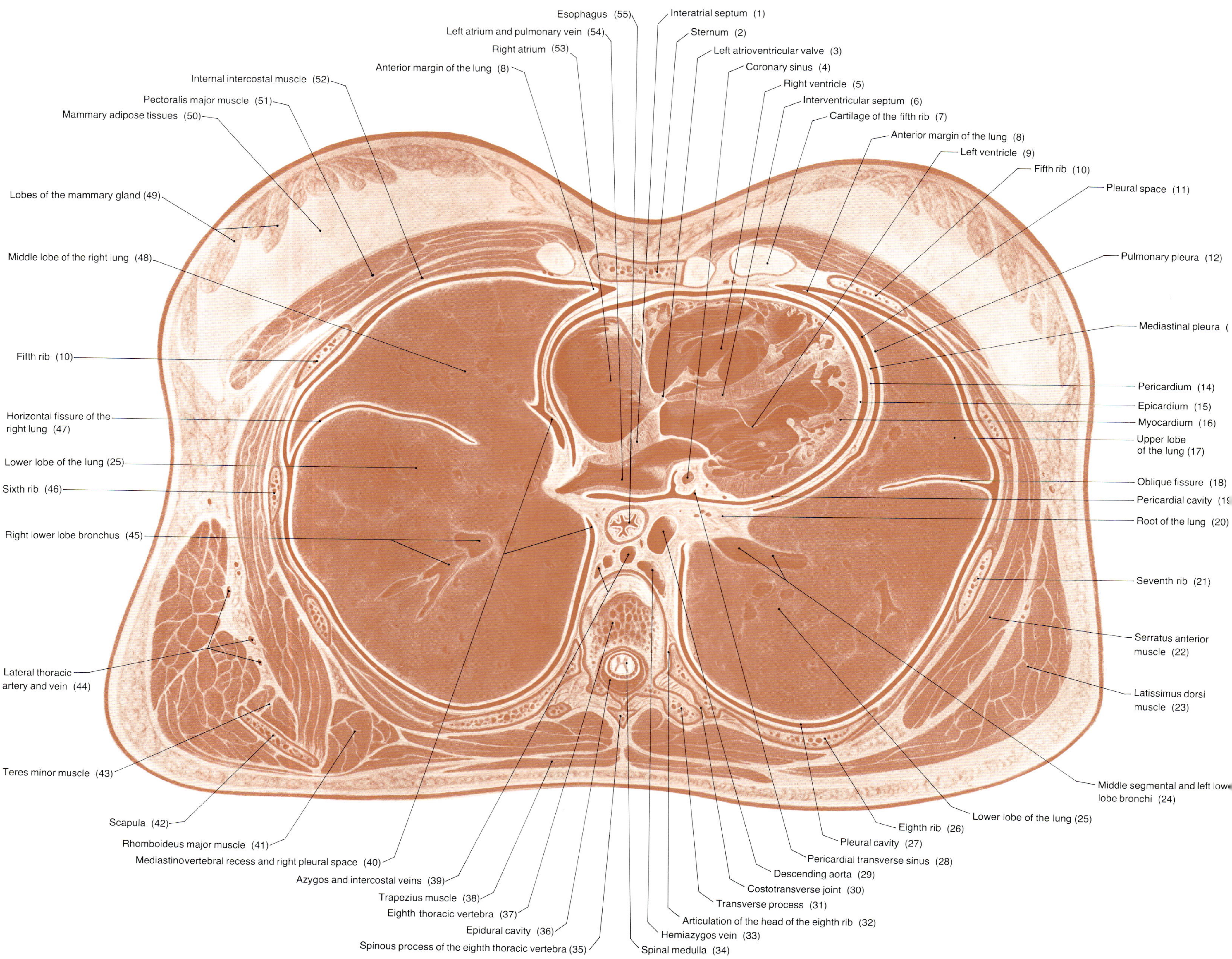

1 Septum interatriale
2 Sternum
3 Valva atrioventricularis sinistra
4 Sinus coronarius
5 Ventriculus dexter
6 Septum interventriculare
7 Cartilago costa V
8 Margo anterior (pulm.)
9 Ventriculus sinister
10 Costa V
11 Spatium pleurae
12 Pleura pulmonalis
13 Pleura mediastinalis
14 Pericardium
15 Epicardium
16 Myocardium
17 Lobus superior pulmonis
18 Fissura obliqua
19 Cavitas pericardialis
20 Radix pulmonis
21 Costa VII
22 M. serratus anterior
23 M. latissimus dorsi
24 Bronchus segmentalis medialis et Bronchus lobaris inferior sinister
25 Lobus inferior pulmonis
26 Costa VIII
27 Cavitas pleuralis
28 Sinus transversus pericardii
29 Aorta descendens
30 Articulatio costotransversaria
31 Processus transversus
32 Articulatio capitis costae VIII
33 V. hemiazygos
34 Medulla spinalis
35 Processus spinosus (Vert. thor. VIII)
36 Cavitas epiduralis
37 Vertebra thoracica VIII
38 M. trapezius
39 V. azygos et V. intercostalis
40 Recessus mediastinovertebralis et Spatium pleurae dextrae
41 M. rhomboideus major
42 Scapula
43 M. teres minor
44 A. et V. thoracica lateralis
45 Bronchus lobaris inferior dexter
46 Costa VI
47 Fissura horizontalis (Pulm. dext.)
48 Costa V
49 Lobi glandulae mammariae
50 Corpus adiposum mammae
51 M. pectoralis major
52 M. intercostalis internus
53 Atrium dextrum
54 Atrium sinistrum et V. pulmonalis
55 Oesophagus

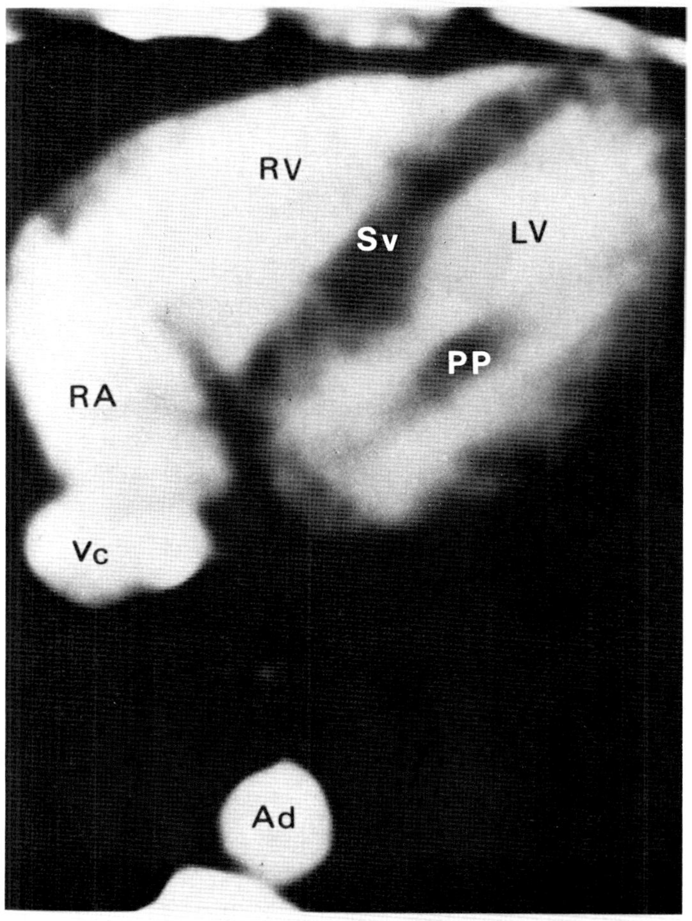

1

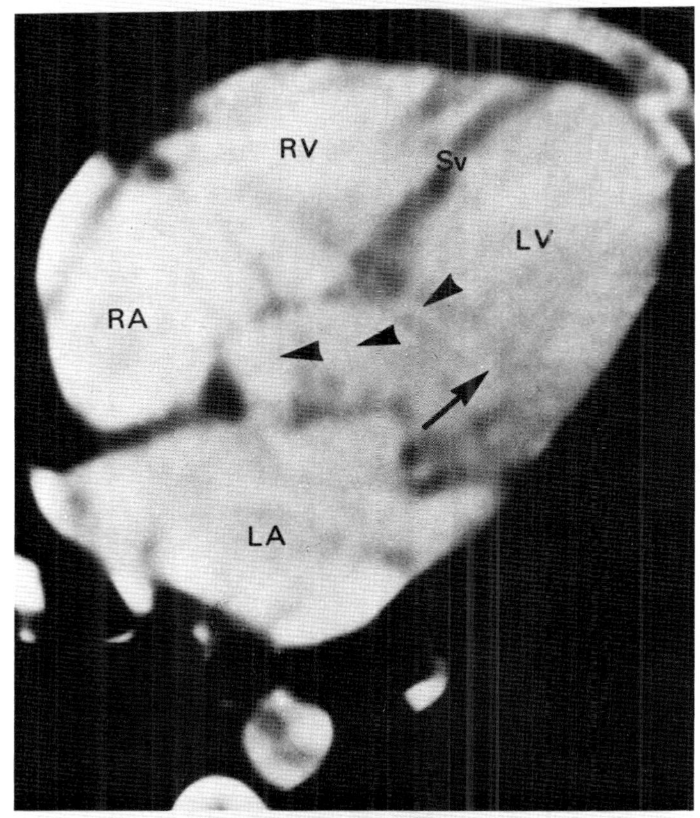

2

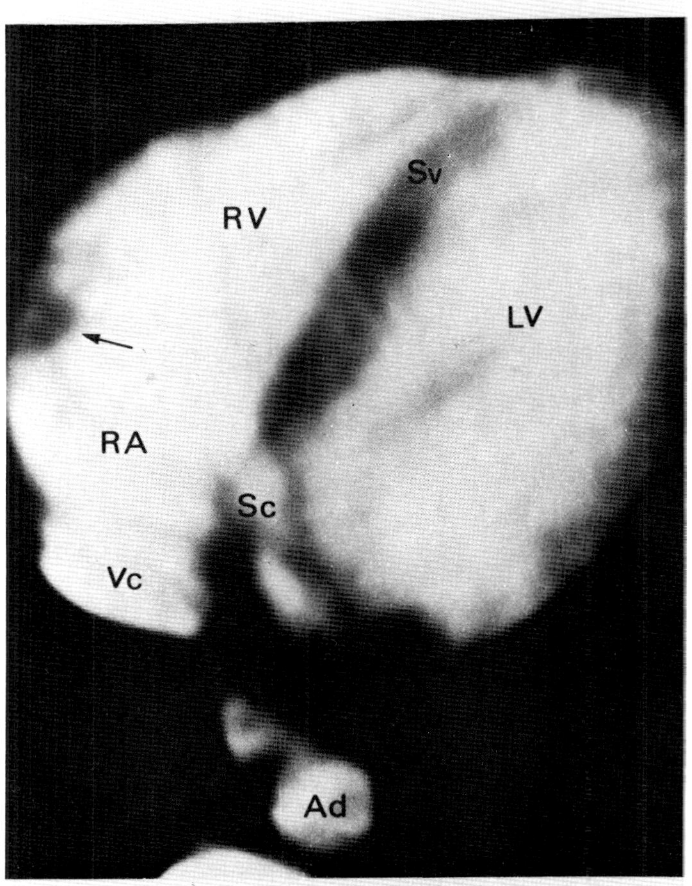

3

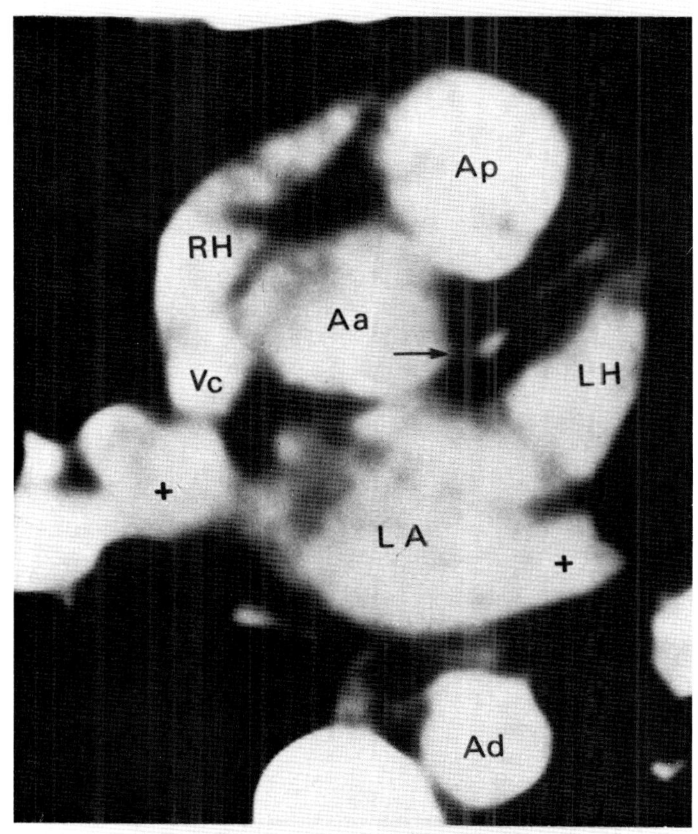

4

1–4: CT, enhanced after bolus injection of contrast medium.
(Reproduced with permission from Lackner, K.: Kardiocomputertomographie. In: Schinz, H. R.: Radiologische Diagnostik in Klinik und Praxis, II. Herz – Große Gefäße. Thieme, Stuttgart 1983.)

RV = Right ventricle,
LV = Left ventricle,
Sv = Interventricular septum,
pp = Papillary muscles,
RA = Right atrium,
Vc = Inferior vena cava,
Ad = Descending aorta,
LA = Left atrium,
Sc = Coronary sinus,
Ap = Pulmonary trunk,
Aa = Ascending aorta,
LH = Left auricle,
RH = Right auricle.
Only in Fig. 4:
Vc = Superior vena cava

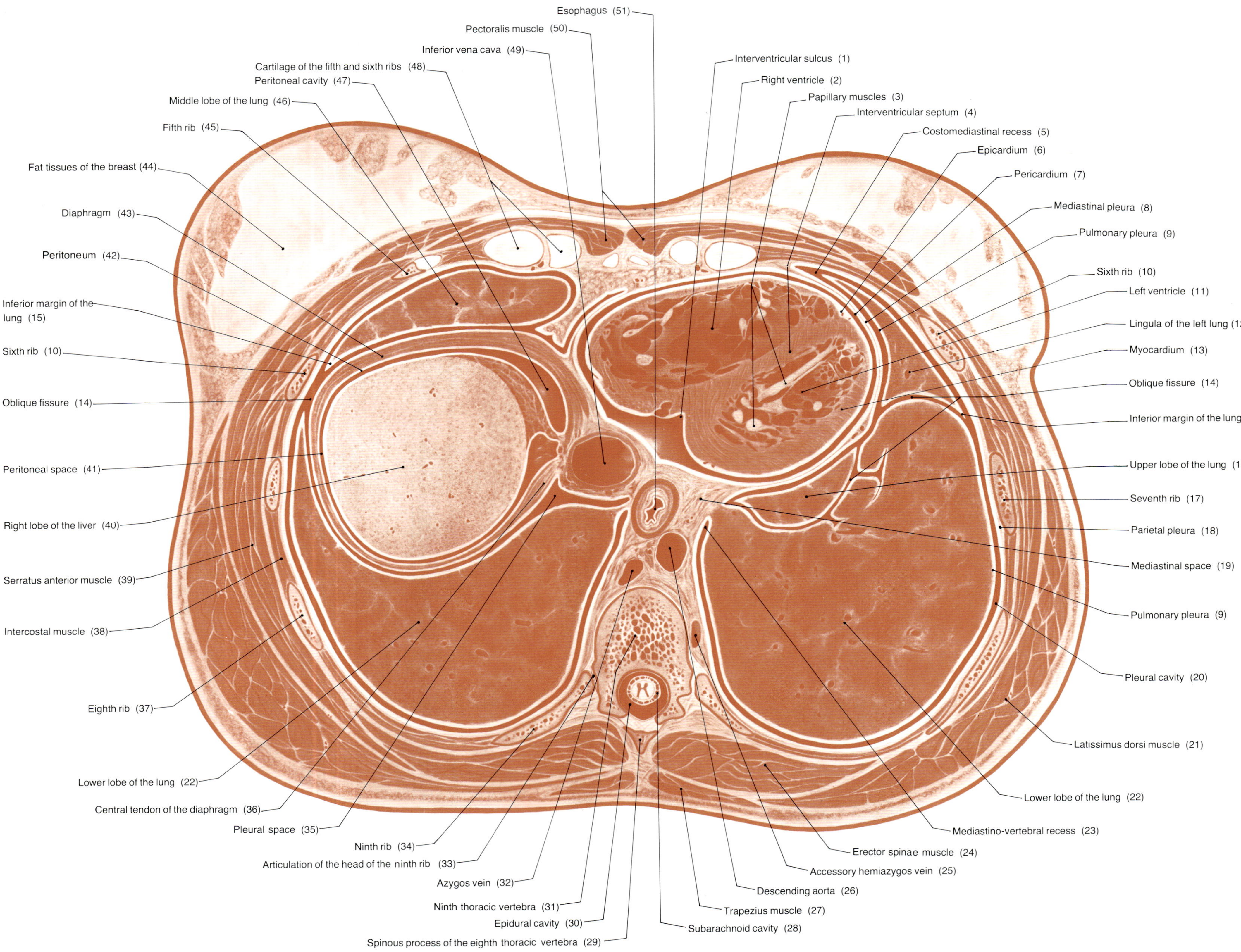

1 Sulcus interventricularis
2 Ventriculus dexter
3 Mm. papillares
4 Septum interventriculare
5 Recessus costomediastinalis
6 Epicardium
7 Pericardium
8 Pleura mediastinalis
9 Pleura pulmonalis
10 Costa VI
11 Ventriculus sinister
12 Lingula pulmonis sinistri
13 Myocardium
14 Fissura obliqua
15 Margo inferior pulmonis
16 Lobus superior pulmonis
17 Costa VII
18 Pleura parietalis
19 Spatium mediastini
20 Cavitas pleuralis
21 M. latissimus dorsi
22 Lobus inferior pulmonis
23 Recessus mediastinovertebralis
24 M. erector spinae
25 V. hemiazygos accessoria
26 Aorta descendens
26.1 Caput costae
27 M. trapezius
28 Cavitas subarachnoidealis
29 Processus spinosus (Vert. thor. VIII)
29.1 Lamina arcus vertebrae
29.2 Corpus vertebrae
30 Cavitas epiduralis
31 Vertebra thoracica IX
32 V. azygos
33 Articulatio capitis costae IX
34 Costa IX
35 Spatium pleurae
36 Diaphragma (Centrum tendineum)
37 Costa VIII
38 M. intercostalis
39 M. serratus anterior
40 Lobus dexter hepatis
41 Spatium peritonaei
42 Peritoneum
43 Diaphragma
44 Corpus adiposum mammae
45 Costa V
46 Lobus medius pulmonis
47 Cavitas peritonealis
48 Cartilago costa V et VI
49 V. cava inferior
50 M. pectoralis
50.1 Atrium dextrum
51 Oesophagus
51.1 Ventriculus

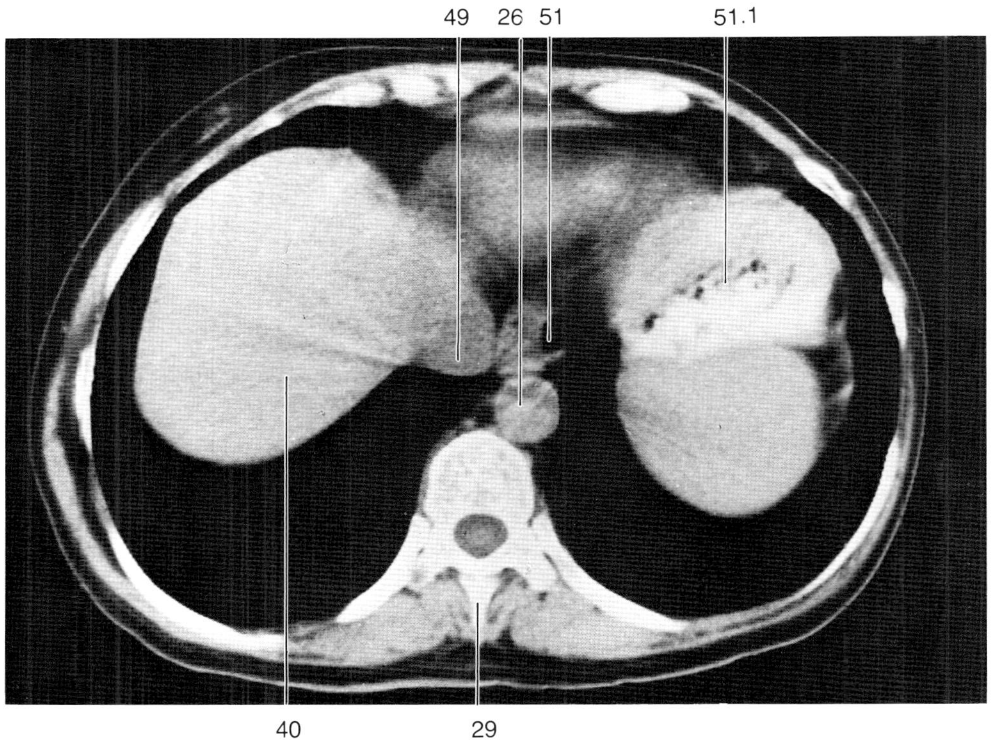

CT with contrast medium in the stomach

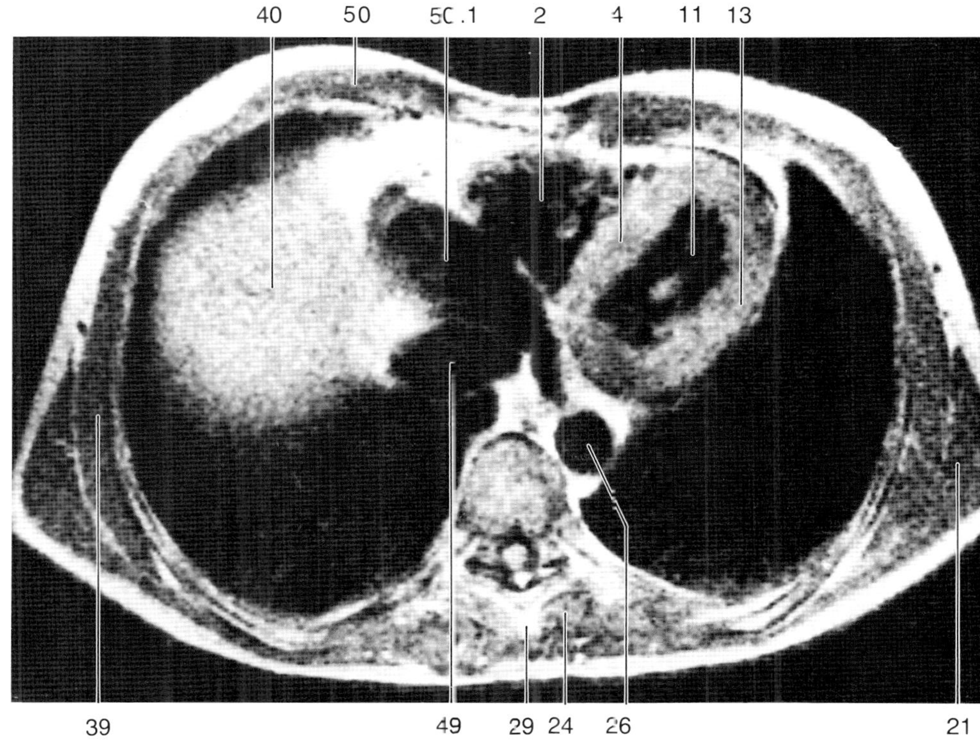

MRI, ECG-triggered, $T_E = 30$ ms

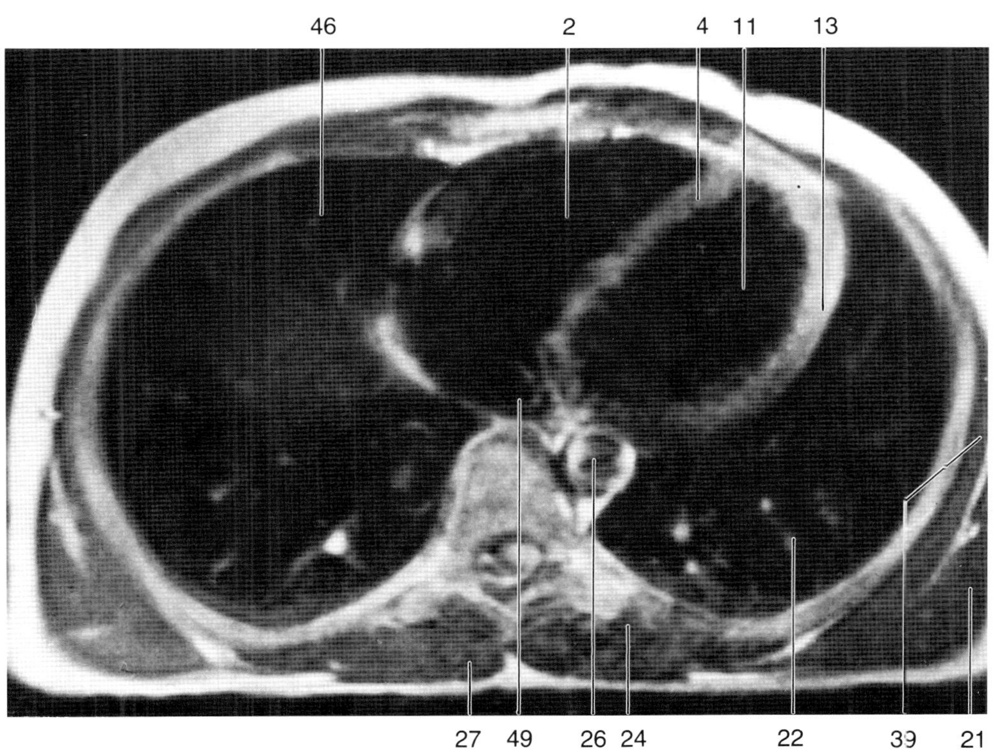

MRI, ECG-triggered, $T_E = 50$ ms

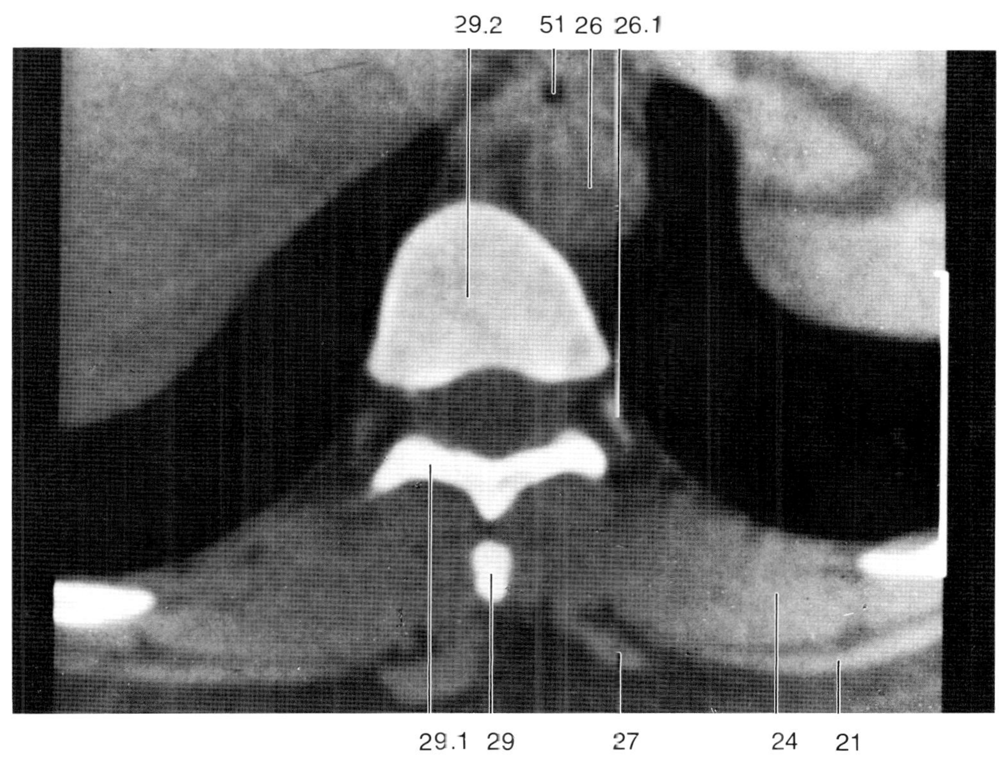

CT scan unenhanced

2 Right ventricle
4 Interventricular septum
11 Left ventricle
13 Myocardium
21 Latissimus dorsi muscle
22 Lower lobe of the lung
24 Erector muscle of spine
26 Descending aorta
26.1 Head of the rib
27 Trapezius muscle
29 Spinous process of the eighth dorsal vertebra
29.1 Vertebral arch
29.2 Vertebral body
39 Serratus anterior muscle
40 Right lobe of the liver
46 Middle lobe of the lung
49 Inferior vena cava
50 Pectoralis muscle
50.1 Right atrium
51 Esophagus
51.1 Stomach

Axial Sections of the Abdomen

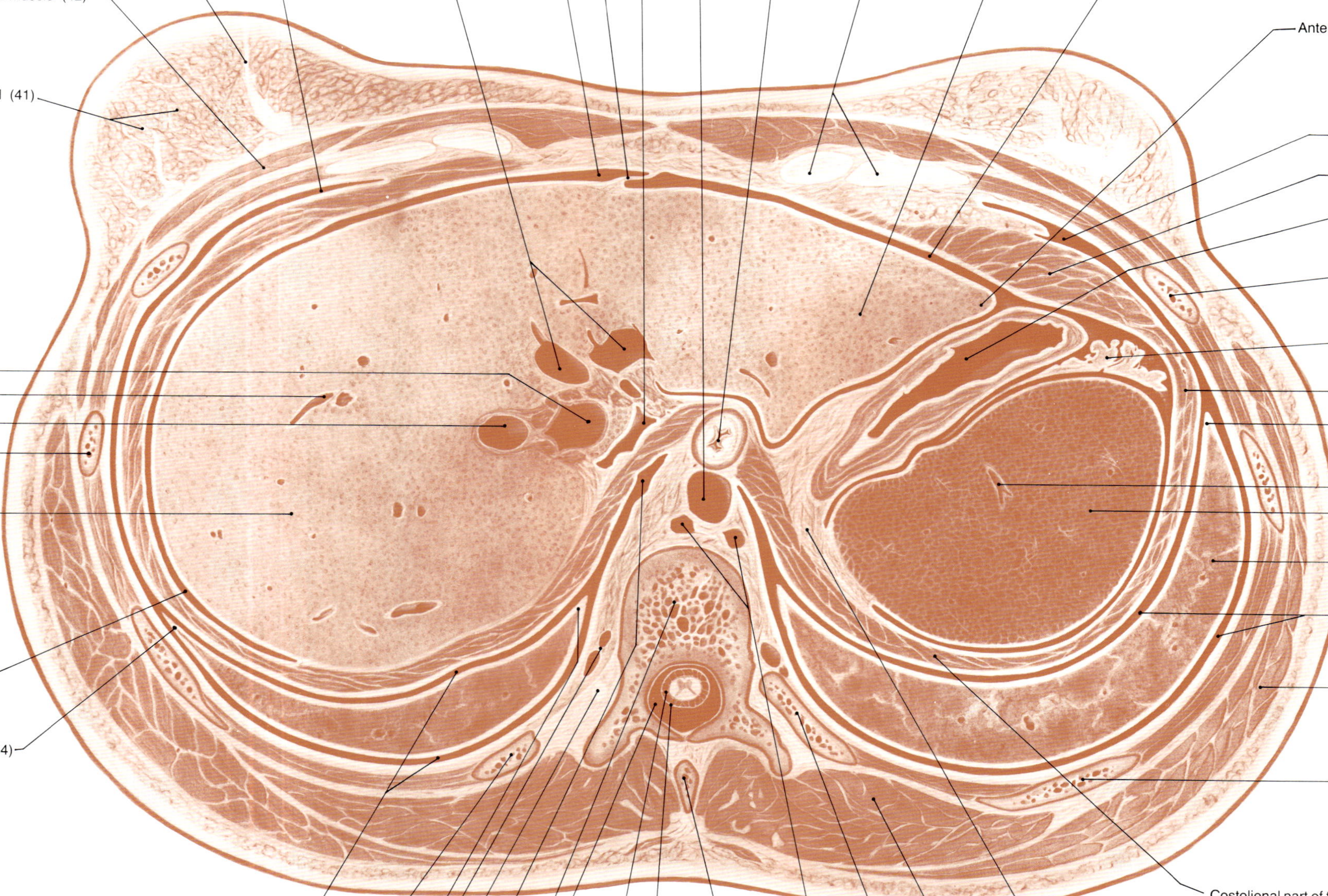

1 Oesophagus
2 Cartilago costae VI et VII
3 Lobus sinister hepatis
4 Cavum peritoneale
5 Margo anterior hepatis
6 Recessus costodiaphragmaticus
7 Pars costalis diaphragmatis
8 Fundus ventriculi
9 Costa VII
10 Omentum lienale
11 Diaphragma
12 Margo inferior pulmonis
13 R. v. lienalis
14 Lien
15 Lobus inferior pulmonis
16 Spatium pleurae sinistrae
17 M. latissimus dorsi
18 Costa IX
19 Diaphragma (Pars costolienalis)
20 Spatium fibrosum lienalis
21 M. erector spinae
22 Costa X
23 V. azygos et V. hemiazygos
24 Processus spinosus (Vert. thor. IX)
25 Dura mater spinalis
26 Cavum subarachnoideale
27 Cavum epidurale
28 Vertebra thoracica X
29 Recessus pleurae phrenicovertebralis
30 Truncus sympathicus
31 A. et V. intercostalis X
32 Margo posterior pulmonis
33 Cavum pleurae
34 Margo anterior pulmonis
35 Spatium peritoneale
36 Lobus hepatis dexter
37 Costa VIII
38 V. hepatica
39 Ductus hepaticus dexter
40 V. cava inferior
41 Lobi glandulae mammariae
42 M. pectoralis major
43 Ligg. suspensoria mammae
44 Rr. v. portae
45 Lig. falciforme hepatis
46 Vestibulum bursae omentalis
47 Aorta descendens

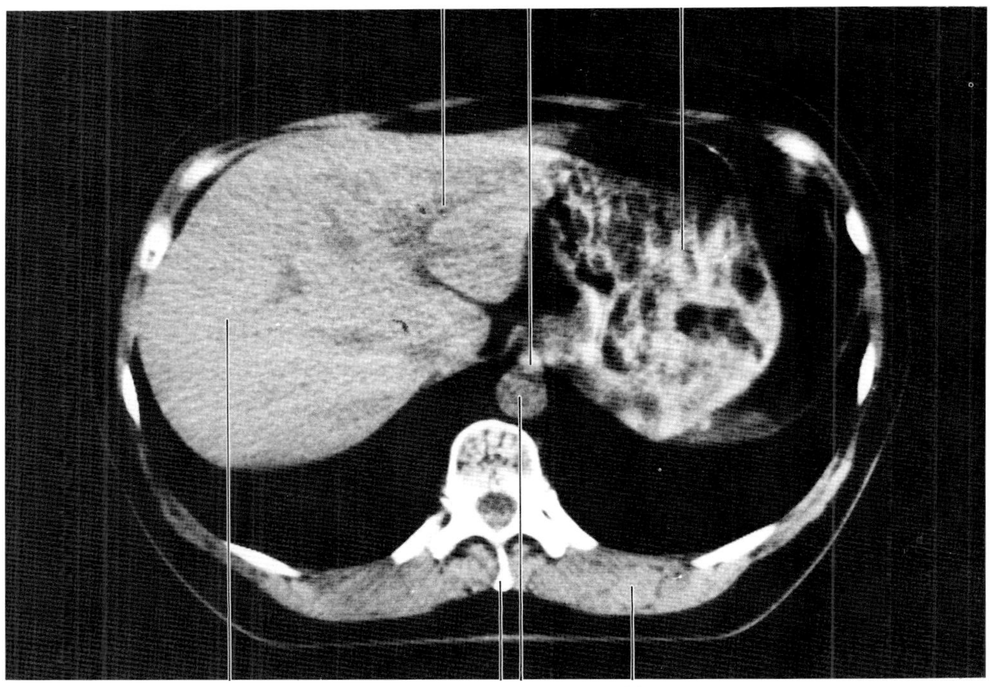

CT with contrast medium in the stomach

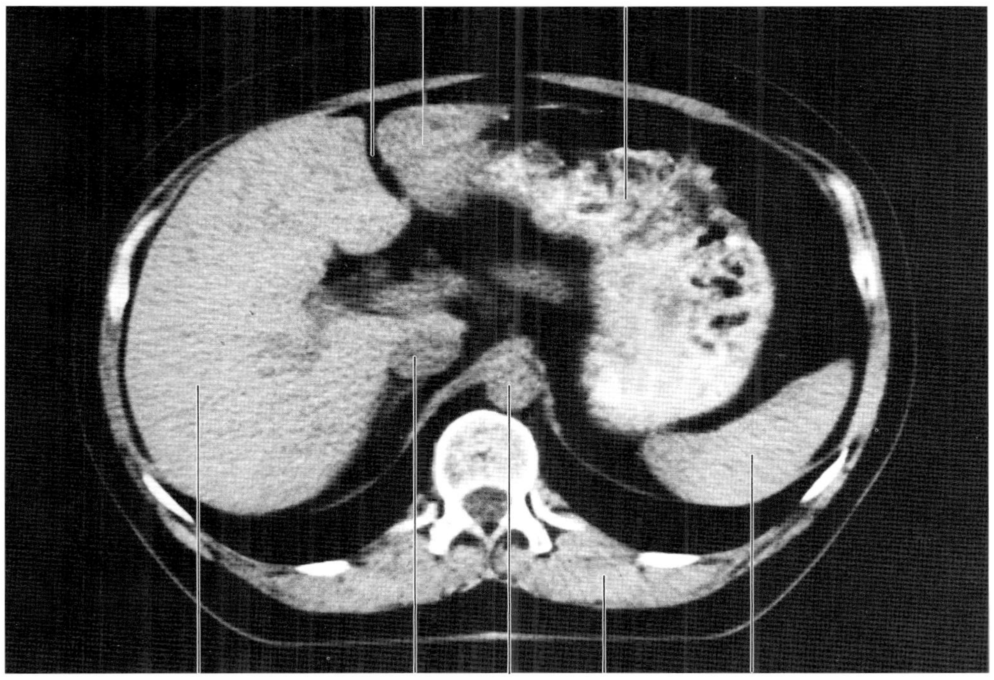

CT with contrast medium in the stomach

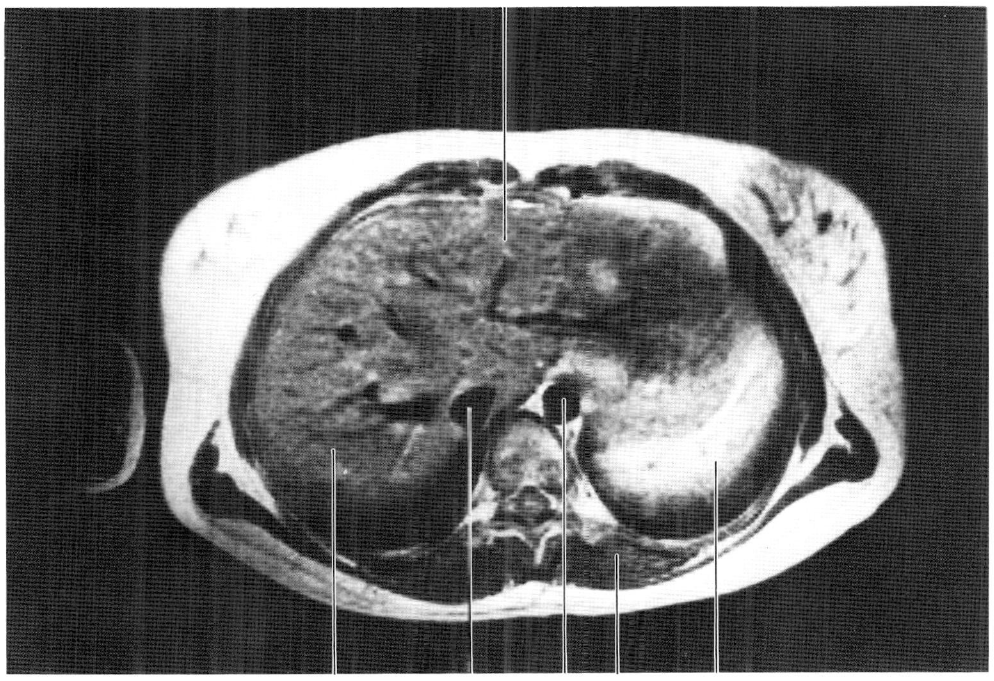

MRI, SE 600/30

1 Esophagus
3 Left lobe of the liver
8 Fundus of the stomach
14 Spleen
21 Erector spinae muscle
24 Spinous process (of the eighth dorsal vertebra)
36 Right hepatic lobe
40 Inferior vena cava
45 Falciform ligament of the liver
47 Descending aorta

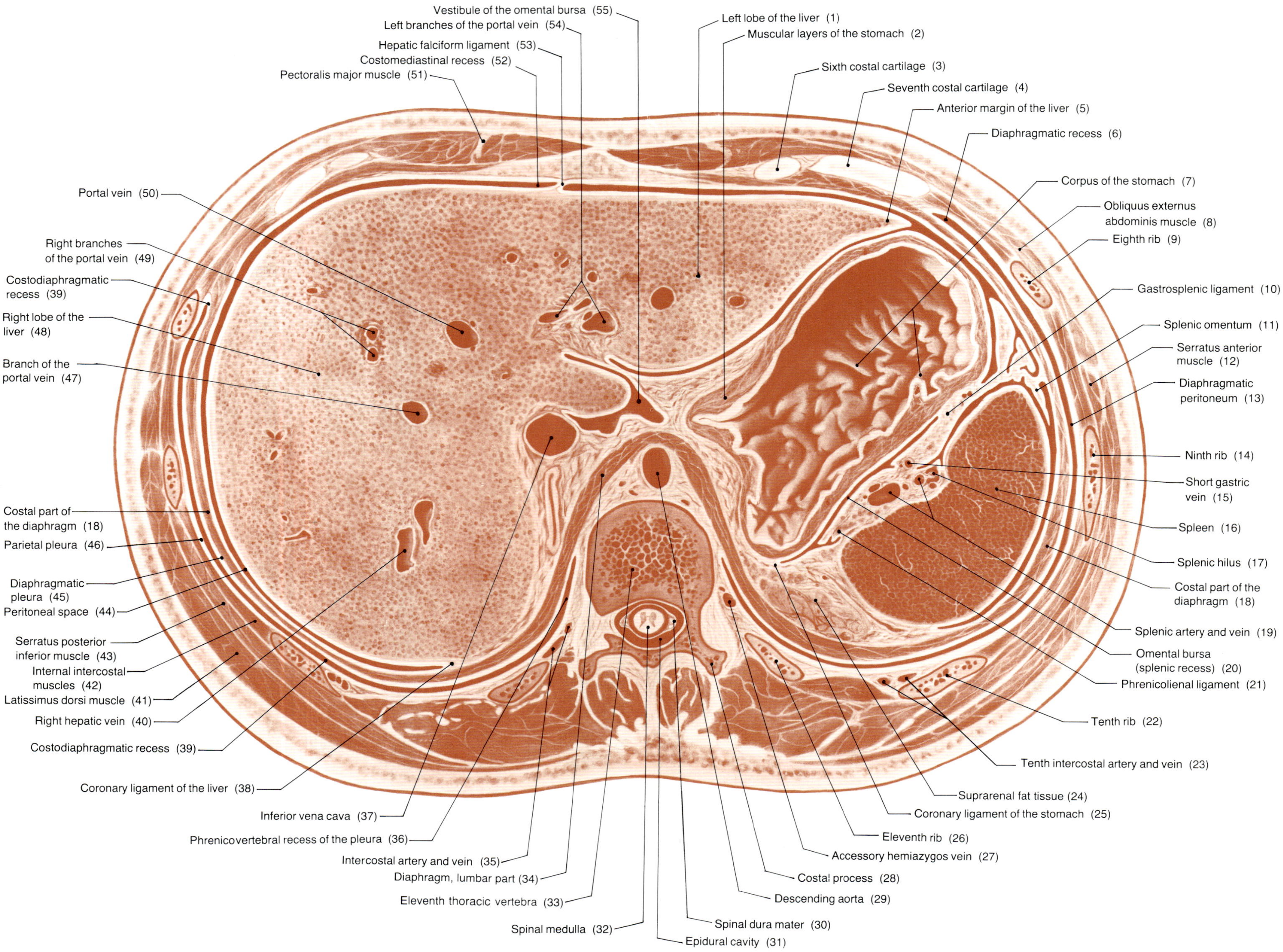

1 Lobus hepatis sinister
2 Tunica muscularis ventriculi
3 Cartilago costae VI
4 Cartilago costae VII
5 Margo anterior hepatis
6 Recessus diaphragmaticus
7 Corpus ventriculi
8 M. obliquus externus abdominis
9 Costa VIII
10 Lig. gastrolienale
11 Omentum lienale
12 M. serratus anterior
13 Peritonaeum diaphragmaticum
14 Costa IX
15 V. gastrica brevis
16 Lien
17 Hilus lienis
18 Pars costalis diaphragmatis
19 A. et V. lienalis
20 Bursa omentalis (Recessus lienalis)
21 Lig. phrenicolienale
22 Costa X
23 A. et V. intercostalis X
24 Capsula adiposa renalis
25 Lig. coronarium ventriculi
26 Costa XI
27 V. hemiazygos accessoria
28 Processus costarius
29 Aorta descendens
30 Dura mater spinalis
31 Cavum epidurale
32 Medulla spinalis
33 Vertebra thoracica XI
34 Diaphragma, pars lumbalis
35 A. et V. intercostalis
36 Recessus phrenicovertebralis pleurae
37 V. cava inferior
38 Lig. coronarium hepatis
39 Recessus costodiaphragmaticus
40 V. hepatica dextra
41 M. latissimus dorsi
42 M. intercostalis internus
43 M. serratus posterior inferior
44 Spatium peritoneale
45 Pleura diaphragmatica
46 Pleura parietalis
47 R. v. portae
48 Lobus hepatis dexter
49 Rr. dextri v. portae
50 V. portae
51 M. pectoralis major
52 Recessus costomediastinalis
53 Lig. falciforme hepatis
54 Rr. sinistri v. portae
55 Vestibulum bursae omentalis

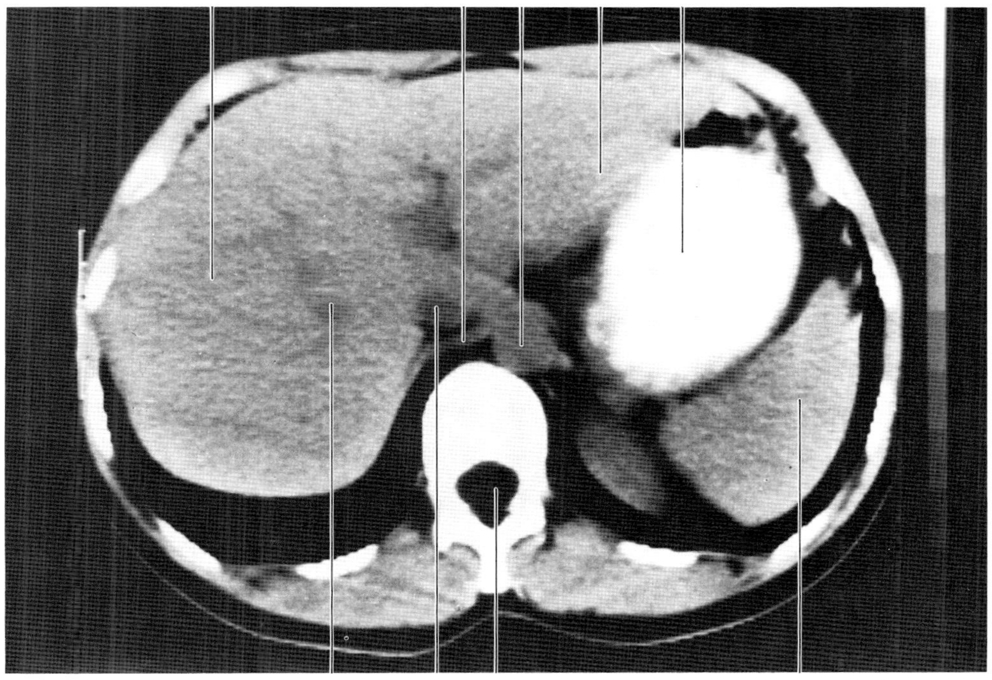

CT with contrast medium in the stomach

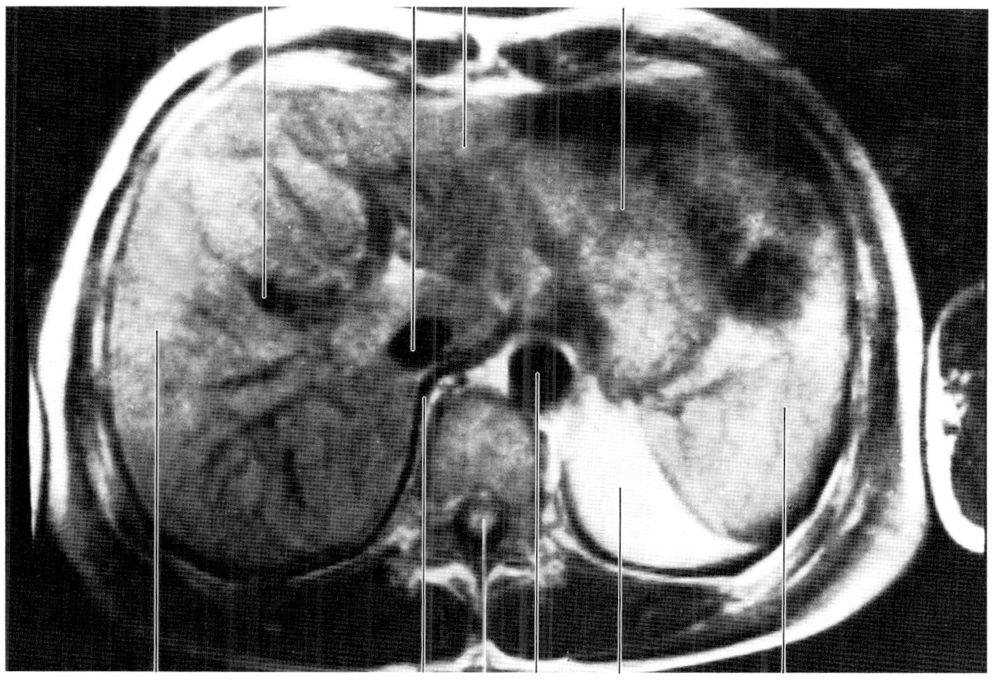

MRI, SE 500/50

1 Left lobe of the liver
7 Corpus of the stomach
16 Spleen
24 Suprarenal fat tissue
29 Descending aorta
32 Spinal medulla
34 Diaphragm, lumbar part
37 Inferior vena cava
47 Branch of the portal vein
48 Right lobe of the liver

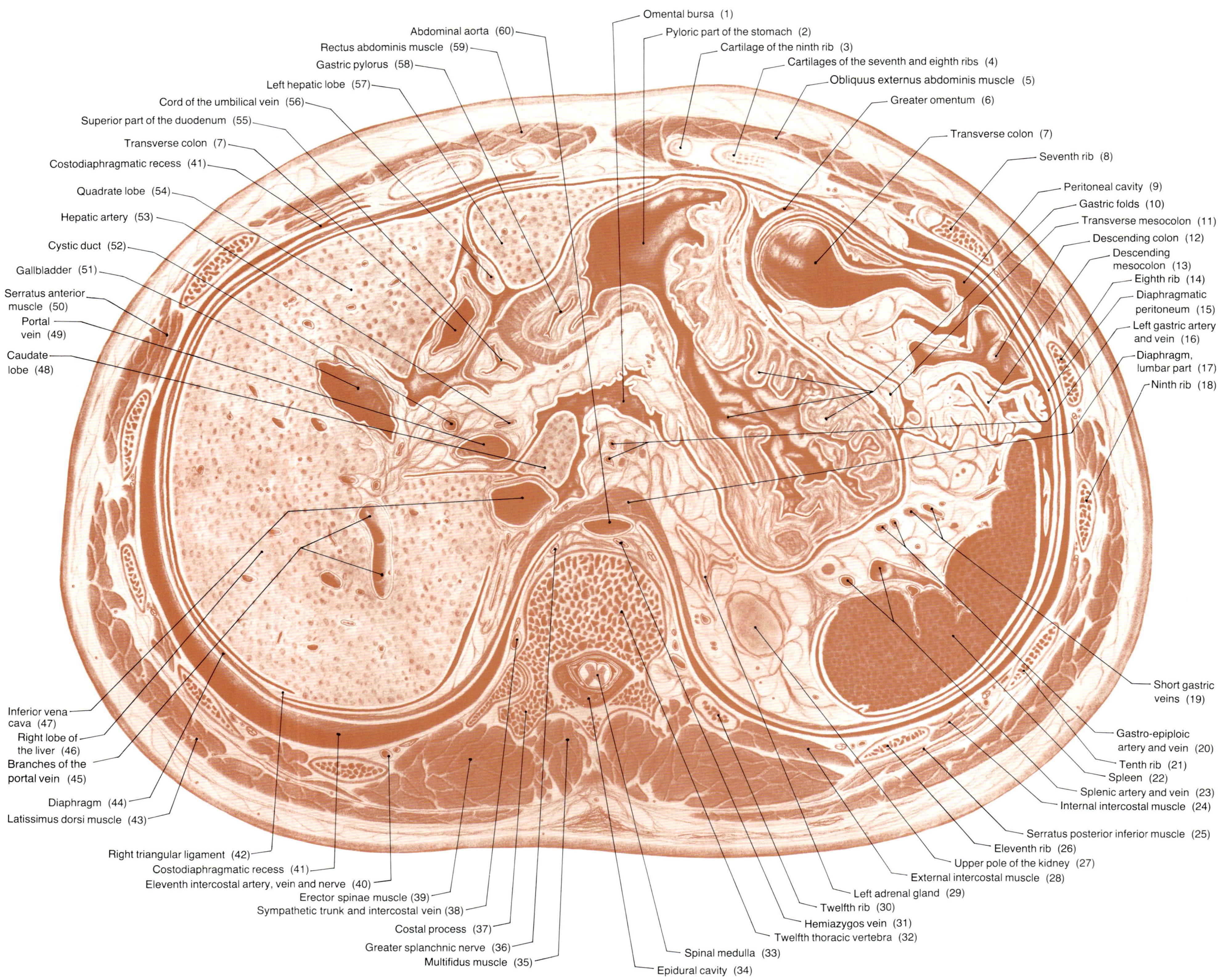

1 Bursa omentalis
2 Pars pylorica ventriculi
2.1 Ventriculus
3 Cartilago costae IX
4 Cartilago costae VII et VIII
5 M. obliquus externus abdominis
6 Omentum majus
7 Colon transversum
7.1 Jejunum
8 Costa VII
9 Cavitas peritonealis
10 Plicae gastricae
11 Mesocolon transversum
12 Colon descendens
13 Mesocolon descendens
14 Costa VIII
15 Peritoneum diaphragmatis
16 A. et V. gastrica sinistra
17 Diaphragma partis lumbalis
18 Costa IX
19 Vv. gastricae breves
20 A. et V. gastroepiploica
21 Costa X
22 Lien
23 A. et V. lienalis
24 M. intercostalis internus
25 M. serratus posterior inferior
26 Costa XI
27 Extremitas superior renis
28 M. intercostalis externus
29 Glandula suprarenalis sinister
30 Costa XII
31 V. hemiazygos
32 Vertebra thoracica XII
33 Medulla spinalis
34 Cavitas epiduralis
35 M. multifidus
36 N. splanchnicus major
37 Processus costarius
38 Truncus sympathicus et V. intercostalis
39 M. erector spinae
40 A. et V. et N. intercostalis XI
41 Recessus costodiaphragmaticus
42 Lig. triangulare dextrum
43 M. latissimus dorsi
44 Diaphragma
45 Vv. hepaticae
46 Lobus hepatis dexter
47 V. cava inferior
48 Lobus caudatus
49 V. portae
50 M. serratus anterior
51 Vesica fellea
52 Ductus cysticus
53 A. hepatica
54 Lobus quadratus
55 Duodenum, Pars superior
56 Chorda v. umbilicalis
57 Lobus hepatis sinister
58 Pylorus ventriculi
59 M. rectus abdominis
60 Aorta abdominalis
60.1 Corpus pancreatis

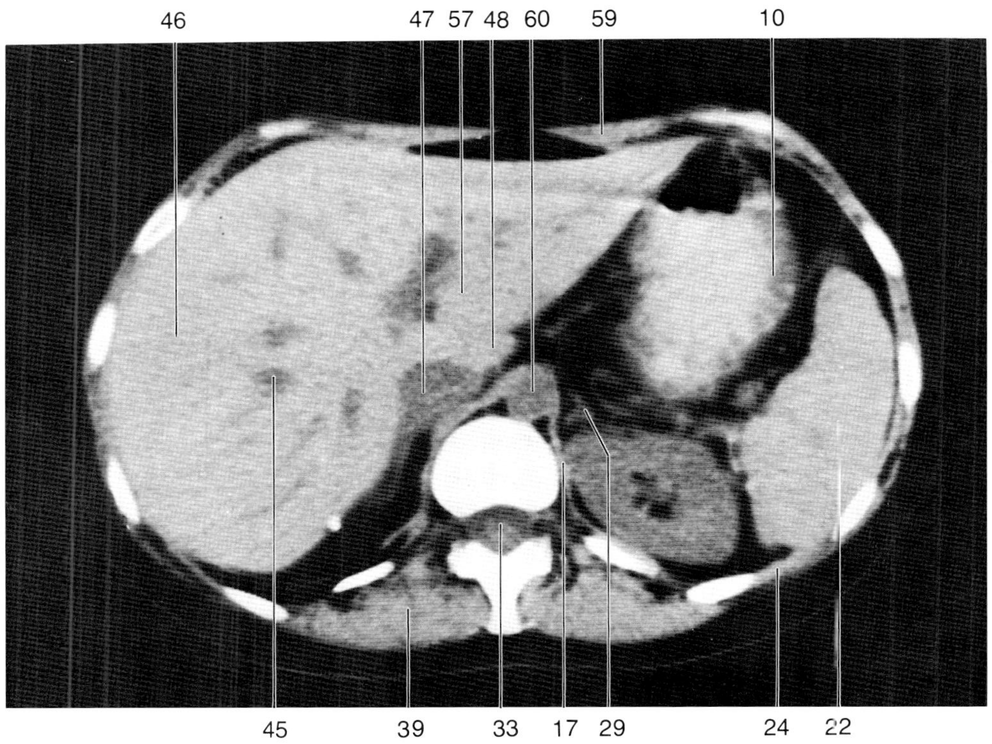

CT with contrast medium in the stomach

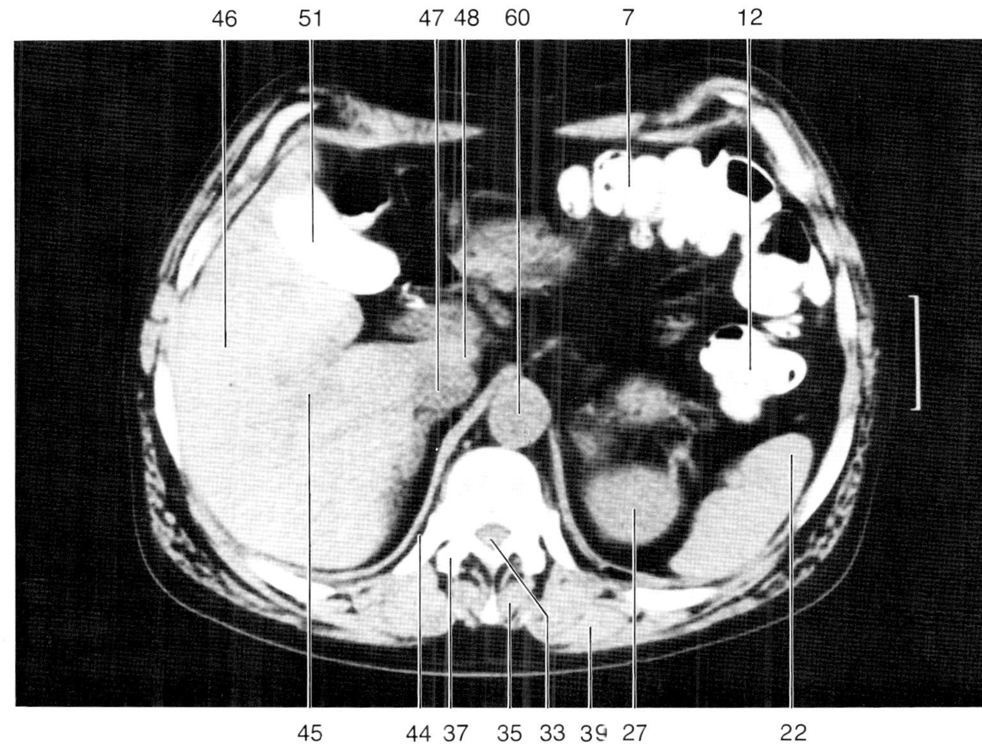

CT with contrast medium in the transverse and descending colon and in the gall bladder

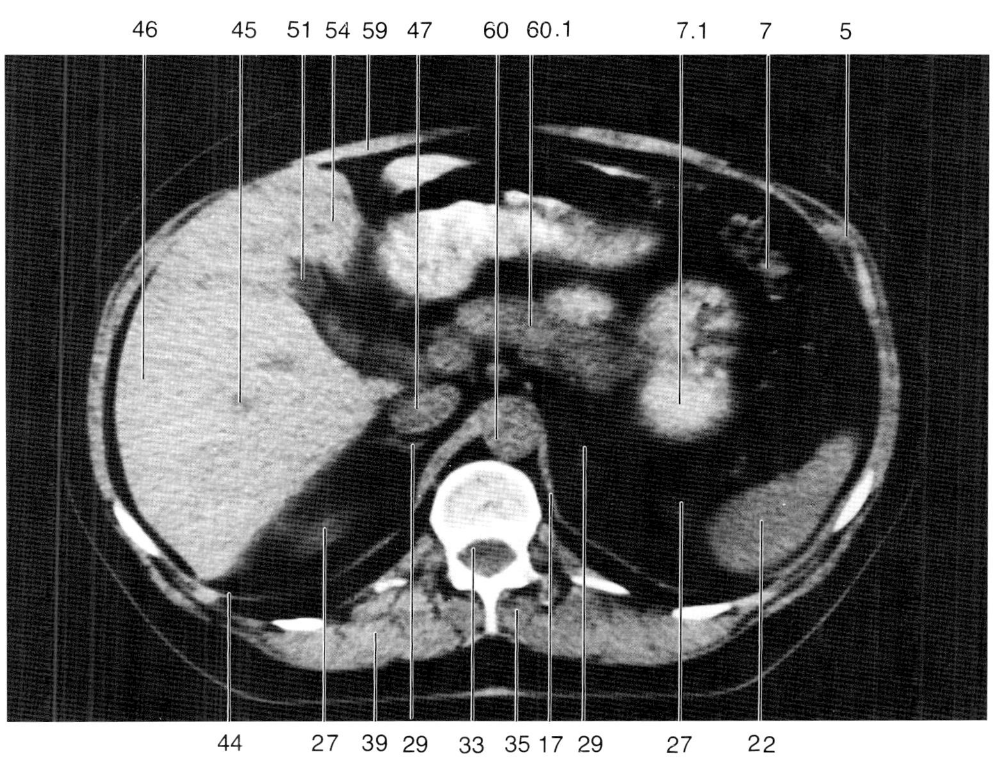

CT with contrast medium in the stomach and small bowel

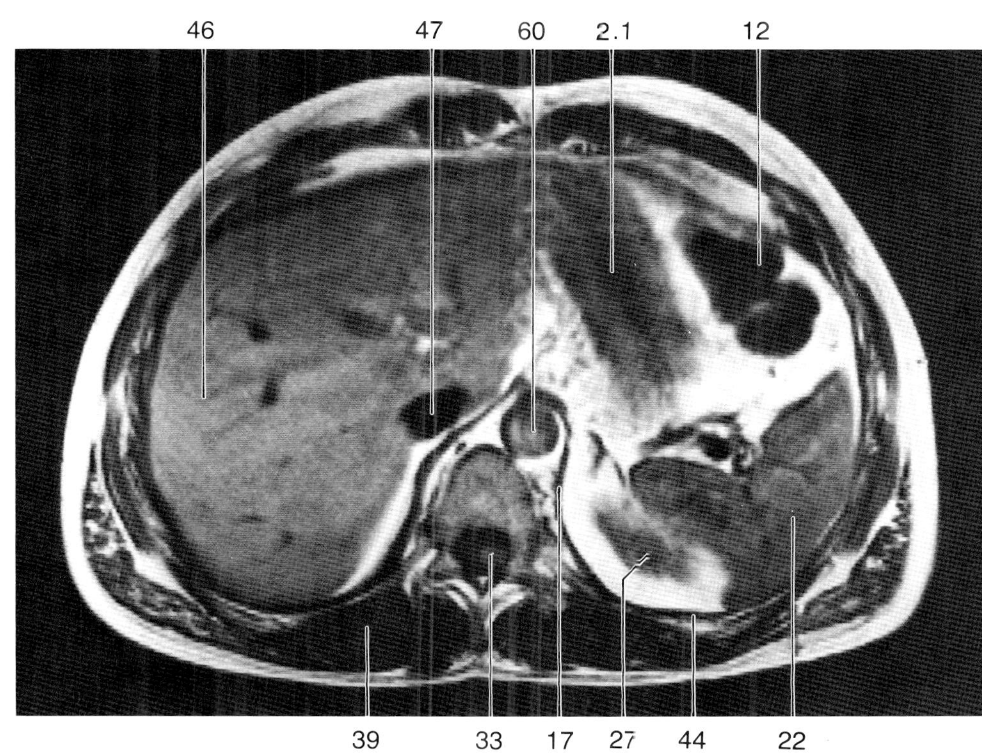

MRI, SE 800/22

2.1 Stomach
5 External oblique muscle of abdomen
7 Transverse colon
7.1 Jejunum
10 Gastric folds
12 Descending colon
17 Diaphragm, lumbar part
22 Spleen
24 Internal intercostal muscle
27 Upper pole of the kidney
29 Left adrenal gland
33 Spinal medulla
35 Multifidus muscle
37 Costal process
39 Erector spinae muscle
44 Diaphragm
45 Hepatic veins
46 Right lobe of the liver
47 Inferior vena cava
48 Caudate lobe of the liver
51 Gallbladder
54 Quadrate lobe
57 Left hepatic lobe
59 Rectus abdominis muscle
60 Abdominal aorta
60.1 Pancreas

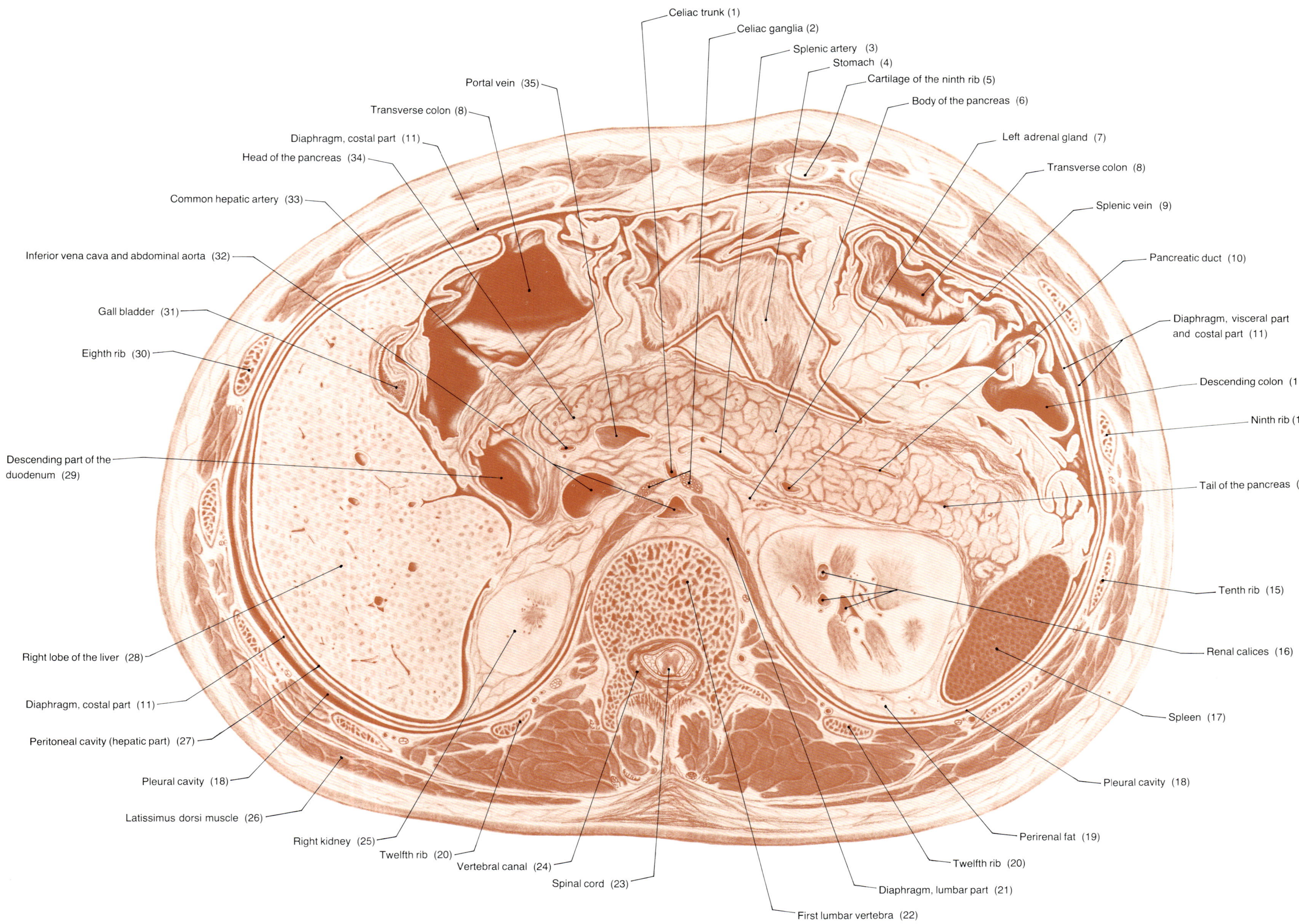

1 Truncus coeliacus
2 Ganglia coeliaca
2.1 V. cava inferior
2.2 Aorta abdominalis
3 A. lienalis
4 Ventriculus
5 Cartilago costae IX
6 Corpus pancreaticum
7 Glandula suprarenalis sinistra
8 Colon transversum
9 V. lienalis
10 Ductus pancreaticus
10.1 Jejunum
11 Diaphragma (Pars costalis et visceralis)
12 Colon descendens
13 Costa IX
14 Cauda pancreatis
15 Costa X
16 Calices renales
17 Lien
18 Cavitas pleuralis
19 Capsula adiposa renalis
20 Costa XII
21 Diaphragma (Pars lumbalis)
22 Vertebra lumbalis I
23 Medulla spinalis
24 Canalis vertebralis
25 Ren dexter
26 M. latissimus dorsi
27 Cavitas peritonealis (Pars hepatis)
28 Lobus hepatis dexter
29 Duodenum (Pars descendens)
30 Costa VIII
31 Vesica fellea
32 A. cava inferior et Aorta abdominis
33 A. hepatica communis
34 Caput pancreatis
35 V. portae

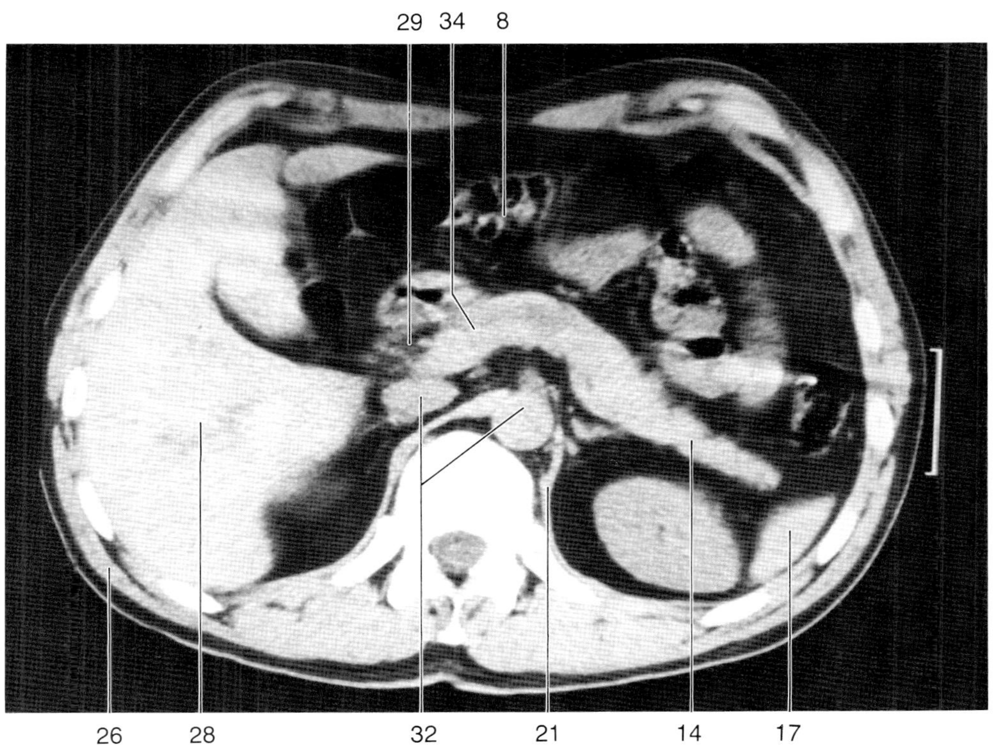

CT scan

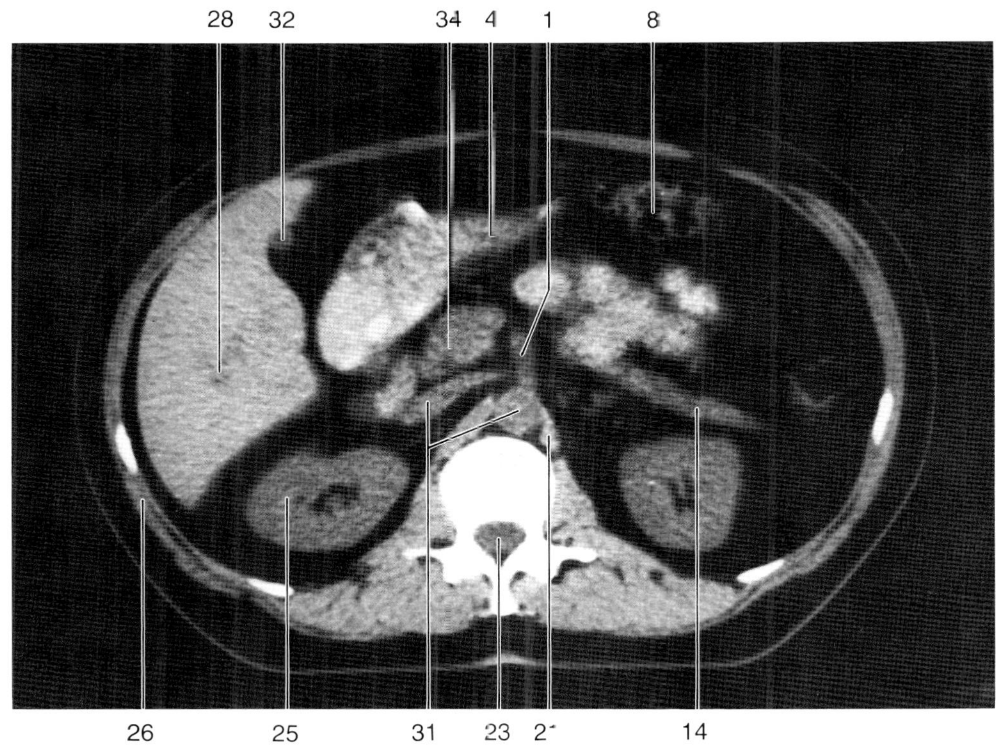

CT with contrast medium in the stomach and small bowel

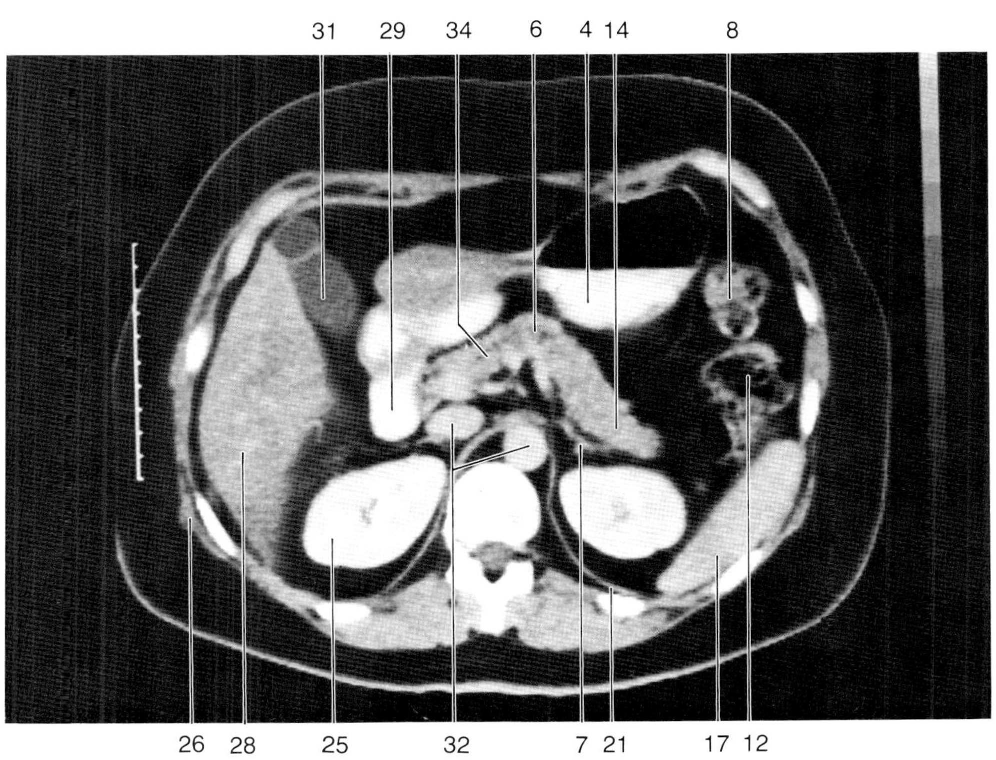

CT, enhanced after injection of contrast medium and with contrast in the stomach and duodenal loop

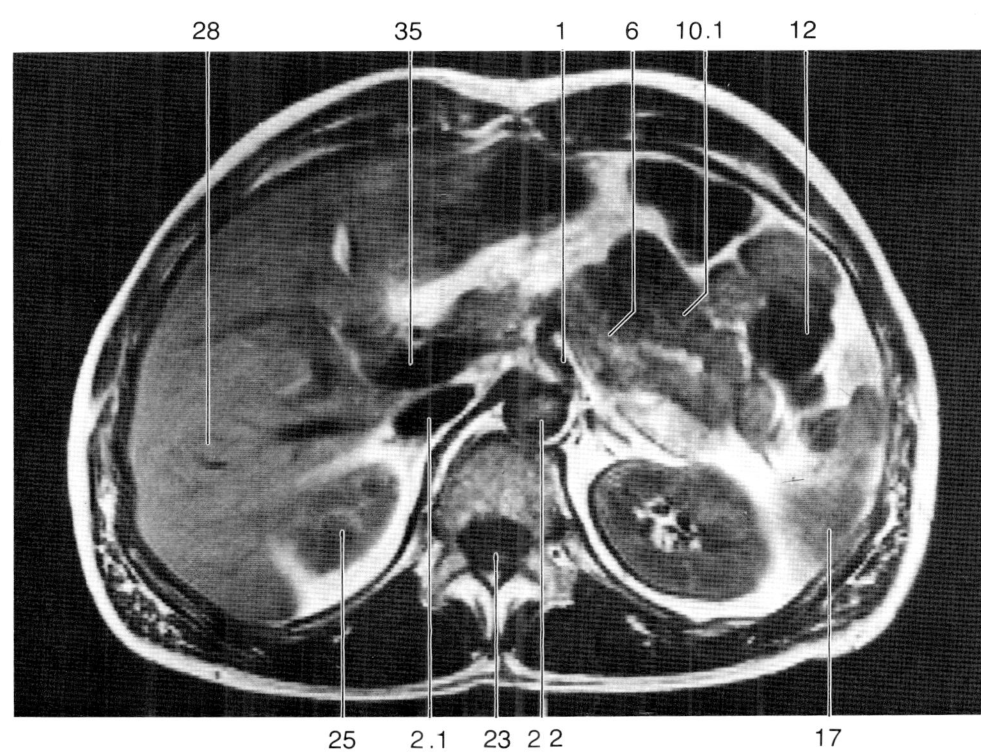

MRI, SE 800/22

1 Coeliac trunk
2.1 Inferior vena cava
2.2 Abdominal aorta
4 Stomach
6 Body of the pancreas
7 Left adrenal gland
8 Transverse colon
10.1 Jejunum
12 Descending colon
14 Tail of the pancreas
17 Spleen
21 Diaphragm, lumbar part
23 Spinal cord
25 Right kidney
26 Latissimus dorsi muscle
28 Right lobe of the liver
29 Descending part of the duodenum
31 Gall bladder
32 Inferior vena cava and abdominal aorta
34 Head of the pancreas
35 Portal vein

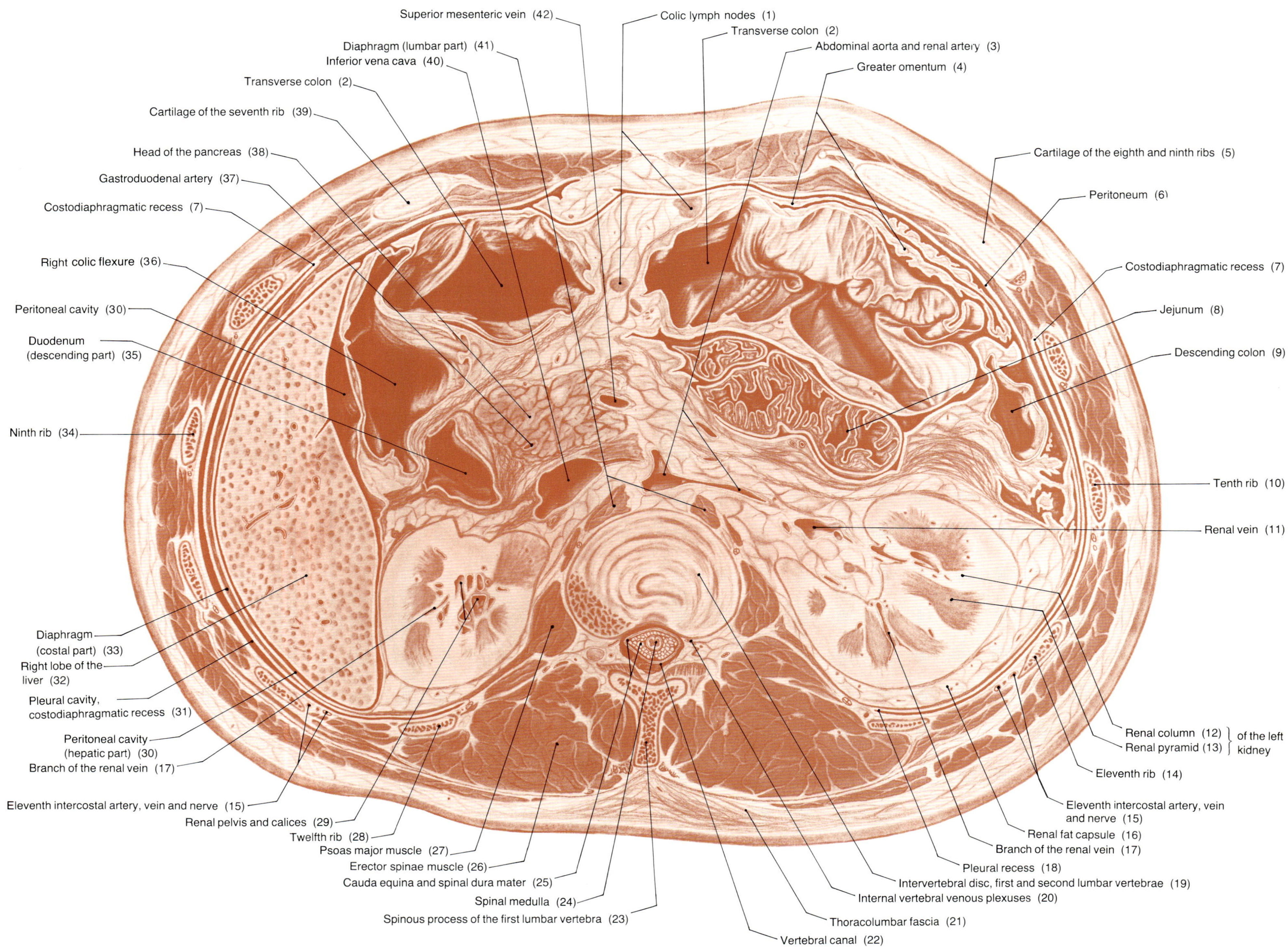

1 Nodi lymphatici colici
1.1 A. mesenterica superior
2 Colon transversum
3 Aorta abdominalis et A. renalis
3.1 Aorta abdominalis
4 Omentum majus
5 Cartilago costae VIII et IX
6 Peritonaeum
7 Recessus costodiaphragmaticus
8 Jejunum
9 Colon descendens
10 Costa X
11 Vena renalis
12 Ren sinister – Columna renalis
13 Ren sinister – Pyramis renalis
14 Costa XI
15 A. et V. et N. intercostalis XI
16 Capsula adiposa renalis
17 R. v. renalis
18 Recessus pleuralis
19 Discus intervertebralis, Vertebrae lumbales I et II
20 Plexus venosi vertebrales interni
21 Fascia thoracolumbalis
22 Canalis vertebralis
23 Processus spinosus vertebrae lumbalis I
24 Medulla spinalis
25 Cauda equina et Dura mater spinalis
26 M. erector spinae
27 M. psoas major
28 Costa XII
29 Pelvis renalis et Calices renales
30 Cavitas peritonealis (Pars hepatis)
31 Cavitas pleuralis, Recessus costodiaphragmaticus
32 Lobus hepatis dexter
33 Diaphragma (Pars costalis)
34 Costa IX
35 Duodenum (Pars descendens)
36 Flexura coli dextra
37 A. gastroduodenalis
38 Caput pancreatis
38.1 Ventriculus
39 Cartilago costae VII
40 V. cava inferior
40.1 V. lienalis
41 Diaphragma (Pars lumbalis)
42 V. mesenterica superior

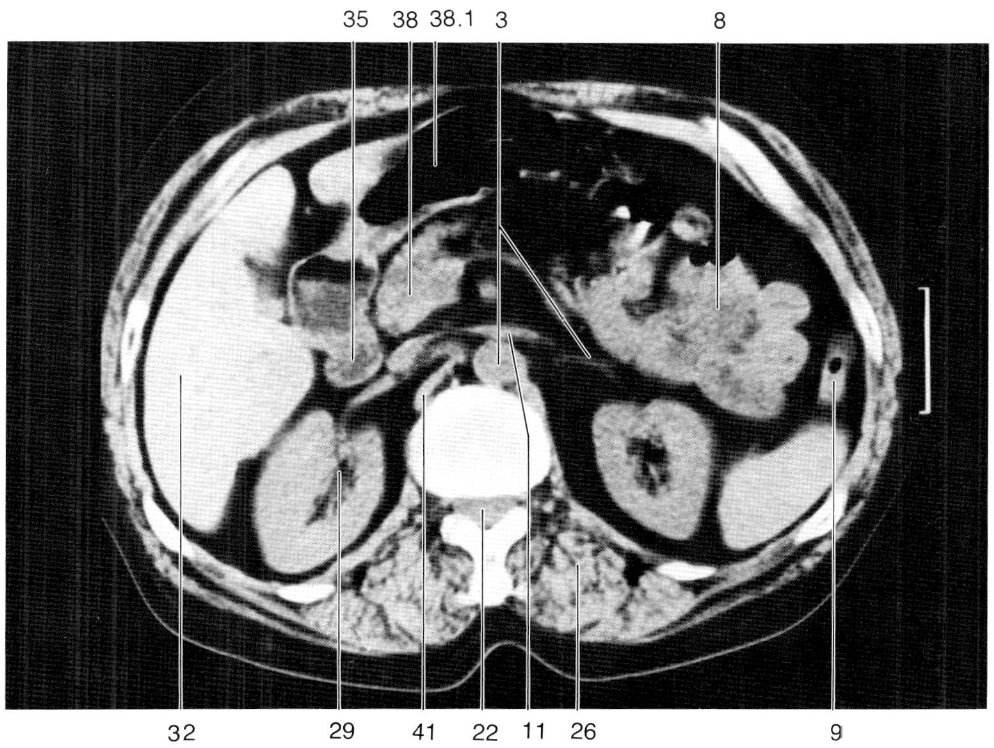

CT without contrast medium

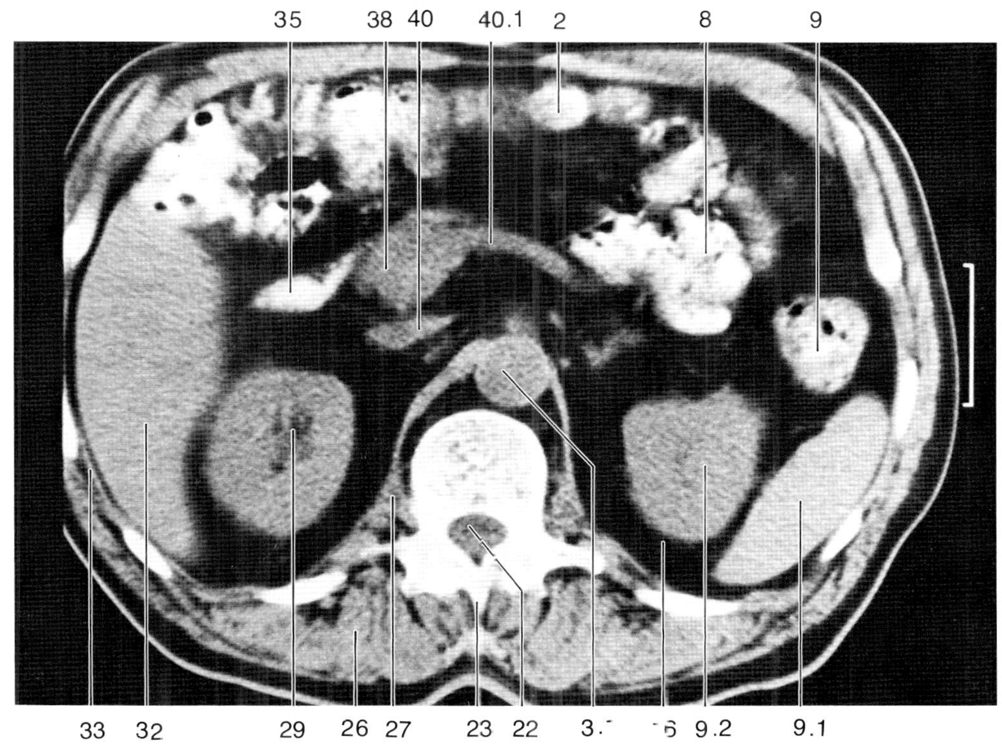

CT with contrast medium in the small bowel and colon

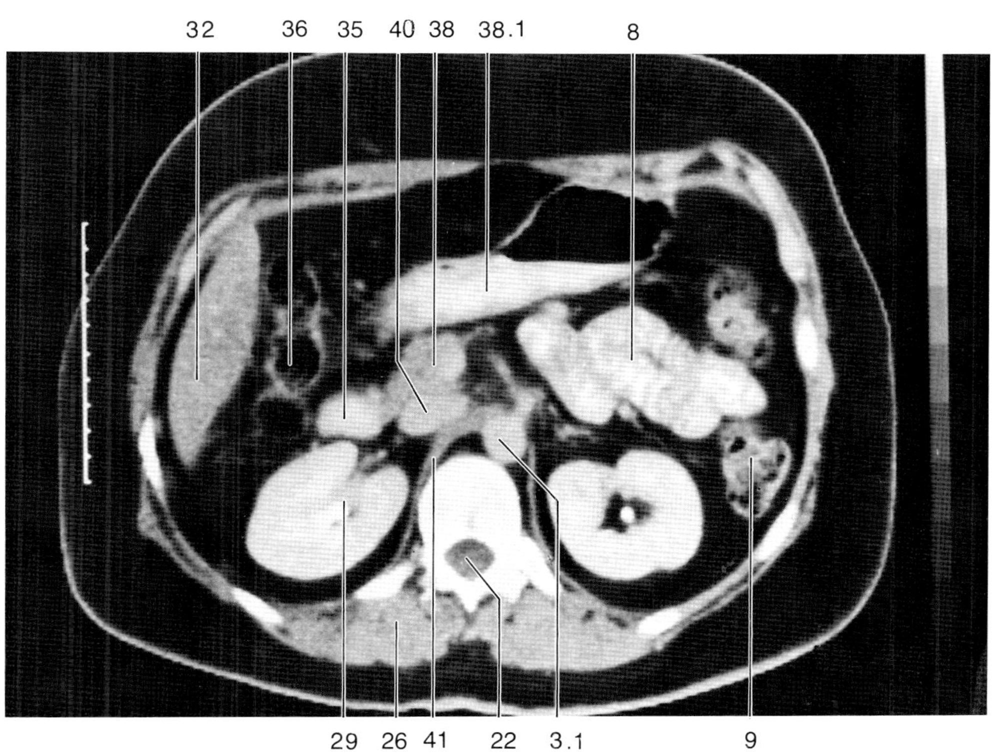

CT, enhanced after bolus injection of contrast medium, and with contrast in the stomach and small bowel

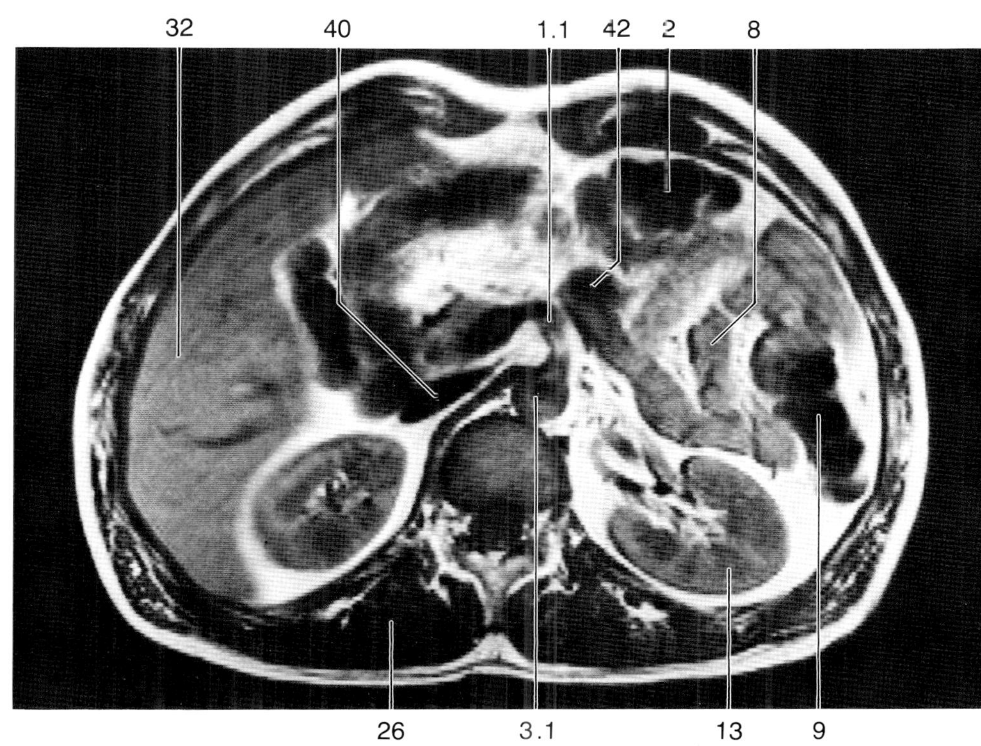

MRI, SE 800/22

- 1.1 Superior mesenteric artery
- 2 Transverse colon
- 3 Abdominal aorta and renal artery
- 3.1 Aorta
- 8 Jejunum
- 9 Descending colon
- 9.1 Spleen
- 9.2 Left kidney
- 11 Renal vein
- 13 Renal pyramid of the left kidney
- 16 Renal fat capsule
- 22 Vertebral canal
- 23 Spinous process of the first lumbar vertebra
- 26 Erector trunci muscle
- 27 Psoas major muscle
- 29 Renal pelvis and calices
- 32 Right lobe of the liver
- 33 Diaphragm (costal part)
- 35 Duodenum (descending part)
- 36 Ascending colon
- 38 Head of the pancreas
- 38.1 Stomach
- 40 Inferior vena cava
- 40.1 Splenic vein
- 41 Diaphragma (lumbar part)
- 42 Superior mesenteric vein

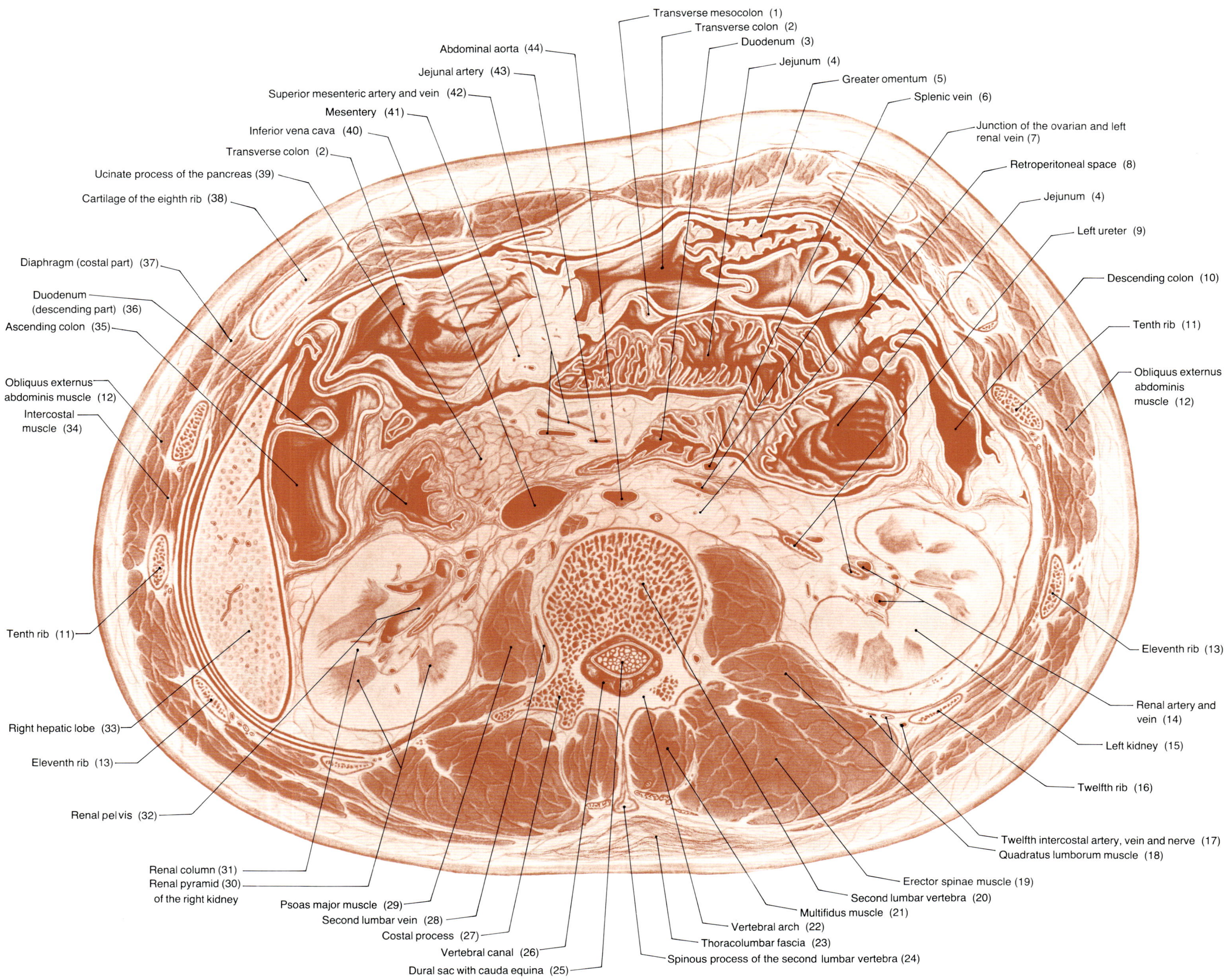

1 Mesocolon transversum
2 Colon transversum
2.1 Ileum
3 Duodenum
4 Jejunum
5 Omentum majus
6 V. lienalis
7 Anastomosis, V. ovarica et V. renalis sinistra
8 Spatium retroperitonaeale
9 Ureter sinister
10 Colon descendens
10.1 Lien
11 Costa X
12 M. obliquus externus abdominis
13 Costa XI
14 A. et V. renalis
15 Ren sinister
15.1 V. renalis sinistra
16 Costa XII
17 A. et V. et N. intercostalis XII
18 M. quadratus lumborum
19 M. erector trunci
20 Vertebra lumbalis II
21 M. multifidus
21.1 A. renalis dextra
22 Arcus vertebrae
23 Fascia thoracolumbalis
24 Processus spinosus vertebrae lumbalis II
25 Spatium subdurale et Cauda equina
26 Canalis vertebralis
27 Processus costarius
28 V. lumbalis II
29 M. psoas major
30 Pyramis renalis (Ren dexter)
31 Columna renalis (Ren dexter)
32 Hilus renalis et A. et V. renalis dexter
32.1 V. renalis dextra
33 Lobus dexter hepatis
34 M. intercostalis
35 Colon ascendens
36 Duodenum (Pars descendens)
37 Diaphragma (Pars costalis)
38 Cartilago costae VIII
39 Processus uncinatus, Caput pancreatis
40 V. cava inferior
41 Mesenterium
42 A. et V. mesenterica superior
43 A. jejunalis
44 Aorta abdominalis
44.1 A. mesenterica superior

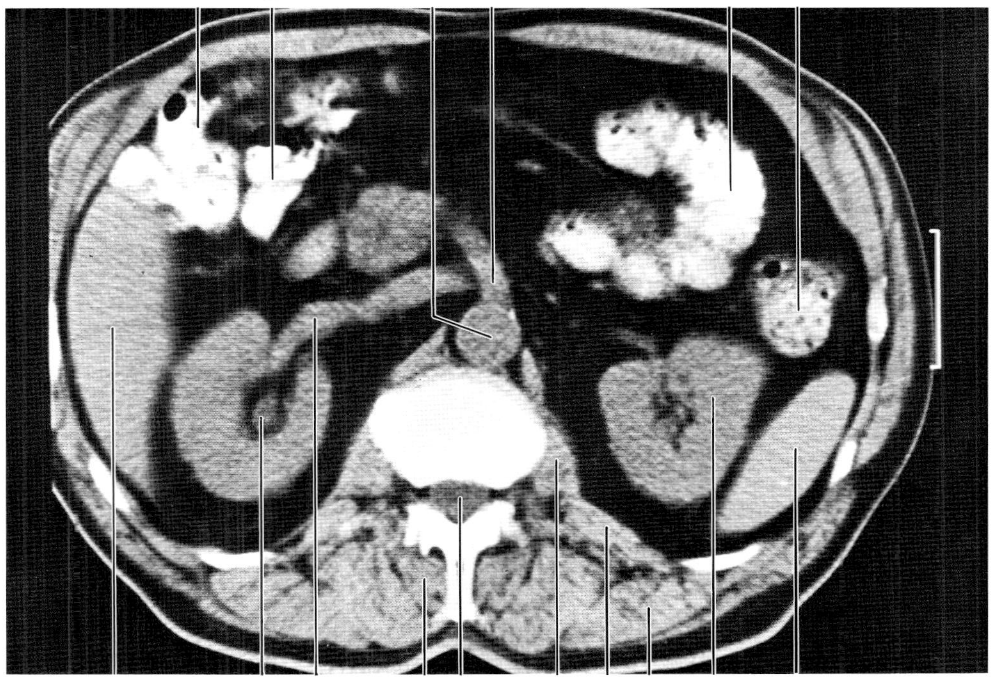

CT with contrast medium in the small bowel and colon

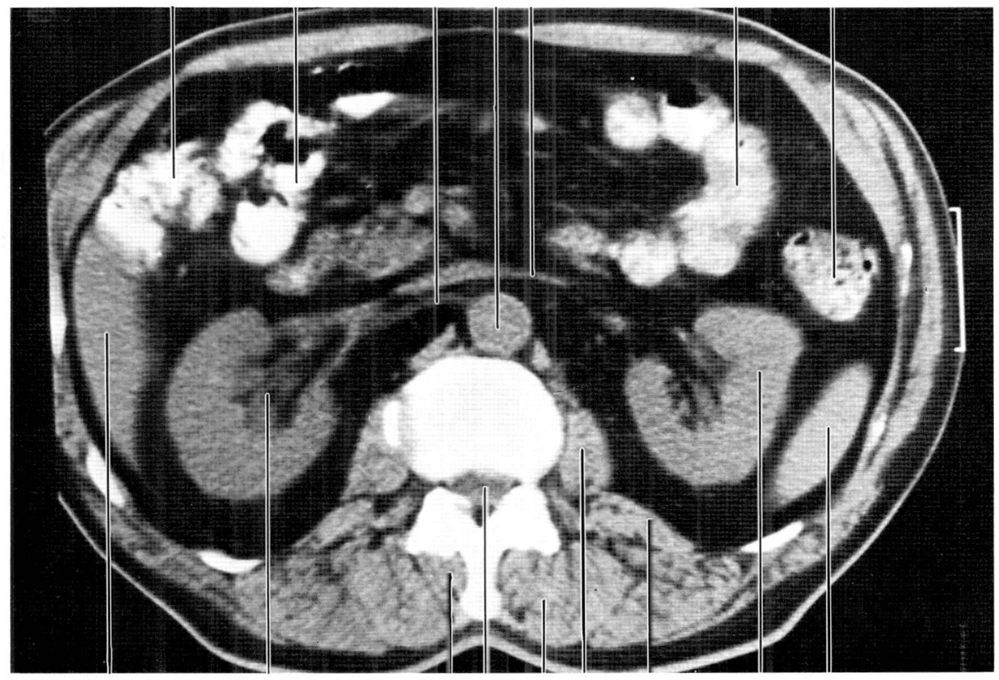

CT with contrast medium in the small bowel and colon

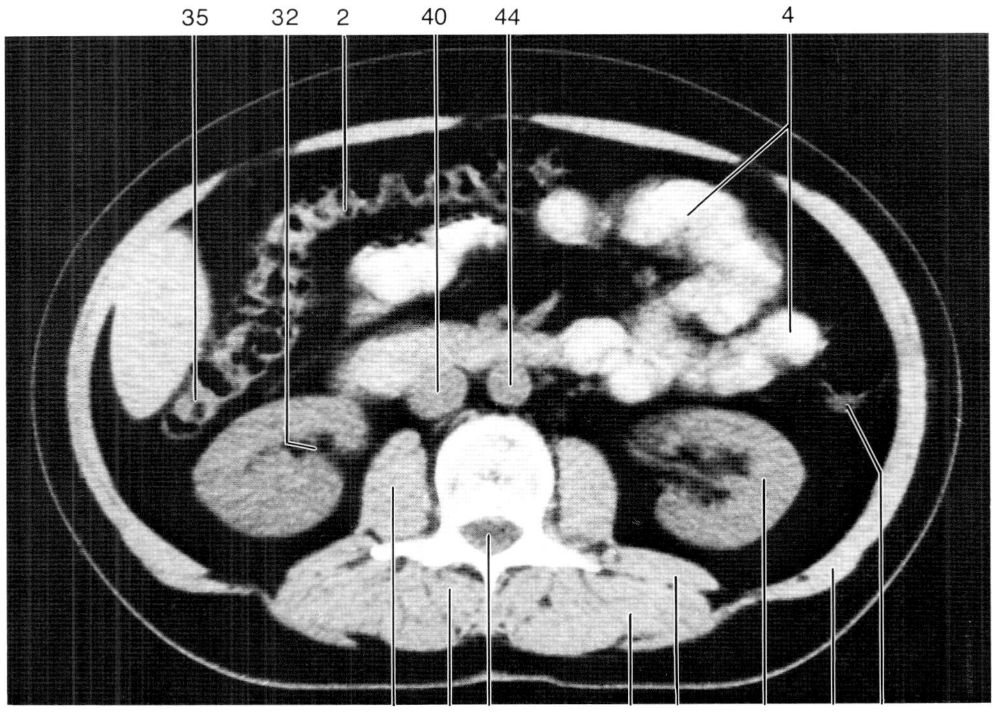

CT with contrast medium in the small bowel

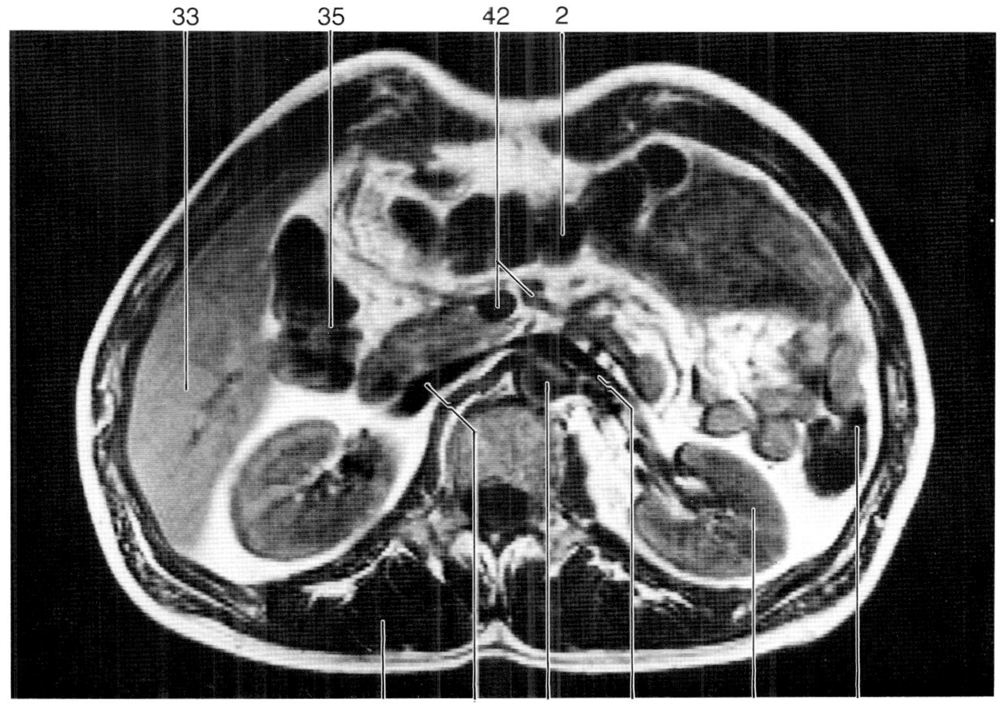

MRI, SE 800/22

2 Transverse colon
2.1 Ileum
4 Jejunum
10 Descending colon
10.1 Spleen
12 Obliquus externus abdominis muscle
15 Left kidney
15.1 Left renal vein
18 Quadratus lumborum muscle
19 Erector spinae muscle
21 Multifidus muscle
21.1 Right renal artery
25 Dural sac with cauda equina
29 Psoas major muscle
32 Renal pelvis
32.1 Right renal vein
33 Right hepatic lobe
35 Ascending colon
40 Inferior vena cava
42 Superior mesenteric artery and vein
44 Abdominal aorta
44.1 Superior mesenteric artery

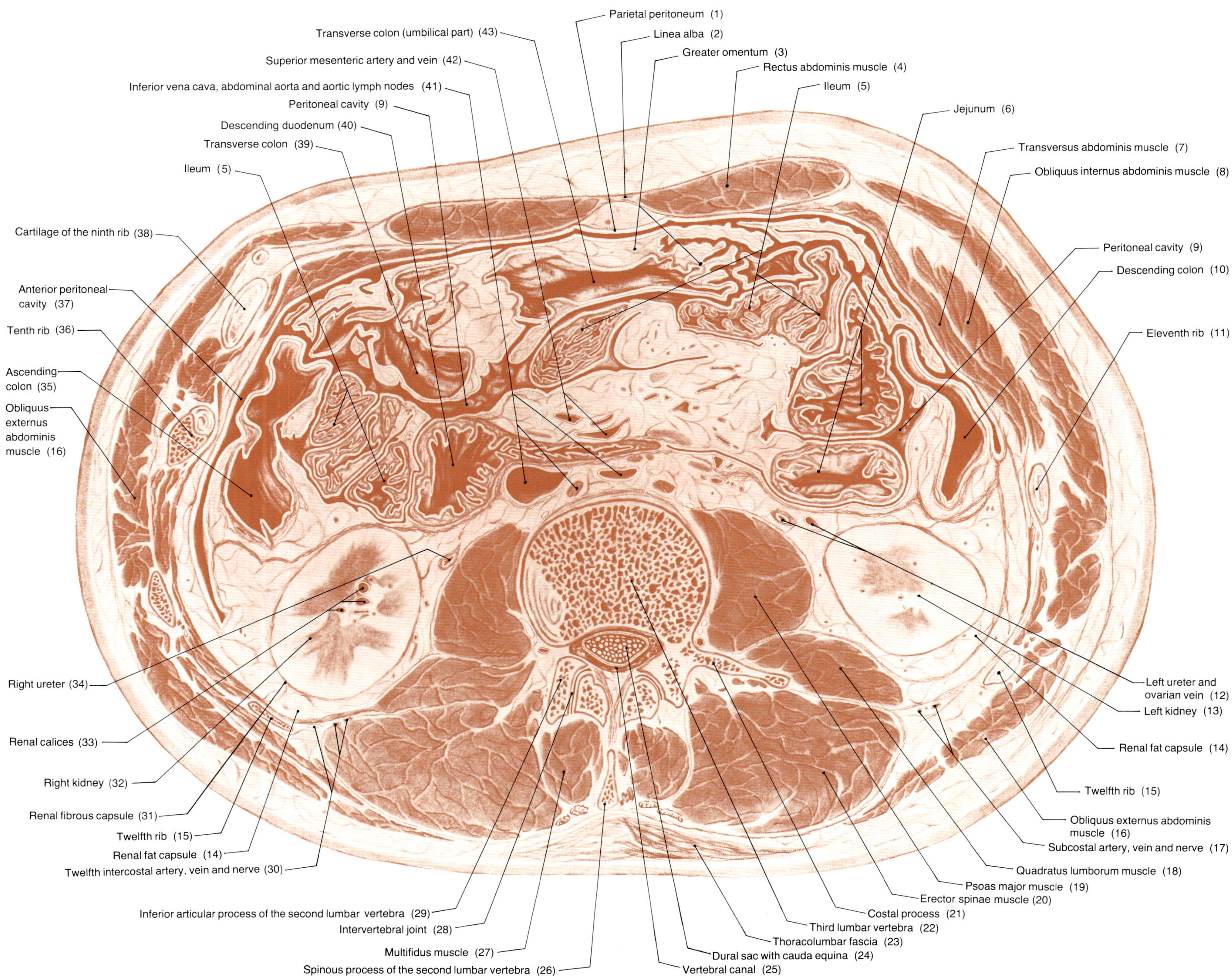

1 Peritoneum parietale
2 Linea alba
3 Omentum majus
4 M. rectus abdominis
5 Ileum
6 Jejunum
7 M. transversus abdominis
8 M. obliquus internus abdominis
9 Cavitas peritonealis
10 Colon descendens
10.1 A. renalis
10.2 V. renalis
11 Costa XI
12 Ureter sinister et V. ovarica
13 Ren sinister
14 Capsula adiposa renalis
14.1 Lobus dexter hepatis
15 Costa XII
16 M. obliquus externus abdominis
17 A. et V. et N. subcostalis
18 M. quadratus lumborum
19 M. psoas major
20 M. erector spinae
21 Processus costarius
22 Vertebra lumbalis III
23 Fascia thoracolumbalis
24 Saccus duralis, Cauda equina
25 Canalis vertebralis
26 Processus spinosus vertebrae lumbalis II
27 M. multifidus
28 Articulus intervertebralis
29 Processus articularis inferior vertebrae lumbalis II
30 A. et V. et N. intercostalis XII
31 Capsula fibrosa renis
32 Ren dexter
33 Calices renales
34 Ureter dexter
35 Colon ascendens
36 Costa X
37 Cavitas peritonealis anterior
38 Cartilago costae IX
39 Colon transversum
40 Duodenum (Pars descendens)
41 V. cava inferior et Aorta abdominalis et Nodi lymphatici aortici
41.1 V. cava inferior
41.2 Aorta abdominalis
42 A. et V. mesenterica superior
43 Colon transversum (Pars umbilicalis)

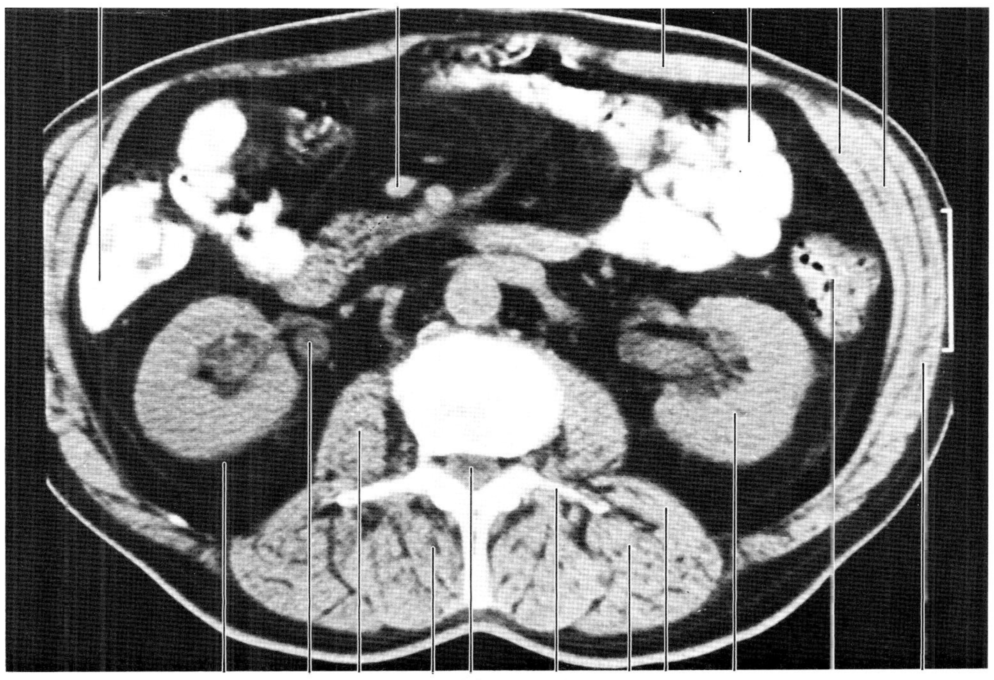

CT with contrast medium in the small bowel and colon

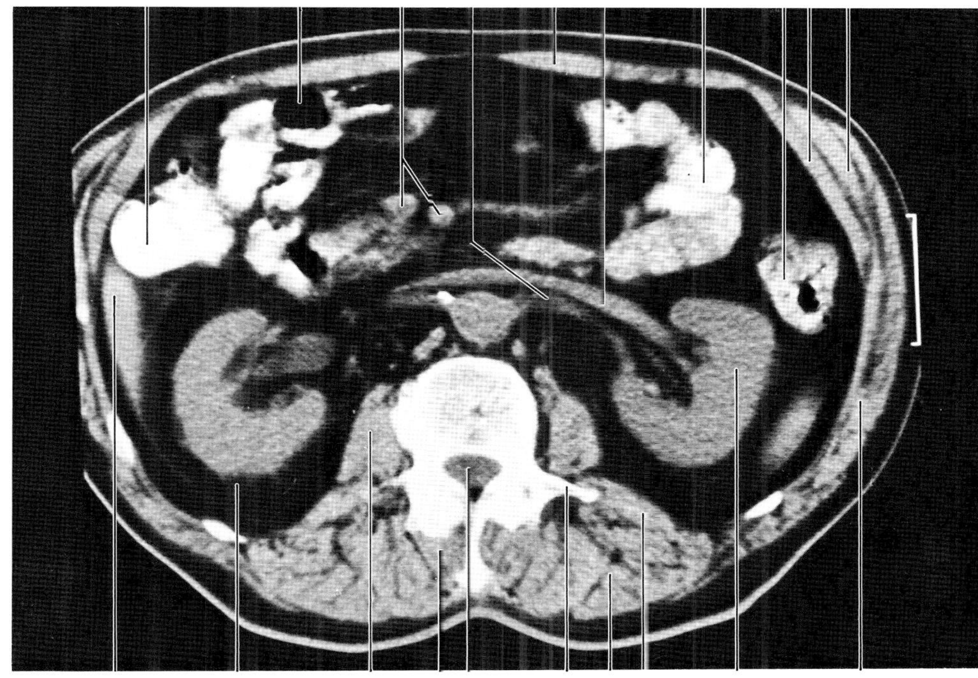

CT with contrast medium in the small bowel and colon

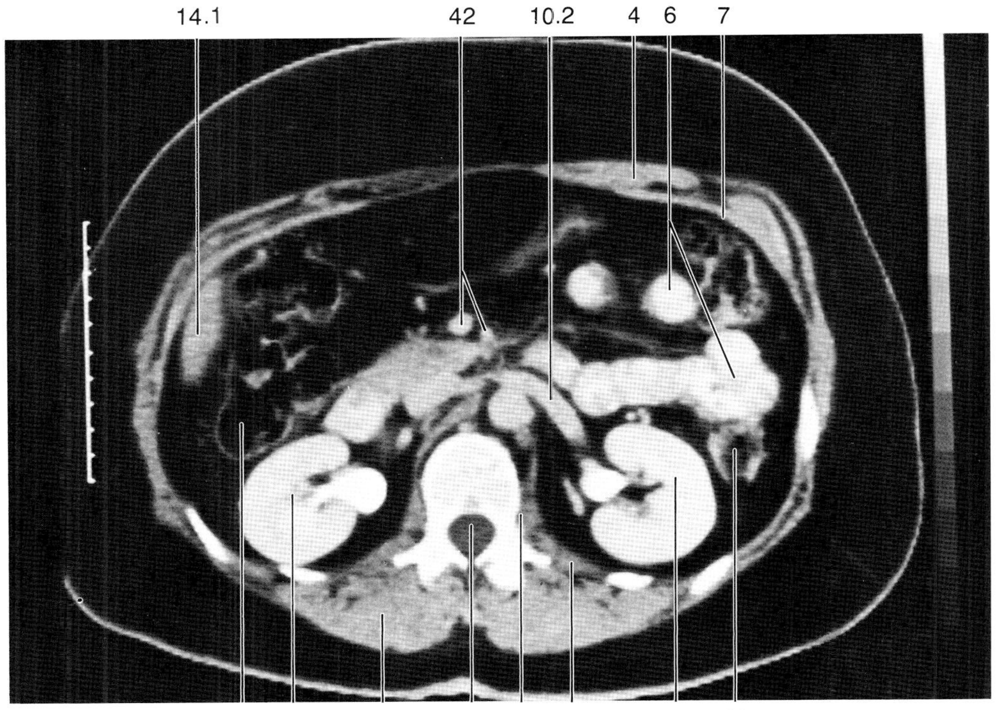

CT, enhanced after bolus injection of contrast medium, and with contrast in the small bowel

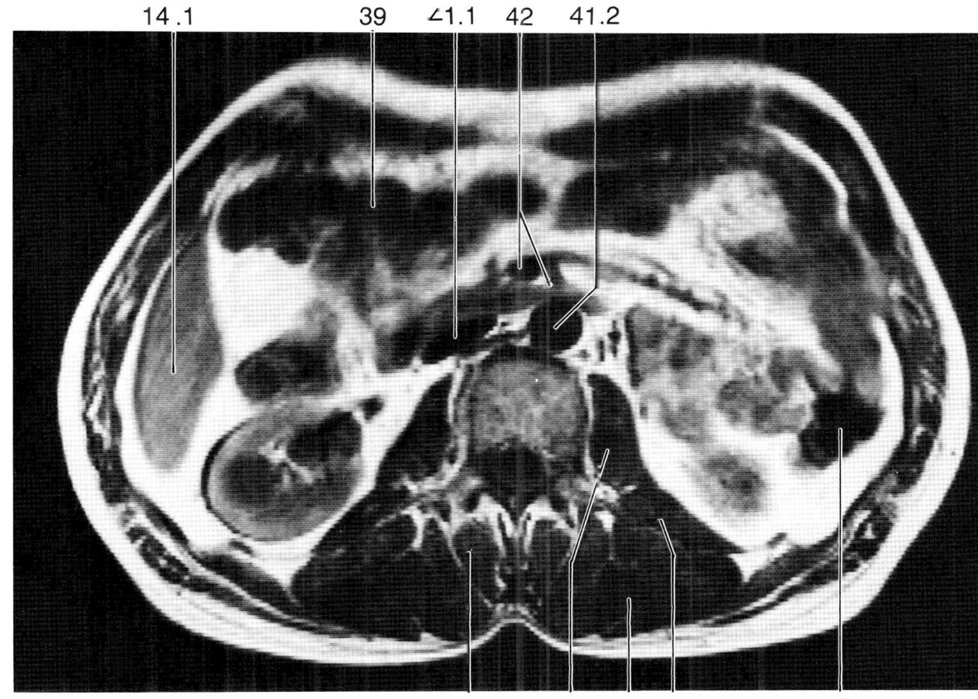

MRI, SE 800/22

- 4 Rectus abdominis muscle
- 6 Jejunum
- 7 Transversus abdominis muscle
- 8 Obliquus internus abdominis muscle
- 10 Descending colon
- 10.1 Renal artery
- 10.2 Renal vein
- 13 Left kidney
- 14 Renal fat capsule
- 14.1 Right hepatic lobe
- 16 Obliquus externus abdominis muscle
- 18 Quadratus lumborum muscle
- 19 Psoas major muscle
- 20 Erector spinae muscle
- 21 Costal process
- 24 Dural sac with cauda equina
- 27 M. multifidus
- 33 Renal calices
- 34 Right ureter
- 35 Ascending colon
- 39 Transverse colon
- 41.1 Inferior vena cava
- 41.2 Abdominal aorta
- 42 Superior mesenteric artery and vein

Coronal Sections of the Female Pelvis

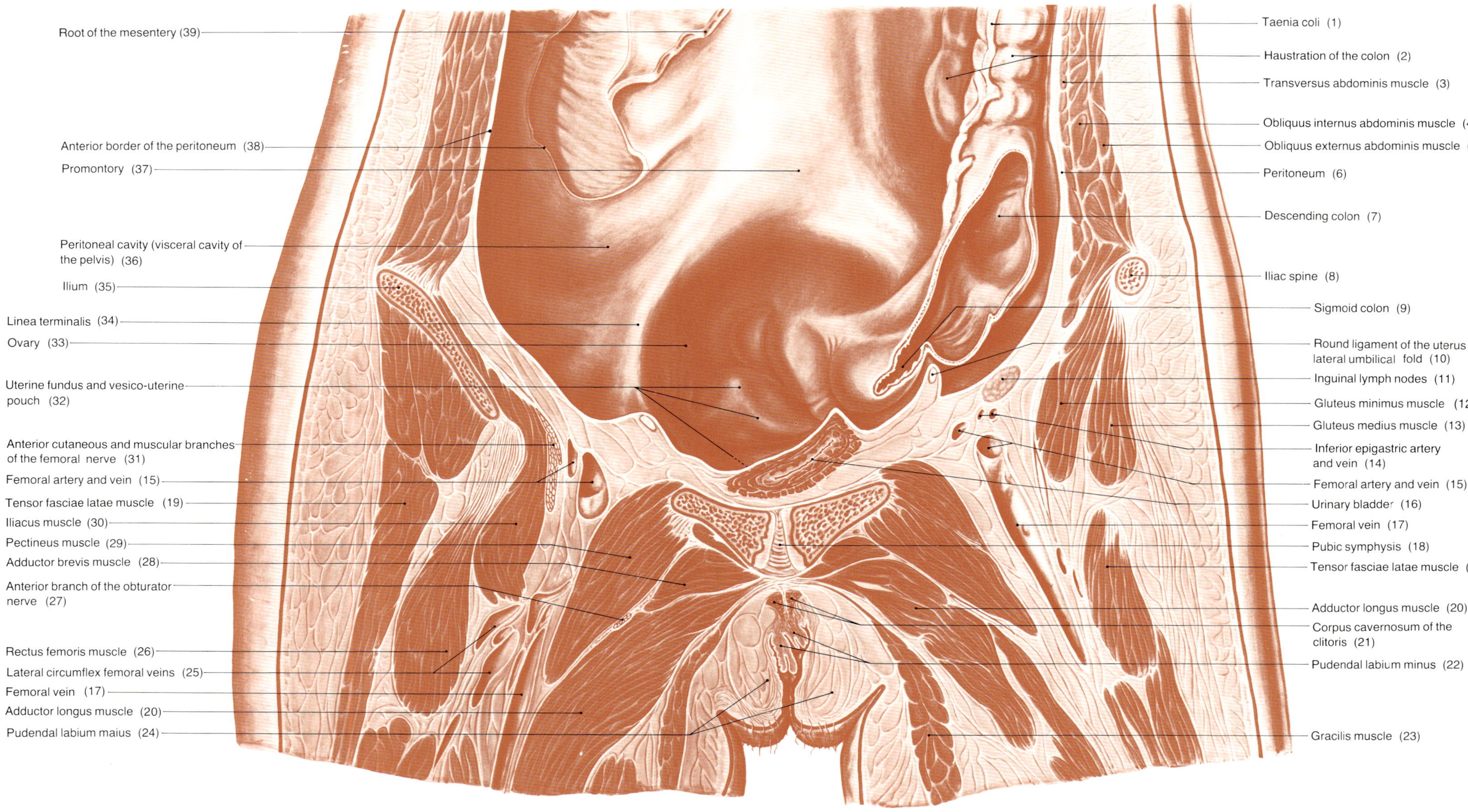

1 Taenia coli
2 Haustra coli
3 M. transversus abdominis
4 M. obliquus internus abdominis
5 M. obliquus externus abdominis
6 Peritoneum
7 Colon descendens
8 Spina iliaca
9 Colon sigmoideum
10 Lig. teres uteri et Plica umbilicalis lateralis
11 Nodi lymphatici inguinales
12 M. glutaeus minimus
13 M. glutaeus medius
14 A. et V. epigastrica inferior
15 A. et V. femoralis
16 Vesica urinaria
17 V. femoralis
18 Symphysis pubica
19 M. tensor fasciae latae
20 M. adductor longus
21 Corpus cavernosum clitoridis
22 Labium minus pudendi
23 M. gracilis
24 Labium majus pudeni
25 Vv. circumflexae femoris laterales
26 M. rectus femoris
27 R. anterior n. obturatorius
28 M. adductor brevis
29 M. pectineus
30 M. iliacus
31 Rr. cutanei anteriores et musculares n. femoralis
32 Fundus uteri et Excavatio vesicouterina
33 Ovarium
34 Linea terminalis
35 Os ilium
36 Cavum peritoneale (Cavum viscerale pelvis)
37 Promontorium
38 Peritoneum
39 Radix mesenterii

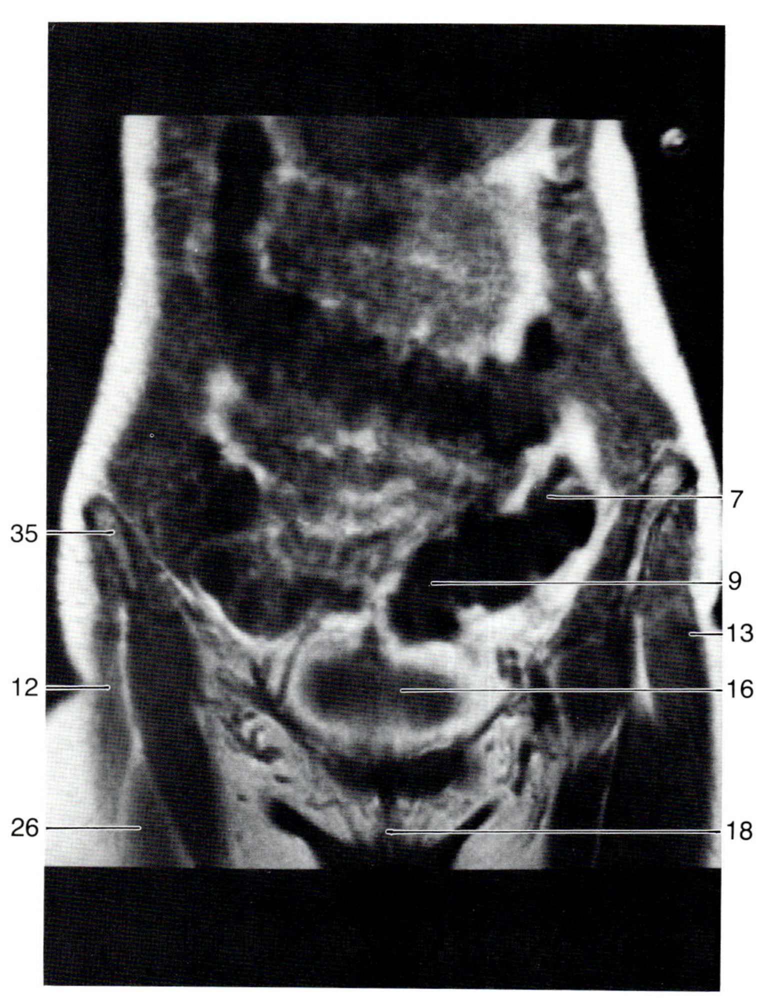

MRI, SE 2000/22

7 Descending colon
9 Sigmoid colon
12 Gluteus minimus muscle
13 Gluteus medius muscle
16 Urinary bladder
18 Pubic symphysis
26 Rectus femoris muscle
35 Ilium

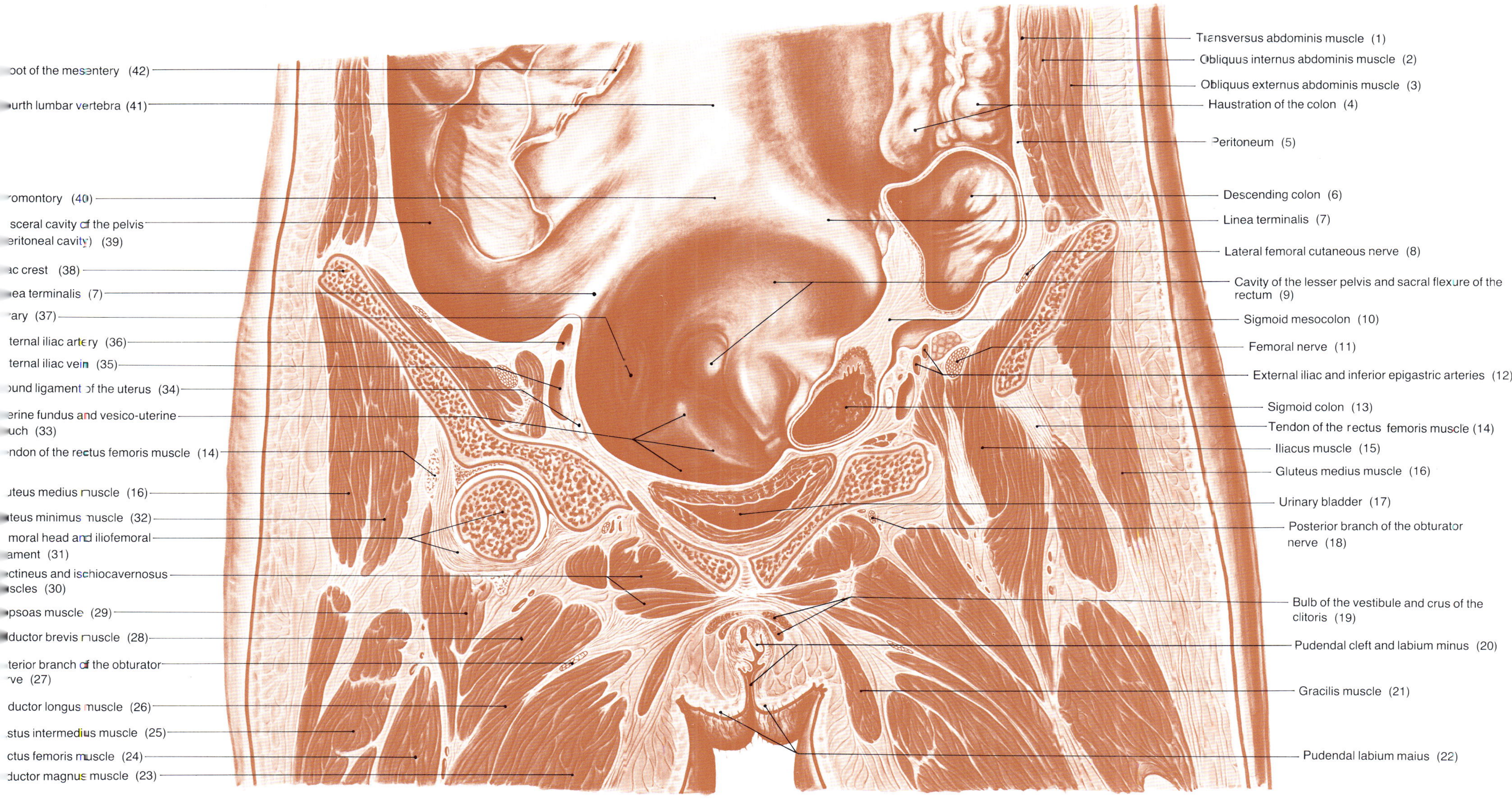

1 M. transversus abdominis
2 M. obliquus internus abdominis
3 M. obliquus externus abdominis
3.1 Aorta abdominalis
4 Haustra coli
5 Peritoneum
6 Colon descendens
6.1 A. iliaca communis
7 Linea terminalis
8 N. cutaneus femoris lateralis
9 Cavum pelvis minoris et Flexura sacralis recti
10 Mesocolon sigmoideum
11 N. femoralis
12 A. iliaca externa et A. epigastrica inferior
13 Colon sigmoideum
14 Tendo m. recti femoris
15 M. iliacus
16 M. glutaeus medicus
17 Vesica urinaria
18 R. posterior n. obturatorii
19 Bulbus vestibuli et Crus clitoridis
20 Labium minus pudendi et Rima pudendi
21 M. gracilis
22 Labium majus pudendi
23 M. adductor magnus
24 M. rectus femoris
25 M. vastus intermedius
26 M. adductor longus
27 R. anterior n. obturatorii
28 M. adductor brevis
29 M. iliopsoas
30 M. pectineus et M. ischiocavernosus
31 Caput femoris et Lig. iliofemorale
32 M. glutaeus minimus
32.1 M. iliacus
33 Fundus uteri et Excavatio vesicouterina
34 Lig. teres uteri
35 V. iliaca externa
36 A. iliaca externa
37 Ovarium
38 Crista iliaca
39 Cavum viscerale pelvis (Cavum peritoneale)
40 Promontorium
41 Vertebra lumbalis IV
42 Radix mesenteri

3 Obliquus externus abdominis muscle
3.1 Abdominal aorta
6 Descending colon
6.1 Common iliac artery
13 Sigmoid colon
16 Gluteus medius muscle
17 Urinary bladder
23 Adductor magnus muscle
25 Vastus intermedius muscle
30 Pectineus and ischiocavernosus muscles
31 Femoral head and iliofemoral ligament
32 Gluteus minimus muscle
32.1 Iliacus muscle
38 Iliac crest
38.1 Inferior vena cava

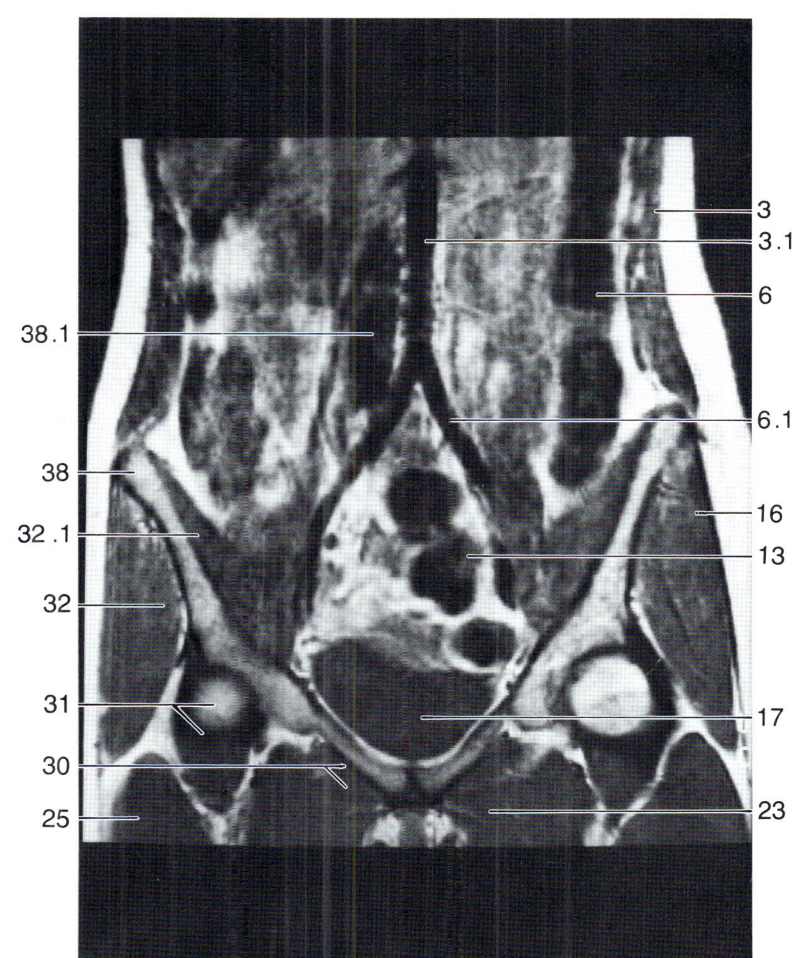

MRI, SE, $T_R/T_E = 0.5$ s/50 ms

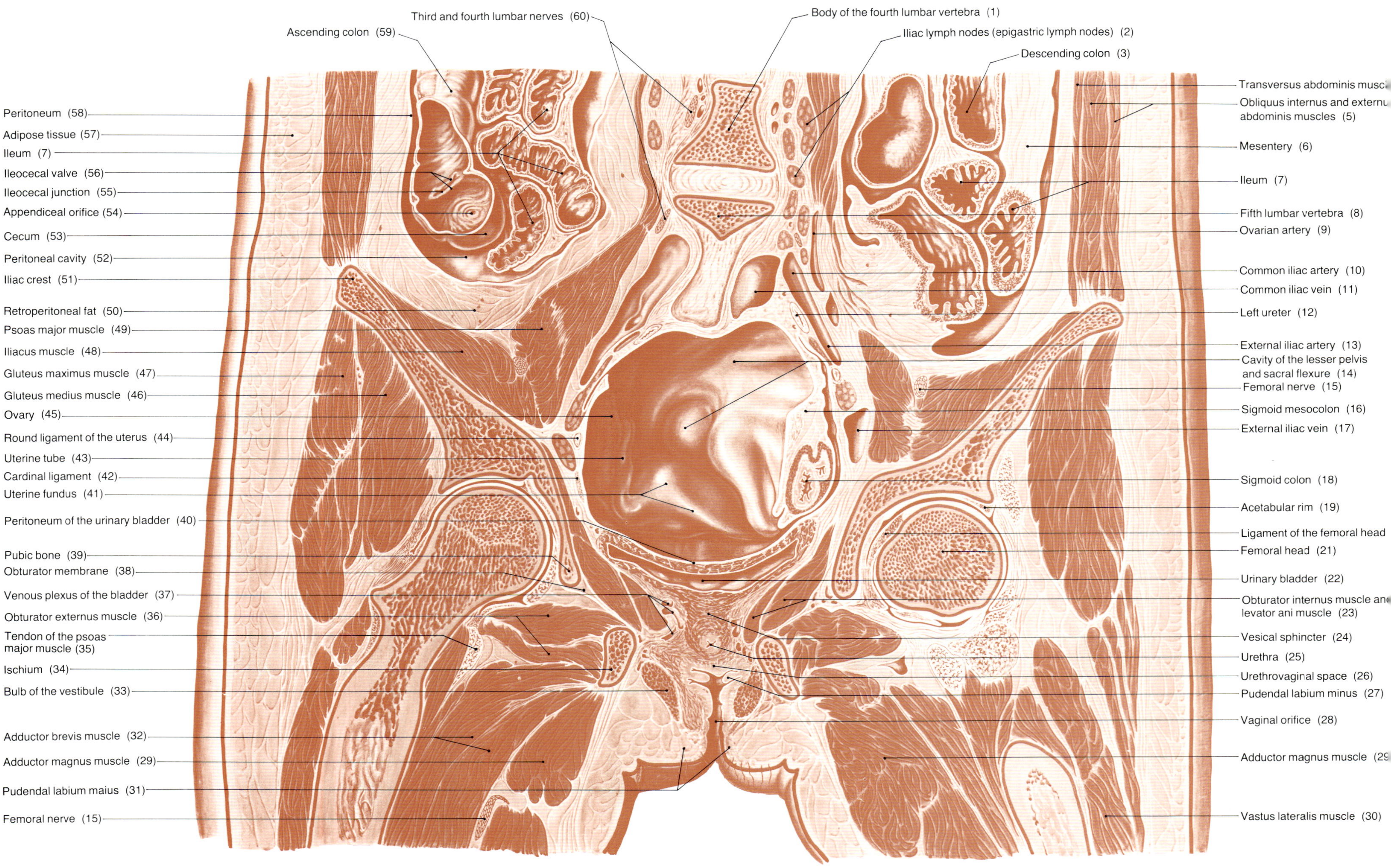

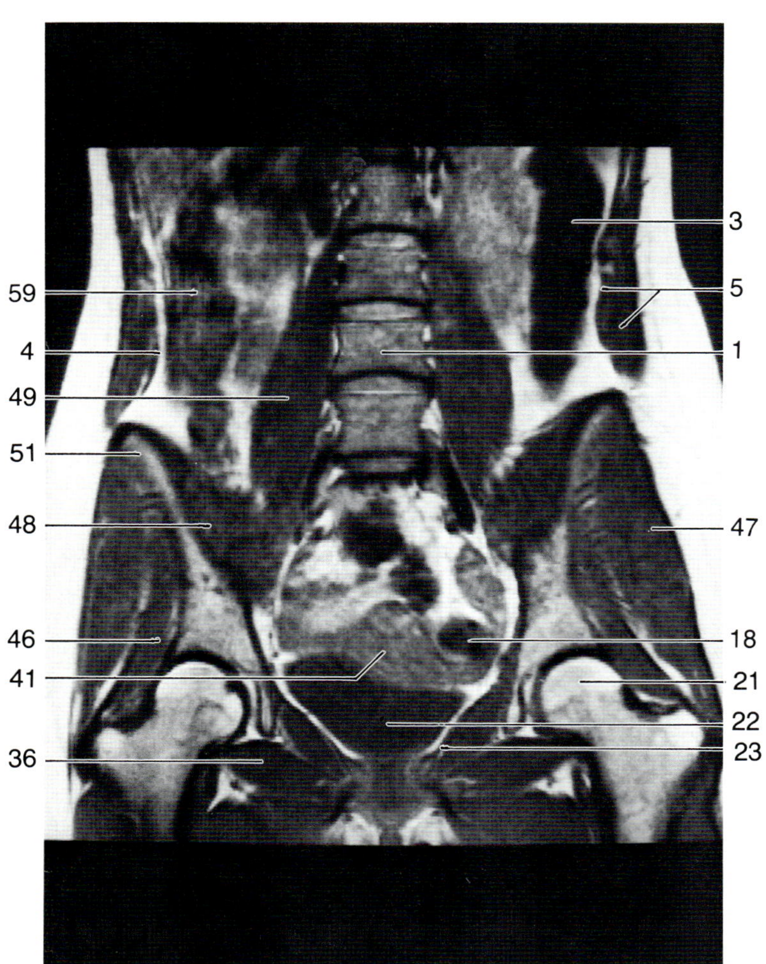

MRI, SE 2000/22

1 Corpus vertebrae lumbalis IV
2 Nodi lymphatici iliaci (Nodi lymphatici epigastrici)
3 Colon descendens
4 M. transversus abdominis
5 Mm. obliquus internus et externus abdominis
6 Mesenterium
7 Ileum
8 Vertebra lumbalis V
9 A. ovarica
10 A. iliaca communis
11 V. iliaca communis
12 Ureter sinister
13 A. iliaca externa
14 Cavum pelvis minoris et Flexura sacralis
15 N. femoralis
16 Mesocolon sigmoideum
17 V. iliaca externa
18 Colon sigmoideum
19 Labrum acetabulare
20 Lig. capitis femoris
21 Caput femoris
22 Vesica urinaria
23 Mm. obturatorius internus et levator ani
24 M. sphincter vesicae
25 Urethra
26 Spatium urethrovaginale
27 Labium minus pudendi
28 Ostium vaginae
29 M. adductor magnus
30 N. vastus lateralis
31 Labium majus pudendi
32 M. adductor brevis
33 Bulbus vestibuli
34 Os ischii
35 Tendo m. psoas majoris
36 M. obturatorius externus
37 Plexus venosus vesicalis
38 Membrana obturatoria
39 Os pubis
40 Peritoneum vesicae urinariae
41 Fundus uteri
42 Lig. cardinale
43 Tuba uterina
44 Lig. teres uteri
45 Ovarium
46 M. glutaeus medius
47 M. glutaeus maximus
48 M. iliacus
49 M. psoas major
50 Substantia adiposa retroperitonealis
51 Crista iliaca
52 Cavum peritonaeale
53 Caecum
54 Ostium appendicis vermiformis
55 Ostium ileocaecale
56 Valva ileocaecalis
57 Panniculus adiposus
58 Peritoneum
59 Colon ascendens
60 N. lumbalis III et IV

1 Body of the fourth lumbar vertebra
3 Descending colon
4 Transversus abdominis muscle
5 Obliquus internus and externus abdominis muscles
18 Sigmoid colon
21 Femoral head
22 Urinary bladder
23 Obturator internus muscle and levator ani muscle
36 Obturator externus muscle
41 Uterine fundus
46 Gluteus medius muscle
47 Gluteus maximus muscle
48 Iliacus muscle
49 Psoas major muscle
51 Iliac crest
59 Ascending colon

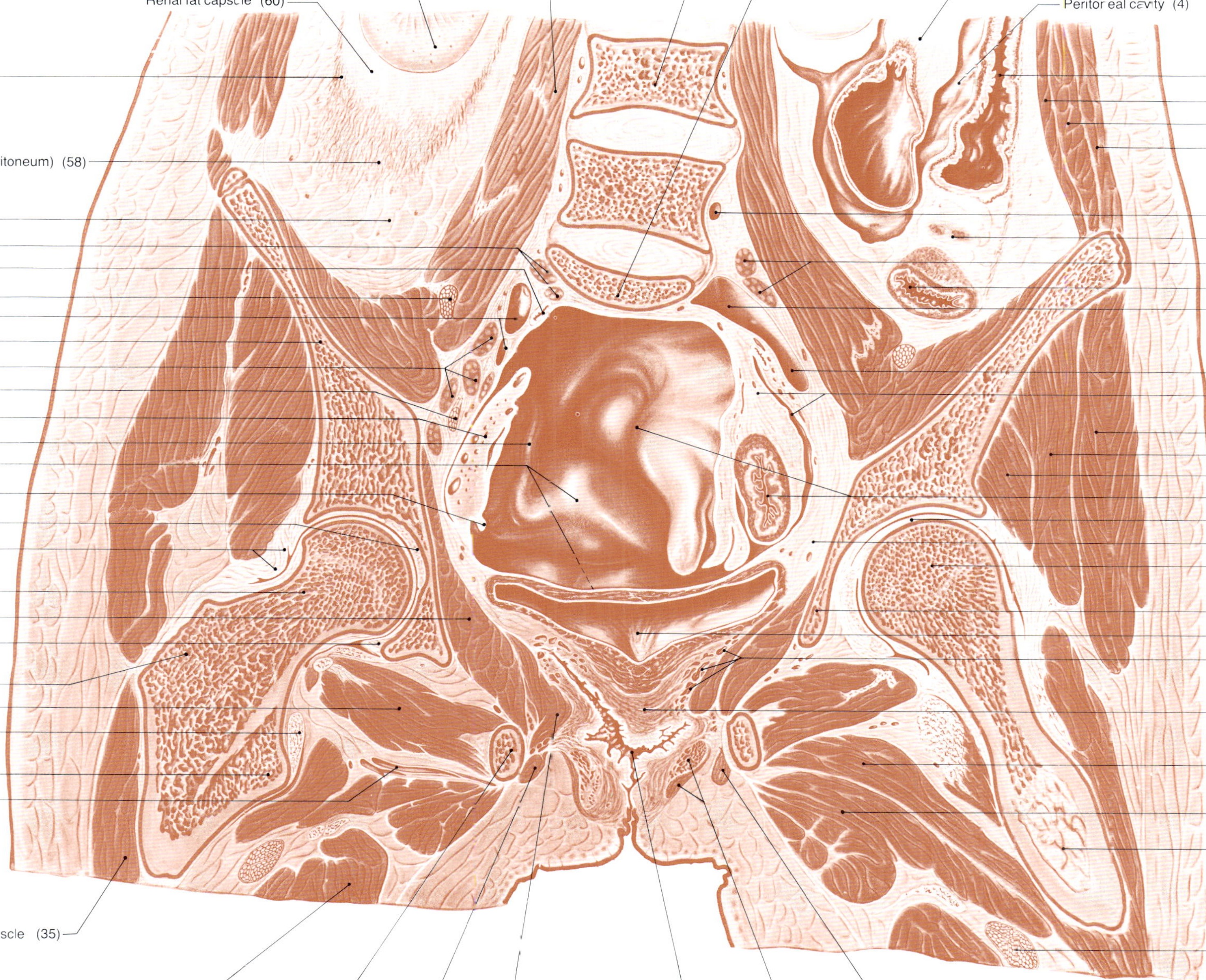

1 Vertebra lumbalis IV
2 Vertebra sacralis I, Os sacrum
3 Mesenterium
4 Cavum peritonaei
5 Colon descendens
6 M. transversus abdominis
7 M. obliquus internus abdominis
8 M. obliquus externus abdominis
9 V. lumbalis
10 Mesocolon descendens
11 Nodi lymphatici iliaci communes
12 V. iliaca communis
13 V. iliaca externa
14 Mesocolon sigmoideum et Recessus intersigmoideus
15 M. glutaeus maximus
16 M. glutaeus medius
17 M. glutaeus minimus
18 Colon sigmoideum
19 Capsula articularis coxae
20 Spatium vesicopudendale
21 Caput femoris
22 Os ischii
23 Vesica urinaria
24 Plexus venosus vesicalis
25 Spatium urethrovaginale
26 M. adductor brevis
27 M. adductor longus
28 Femur
29 N. ischiadicus
30 M. transversus perinei superficialis
31 Bulbus vestibuli et M. ischiocavernosus
32 Vagina
33 M. levator ani
34 M. adductor magnus
35 M. vastus lateralis
36 A. et V. circumflexa femoris medialis
37 Trochanter minor
38 Tendo m. psoas majoris
39 M. obturatorius externus
40 Trochanter major
41 Labium acetabulare
42 M. obturatorius internus
43 Collum femoris
44 Zona orbicularis et Lig. iliofemorale
45 Lig. capitis femoris
46 Lig. teres uteri
47 Fundus uteri et Excavatio vesicouterina
48 Tuba uterina
49 Ovarium
50 N. obturatorius
51 Nodi lymphatici iliaci
52 Os ilium
53 A. et V. iliaca interna
54 N. femoralis
55 Ureter
56 Nodus lymphaticus sacralis
57 Substantia adiposa retroperitonealis
58 Spatium fibrosum retroperitonealis (Retroperitoneum)
59 Fascia anterior renis
60 Capsula adiposa renis
61 Ren dexter
62 M. psoas major

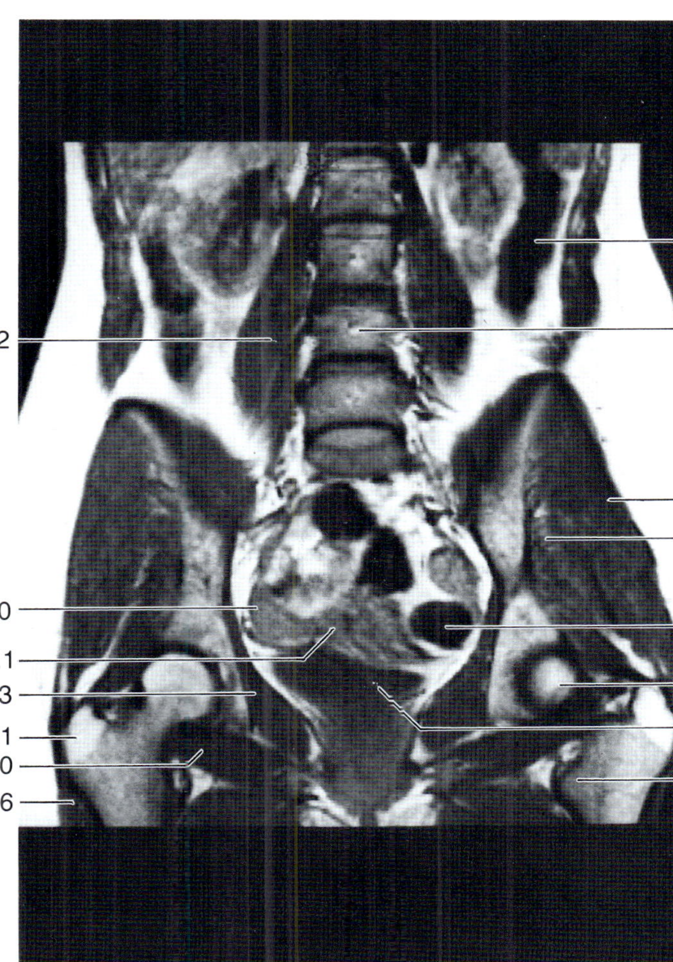

MRI, SE 2000/22

1 Fourth lumbar vertebra
5 Descending colon
15 Gluteus maximus muscle
17 Gluteus minimus muscle
18 Sigmoid colon
21 Head of the femur
22 Ischial bone
23 Urinary bladder
36 Vastus lateralis muscle
38 Lesser trochanter
40 Obturator externus muscle
41 Greater trochanter
43 Obturator internus muscle
43.1 Uterus
50 Ovary
62 Psoas major muscle

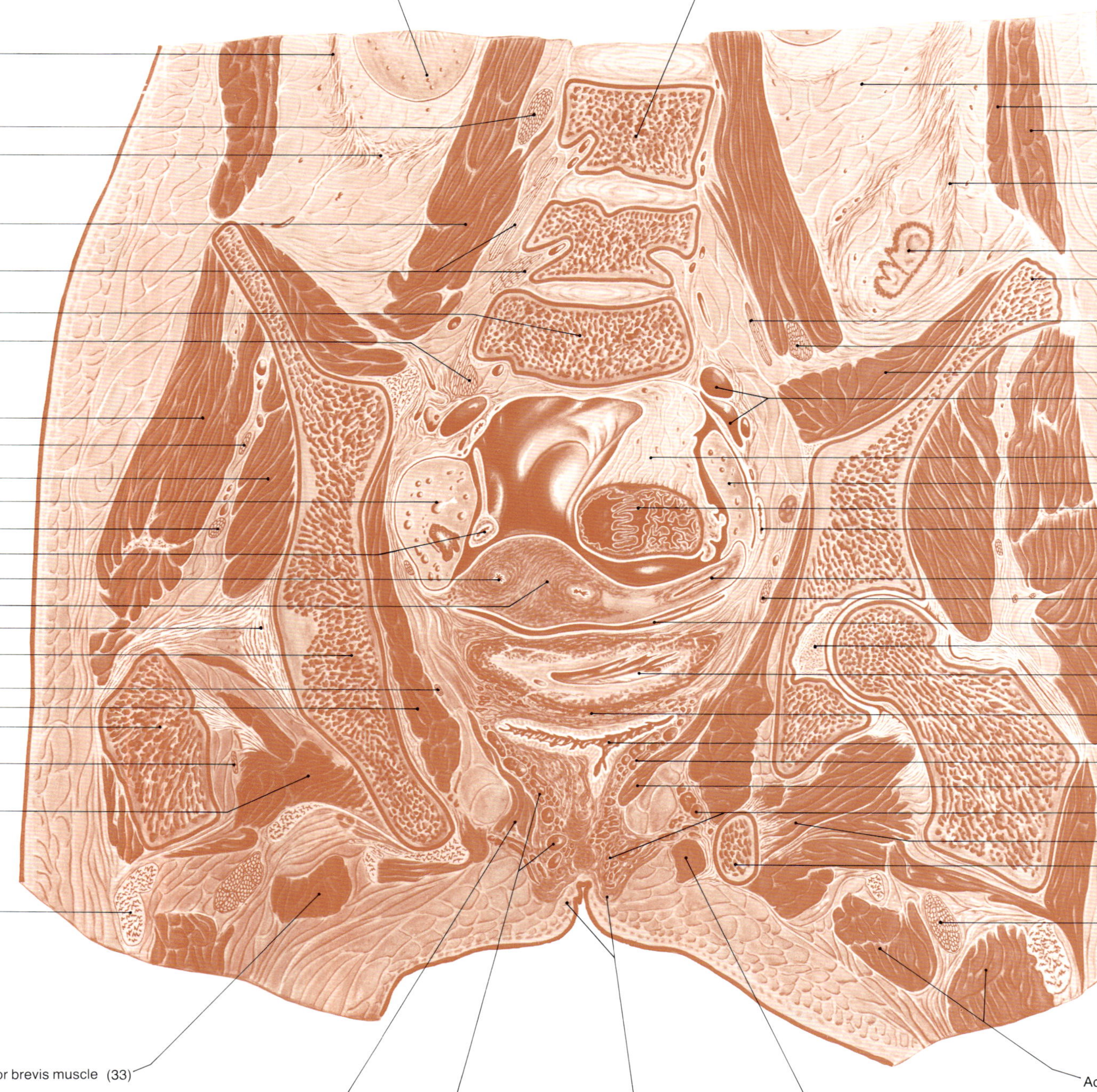

1 Vertebra lumbalis IV
2 Substantia adiposa retroperitonealis
3 M. transversus abdominis
4 M. obliquus internus
5 Area fibrosa (c. descendens)
6 Colon descendens
7 Crista iliaca
7.1 Cauda equina
8 N. genitofemoralis
9 N. femoralis
10 M. iliacus
11 A. et V. iliaca interna
12 Mesocolon sigmoideum
13 Ovarium sinistrum
14 Colon sigmoideum et Ampulla recti
15 Ureter sinister
16 Isthmus tubae uterinae
17 N. obturatorius
18 Excavatio vesicouterina
19 Lig. capitis femoris
20 Fornix vaginae
21 Tunica muscularis vaginae
22 Vagina
23 Plexus venosus bulbi vestibuli
24 Diaphragma pelvis
25 Corpus cavernosum clitoridis
26 M. obturatorius externus
27 Tuber ischiadicum
28 N. ischiadicus
29 Mm. adductor longus et brevis
30 M. transversus perinei superficialis
31 Perineum
32 M. levator ani
33 M. adductor brevis
34 Tendo m. vasti lateralis
35 M. piriformis
36 R. muscularis n. femoralis
37 Trochanter major
38 M. obturatorius internus
39 Corpus ossis ilii
40 Lig. iliofemorale
41 Corpus uteri
42 Ostium uterinum tubae
43 Ureter dexter
44 N. glutaeus inferior
45 Ovarium dextrum
46 M. glutaeus medius
47 N. glutaeus superior
48 M. glutaeus maximus
49 Nn. genitofemoralis et femoralis
50 Sacrum
51 Nn. lumbalis III et IV
52 M. psoas major
53 Spatium fibrosum retroperitoneale
54 N. lumbalis II
55 Fascia anterior renis
56 Ren dexter

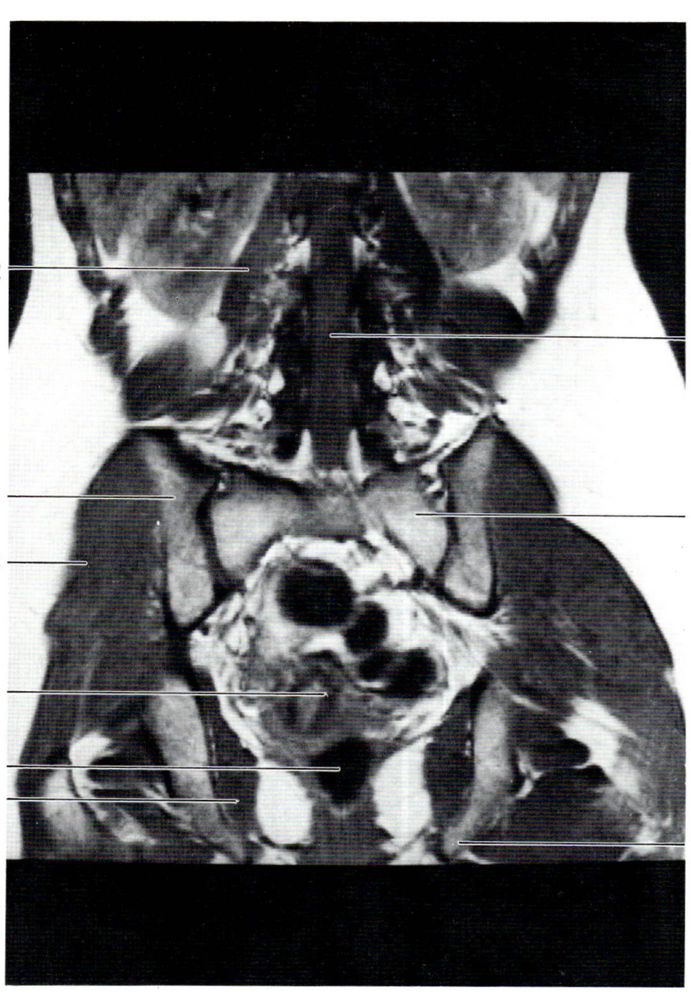

MRI, SE 2000/22

7.1 Cauda equina
20.1 Rectum
27 Ischial tuberosity
38 Obturator internus muscle
39 Body of the ilium
41 Corpus uteri
48 Gluteus maximus muscle
50 Sacrum
52 Psoas major muscle

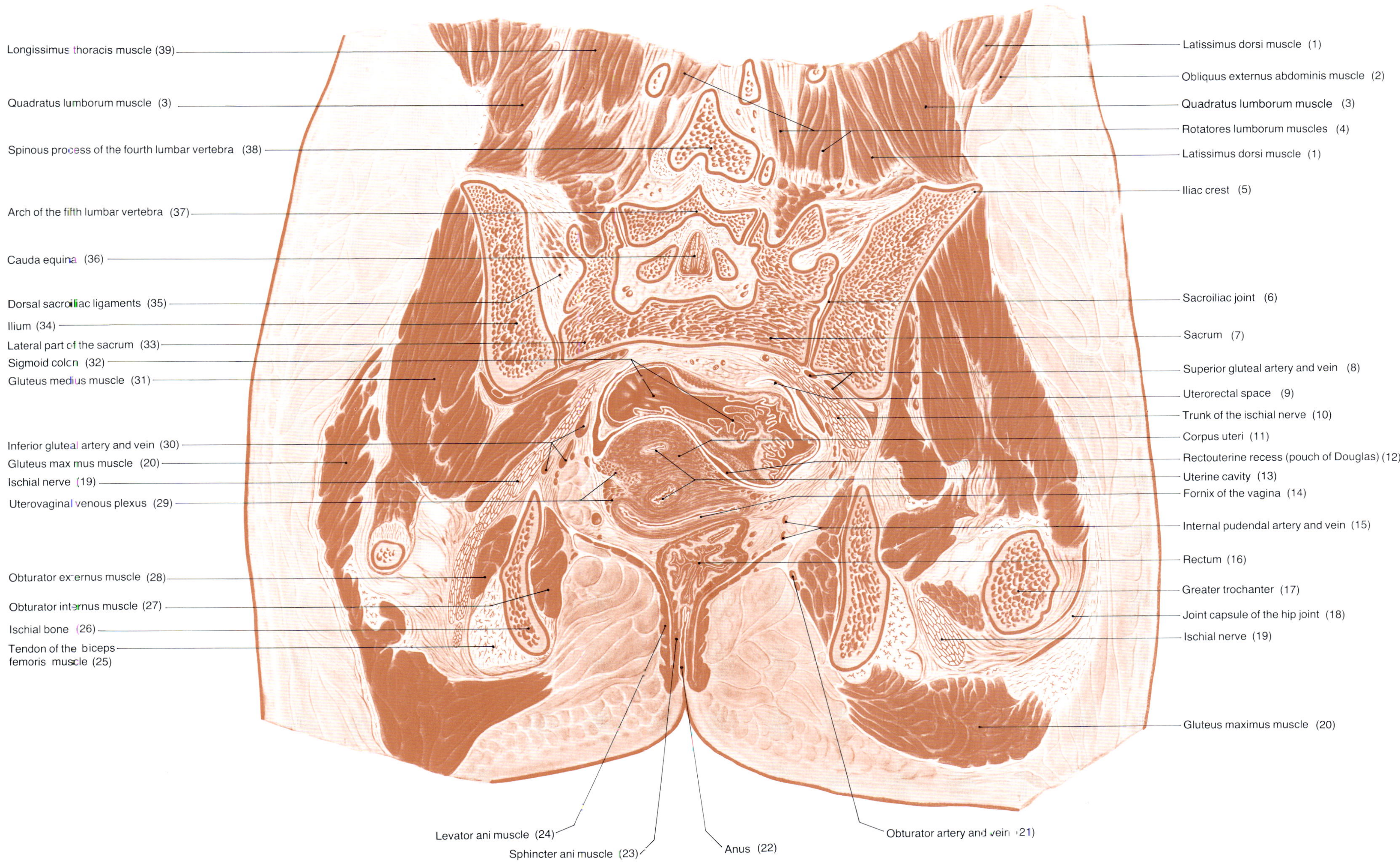

1 M. latissimus dorsi
2 M. obliquus externus abdominis
3 M. quadratus lumborum
4 Mm. rotatores lumborum
5 Crista iliaca
6 Articulatio sacroiliaca
7 Os sacrum
8 A. et V. glutaea superior
9 Spatium retrorectale
10 Truncus n. ischiadici
11 Corpus uteri
12 Excavatio rectouterina (Cavum Douglasi)
13 Cavum uteri
14 Fornix vaginae
15 A. et V. pudenda interna
16 Rectum
17 Trochanter major
18 Capsula articularis coxae
19 N. ischiadicus
20 M. glutaeus maximus
21 A. et V. obturatoria
22 Anus
23 M. sphincter ani
24 M. levator ani
25 Tendo m. bicipitis femoris
26 Os ischii
27 M. obturatorius internus
28 M. obturatorius externus
29 Plexus venosus uterovaginalis
30 A. et V. glutaea inferior
31 M. glutaeus medius
32 Colon sigmoideum et Ampulla recti
33 Pars lateralis ossis sacri
34 Os ilium
35 Ligg. sacroiliaca dorsalia
36 Cauda equina
37 Arcus vertebrae lumbalis V
38 Processus spinosus vertebrae lumbalis IV
39 M. longissimus thoracis

3 Quadratus lumborum muscle
5 Iliac crest
6 Sacroiliac joint
7 Sacrum
11 Corpus uteri
16 Rectum
27 Obturator internus muscle
28 Obturator externus muscle
31 Gluteus medius muscle
32 Sigmoid colon
34 Ilium
39 Longissimus thoracis muscle

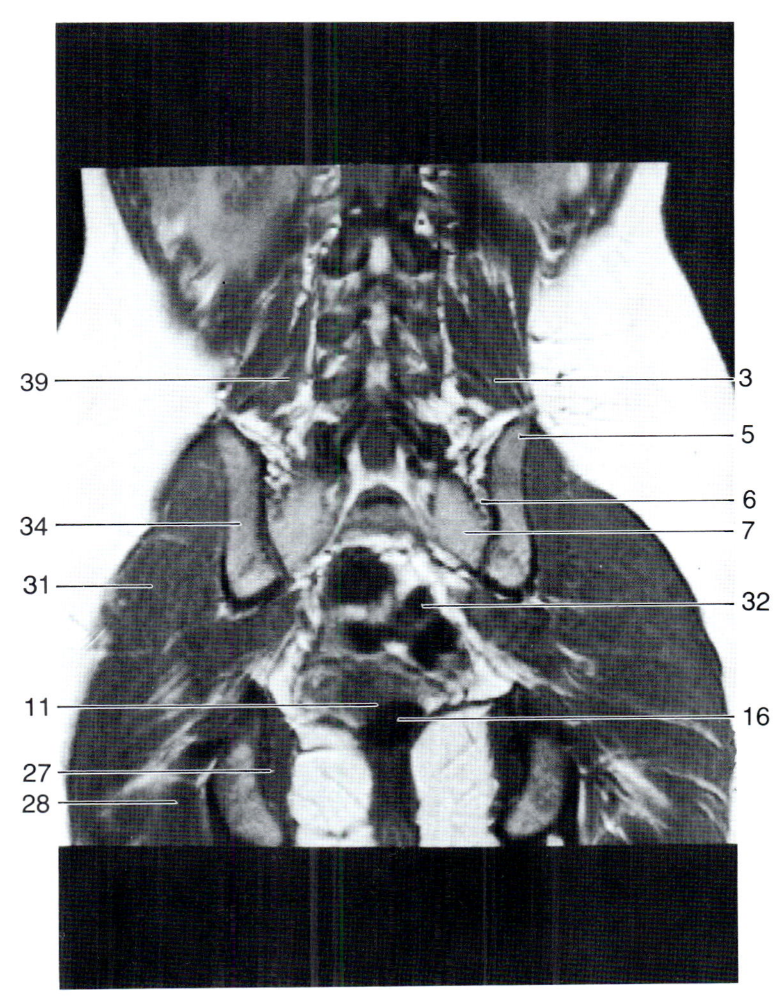

MRI, SE 2000/22

Axial Sections of the Female Pelvis

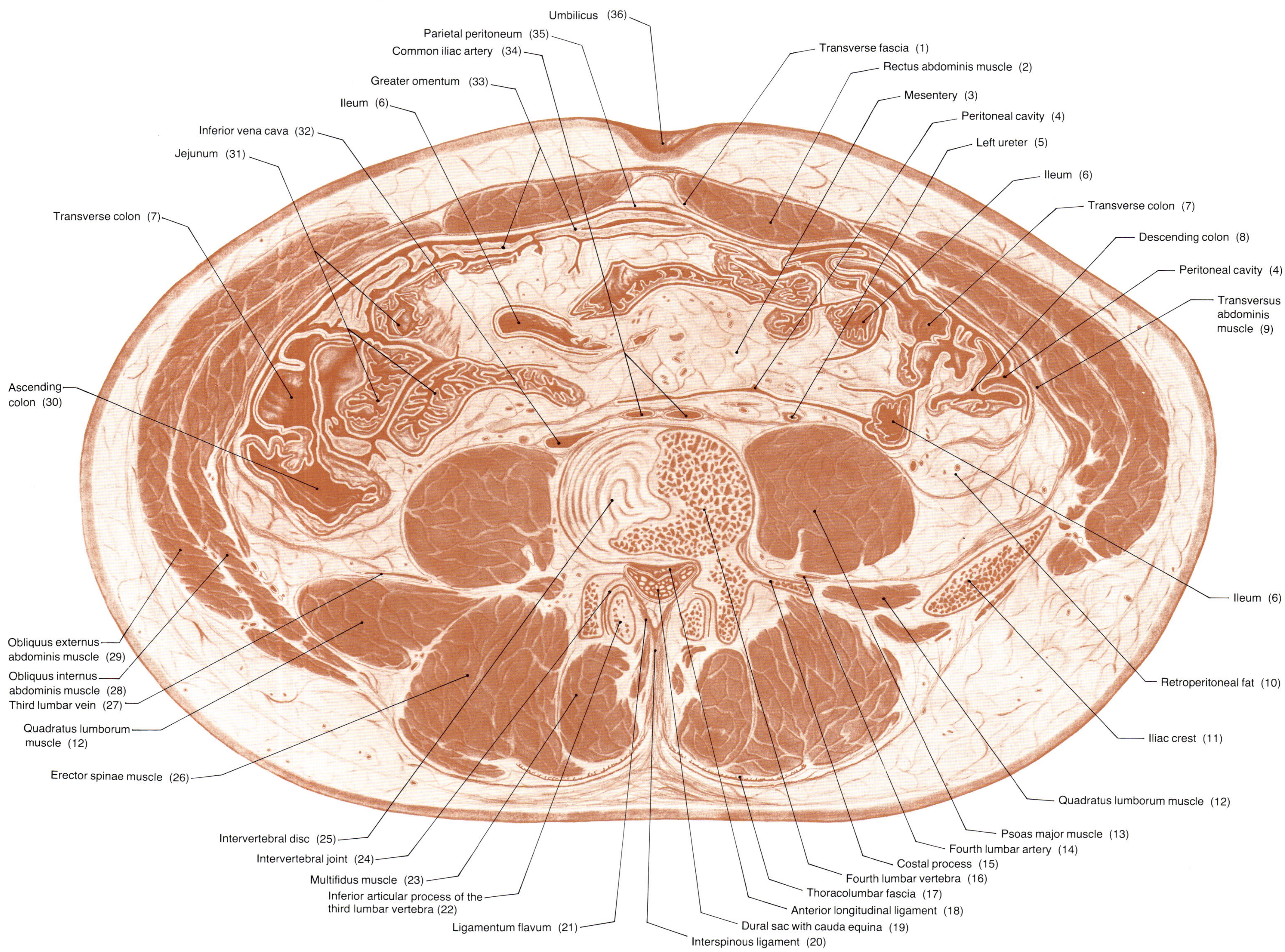

1 Fascia transversalis
2 M. rectus abdominis
3 Mesenterium
4 Cavitas peritonealis
5 Ureter sinister
6 Ileum
7 Colon transversum
8 Colon descendens
9 M. transversus abdominis
10 Corpus adiposum retroperitoneale
11 Crista iliaca
12 M. quadratus lumborum
13 M. psoas major
14 A. lumbalis IV
15 Processus costarius
16 Vertebra lumbalis IV
16.1 Processus transversus
16.2 Corpus vertebrae
16.3 V. basivertebralis
16.4 Radix arcus vertebrae
16.5 Lamina
16.6 Processus spinosus
16.7 Processus articularis inferior
16.8 Processus articularis superior
17 Fascia thoracolumbalis
18 Lig. longitudinale anterius
19 Spatium subdurale et Cauda equina
20 Lig. interspinale
21 Lig. flavum
22 Processus articularis inferior vertebrae lumbalis II
23 M. multifidus
24 Articulus intervertebralis
25 Discus intervertebralis
26 M. erector spinae
27 V. lumbalis III
28 M. obliquus internus abdominis
29 M. obliquus externus abdominis
30 Colon ascendens
31 Jejunum
32 V. cava inferior
33 Omentum majus
34 A. iliaca communis
35 Peritoneum parietale
36 Umbilicus

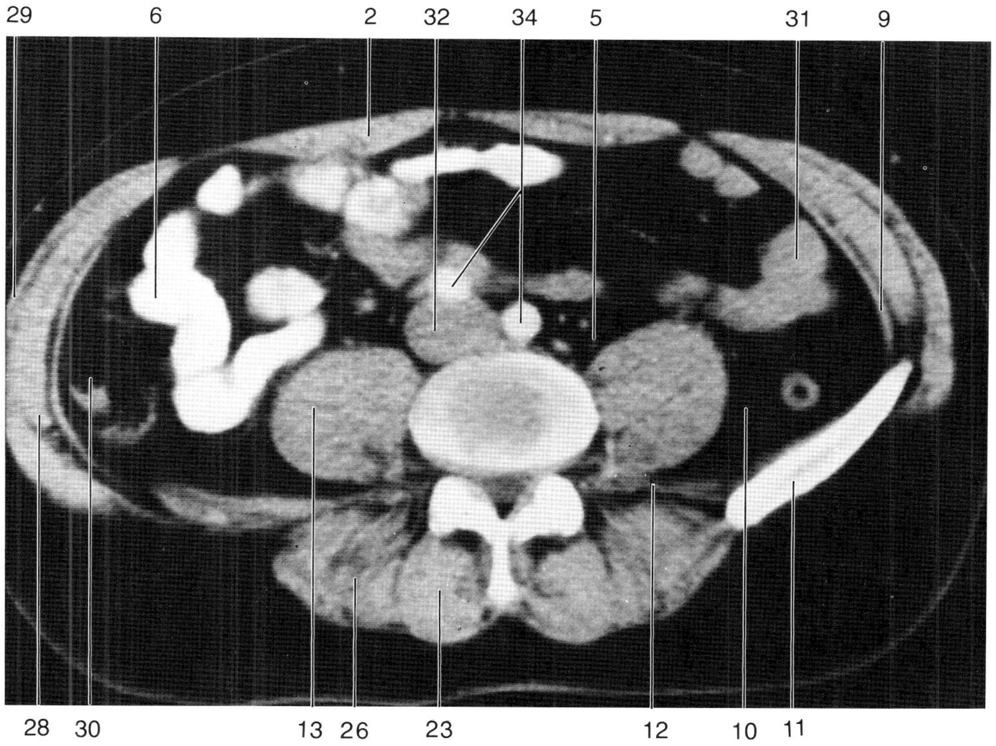

CT with contrast medium in the small bowel and after i.v. bolus injection of contrast medium

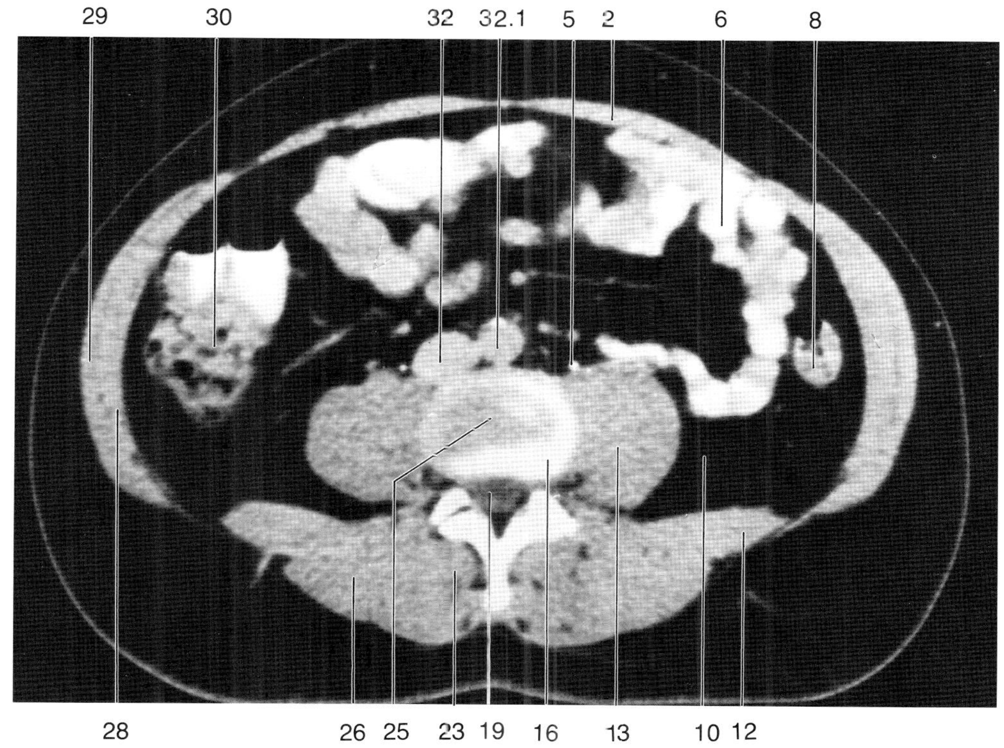

CT with contrast medium in the small bowel and colon

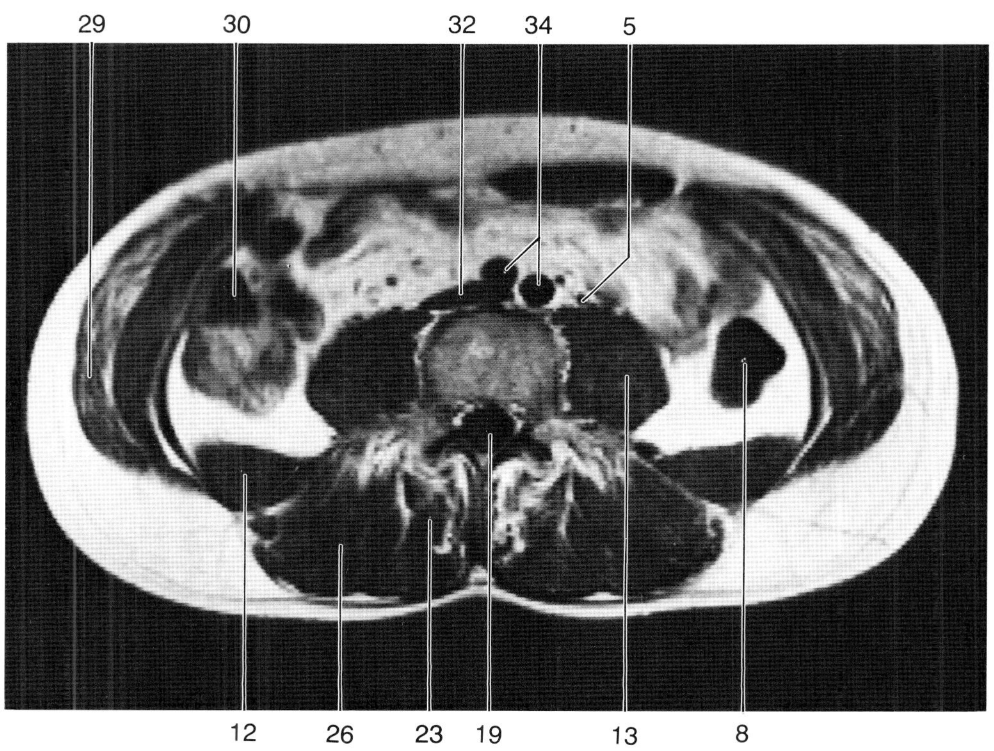

MRI, SE 800/22

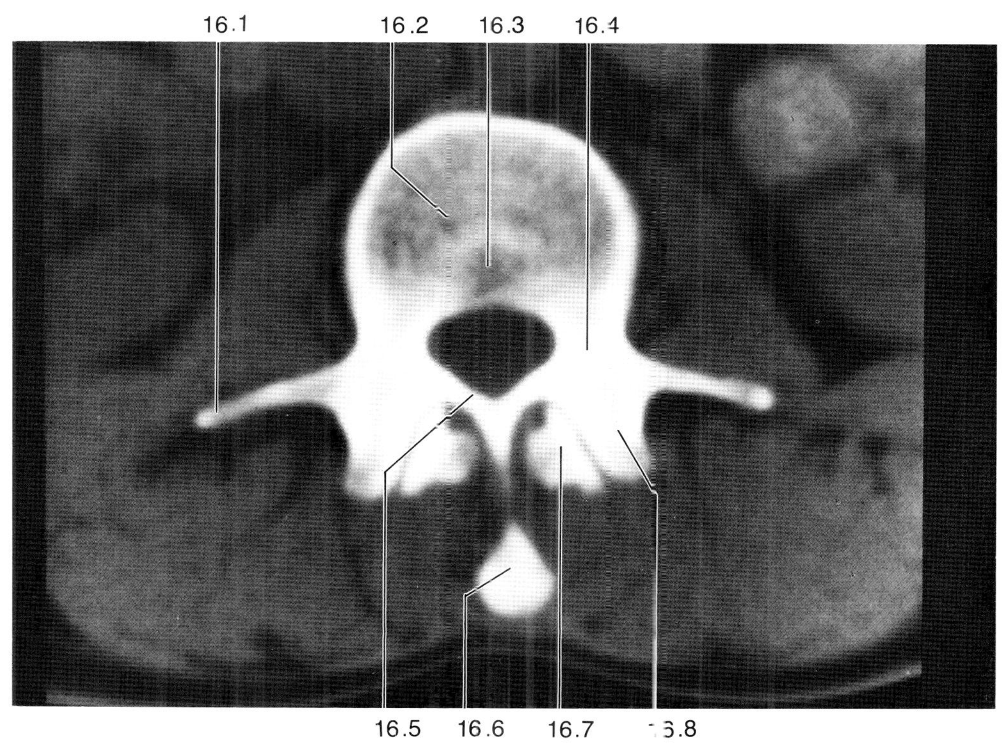

CT section of a lumbar vertebra

2 Rectus abdominis muscle
5 Left ureter
6 Ileum
8 Descending colon
9 Transversus abdominis muscle
10 Retroperitoneal fat
11 Iliac crest
12 Quadratus lumborum muscle
13 Psoas major muscle
16 Fourth lumbar vertebra
16.1 Transverse process
16.2 Vertebral body
16.3 Basivertebral veins
16.4 Vertebral pedicle
16.5 Lamina
16.6 Spinous process
16.7 Inferior articular process
16.8 Superior articular process
19 Dural sac with cauda equina
23 Multifidus muscle
25 Intervertebral disc
26 Erector spinae muscle
28 Obliquus internus abdominis muscle
29 Obliquus externus abdominis muscle
30 Ascending colon
31 Jejunum
32 Inferior vena cava
32.1 Abdominal aorta
34 Common iliac artery

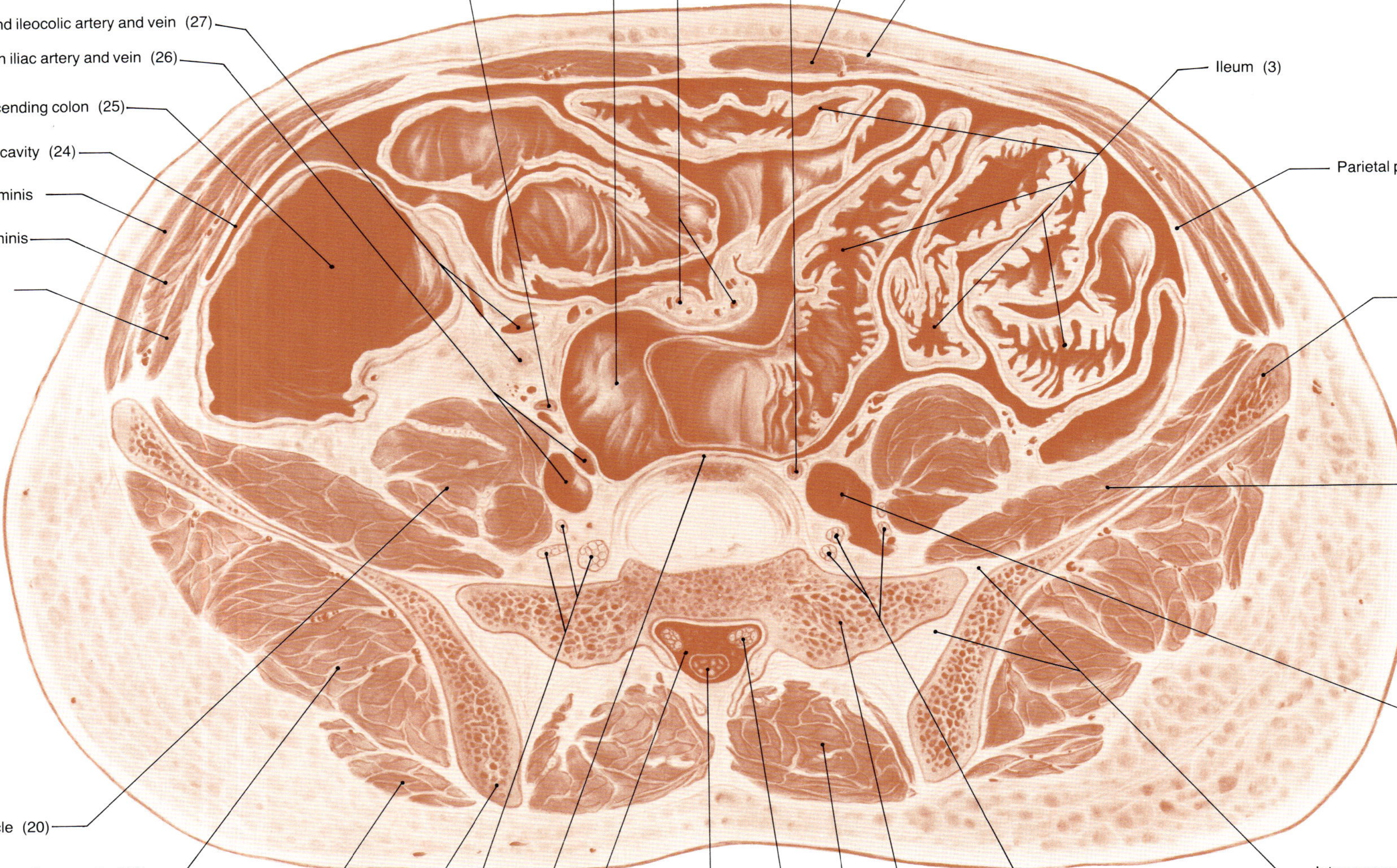

1 M. rectus abdominis
2 Lamina anterior, Vagina m. recti abdominis
3 Ileum
4 Peritoneum parietale
5 Os ilium
6 M. iliacus
7 A. et V. iliaca communis sinistra
8 Ligg. sacroiliaca interossea
9 N. lumbalis III et IV et N. genitofemoralis et N. cutaneus femoris lateralis
10 Os sacrum
11 M. erector spinae
12 Ganglion spinale n. sacralis I
13 Spatium subdurale et Cauda equina
14 Canalis sacralis, Spatium extradurale
15 Promontorium
16 Truncus lumbosacralis et N. femoralis et N. obturatorius
17 Spina iliaca posterior superior
18 M. glutaeus maximus
19 M. glutaeus medius
20 M. psoas major
21 M. transversus abdominis
22 M. obliquus internus abdominis
23 M. obliquus externus abdominis
24 Cavitas peritonealis anterius
25 Colon ascendens
26 A. et V. iliaca communis
27 Radix mesenterii et A. et V. ileocolica
28 Ureter dexter et A. et V. ovarica
29 Mesocolon sigmoideum
30 Mesenterium et Vasa ileocolica
31 Ureter sinister

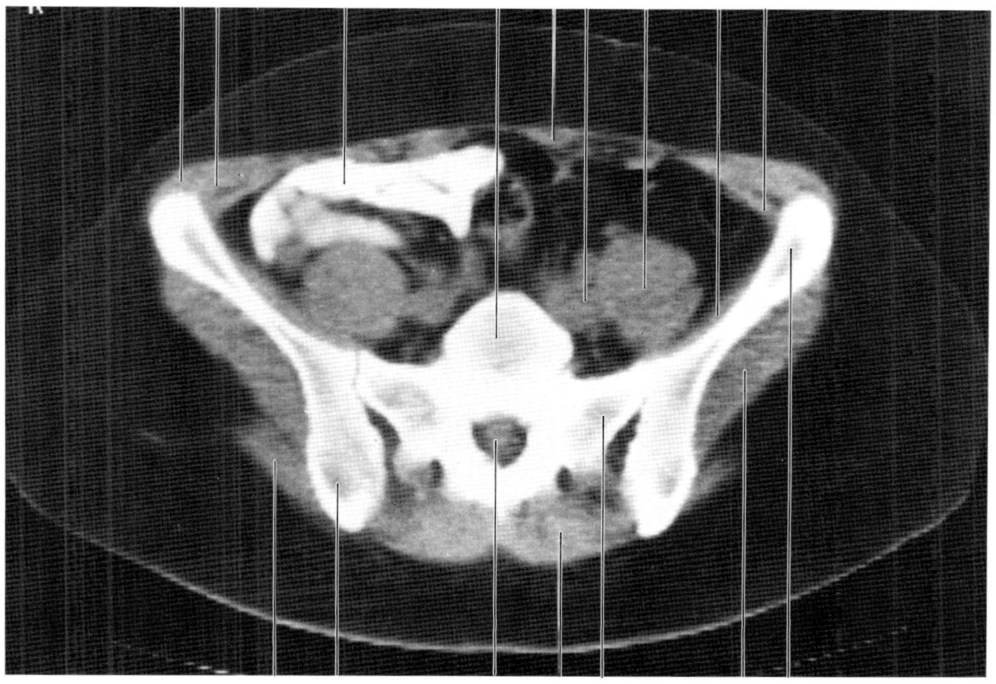

CT with contrast medium in the small bowel

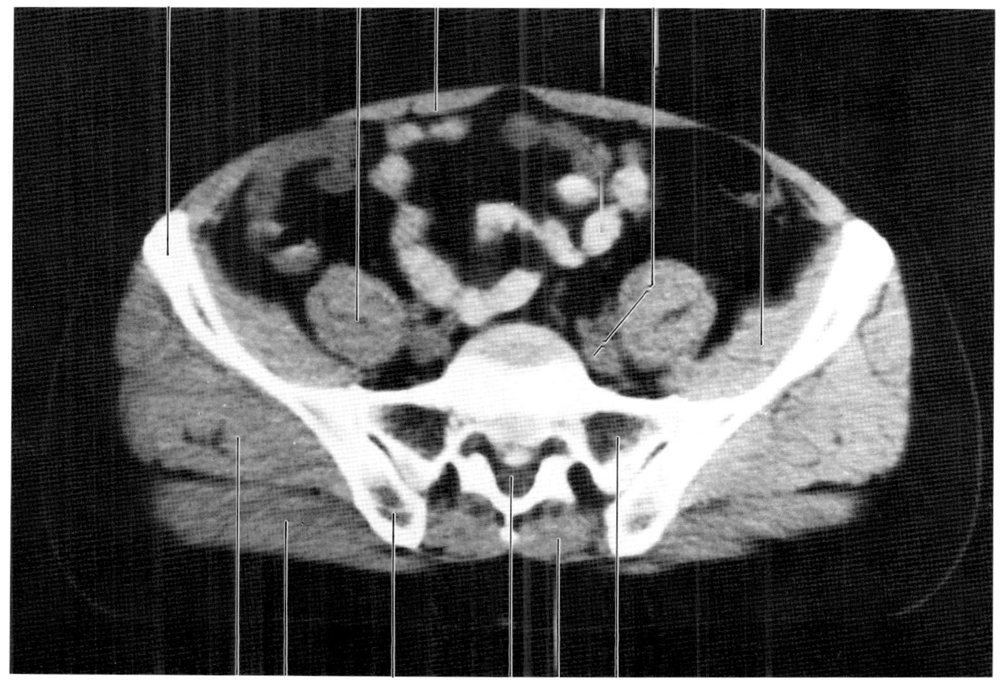

CT with contrast medium in the small bowel

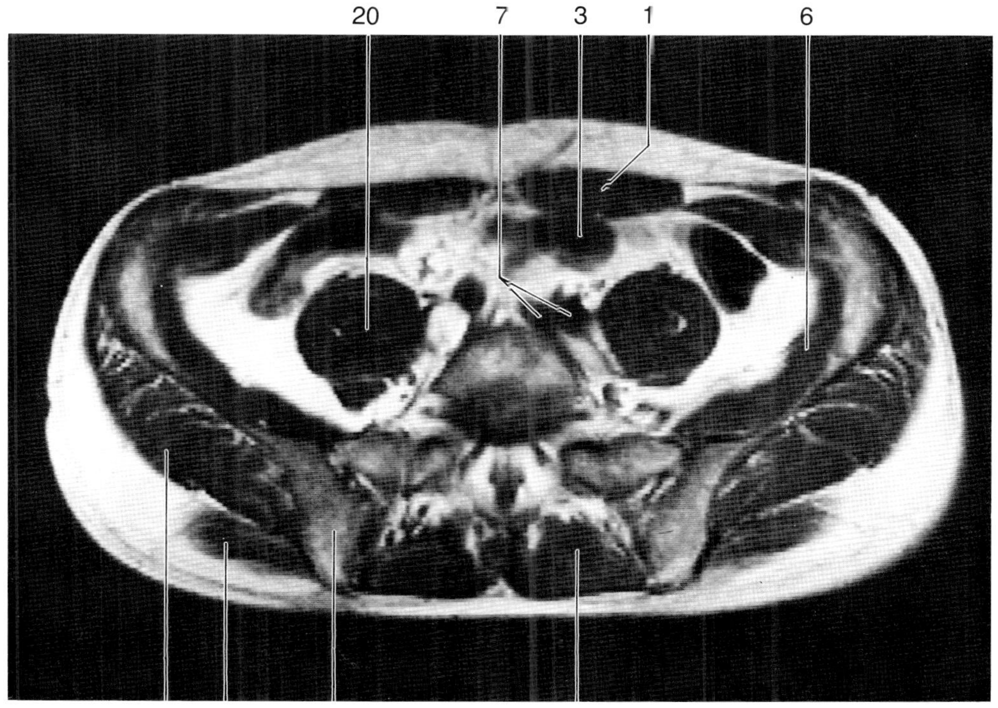

MRI, SE 800/22

1 Rectus abdominis muscle
3 Ileum
5 Ilium
6 Iliacus muscle
7 Left common iliac artery and vein
10 Sacrum
11 Erector spinae muscle
13 Dural sac with cauda equina
15 Promontory
17 Posterior superior iliac spine
18 Gluteus maximus muscle
19 Gluteus medius muscle
20 Psoas major muscle
21 Transversus abdominis muscle
22 Obliquus internus abdominis muscle
23 Obliquus externus abdominis muscle

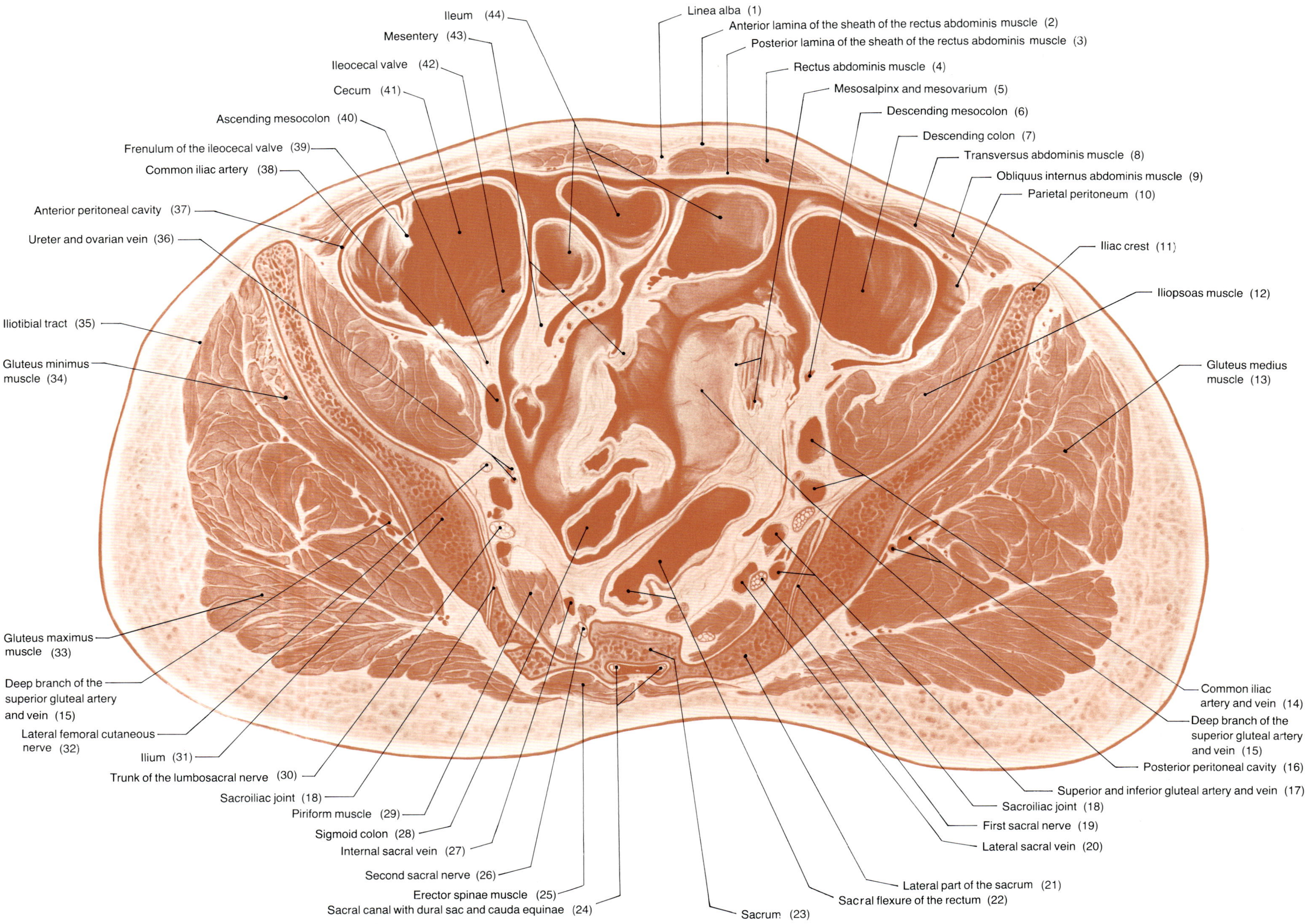

1 Linea alba
2 Vagina m. recti abdominis, Lamina anterior
3 Vagina m. recti abdominis, Lamina posterior
4 M. rectus abdominis
5 Mesosalpinx et Mesovarium
6 Mesocolon descendens
7 Colon descendens
8 M. transversus abdominis
9 M. obliquus internus abdominis
10 Peritoneum parietale
11 Crista iliaca
12 M. iliopsoas
13 M. glutaeus medius
14 A. et V. iliaca communis
15 R. profundus A. et V. glutaea superior
16 Cavitas peritonealis posterior
17 A. et V. glutaea superior et inferior
18 Articulatio sacroiliaca
19 N. sacralis I
20 V. sacralis lateralis
21 Pars lateralis ossis sacri
22 Flexura sacralis recti
23 Os sacrum
24 Canalis sacralis et Cauda equina
25 M. erector spinae
26 N. sacralis II
27 V. sacralis interna
28 Colon sigmoideum
29 M. piriformis
30 Truncus n. lumbosacralis
31 Os ilium
32 N. cutaneus femoris lateralis
33 M. glutaeus maximus
34 M. glutaeus minimus
35 Tractus iliotibialis
36 Ureter et V. ovarica
37 Cavitas peritonealis anterior
38 A. iliaca communis
39 Frenulum valvae ileocaecalis
40 Mesocolon ascendens
41 Caecum
42 Valva ileocaecalis
43 Mesenterium
44 Ileum

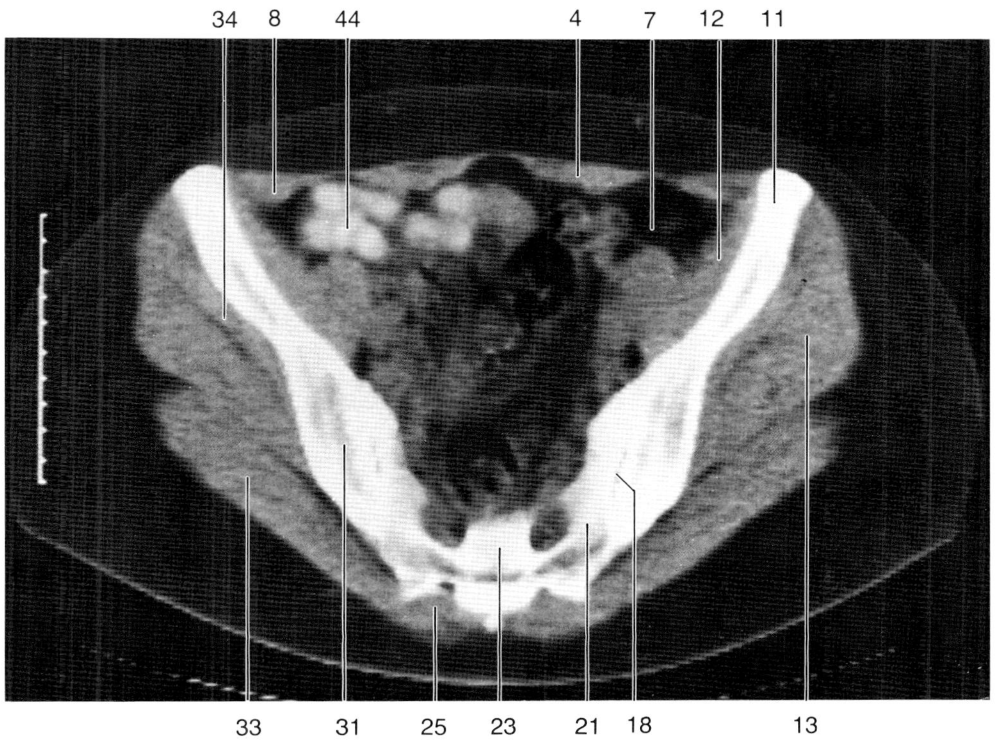

CT with contrast medium in the small bowel

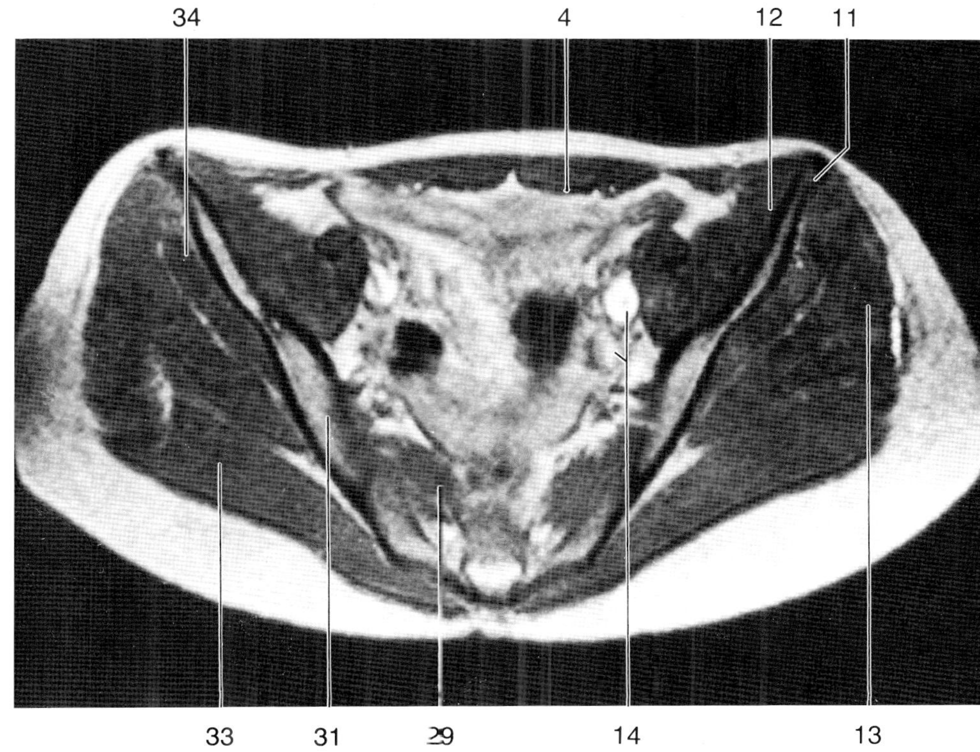

MRI, SE, ECG triggered, $T_E = 30$

4 Rectus abdominis muscle
7 Descending colon
8 Transversus abdominis muscle
11 Iliac crest
12 Iliopsoas muscle
13 Gluteus medius muscle
14 Common iliac artery and vein
18 Sacroiliac joint
21 Lateral part of the sacrum
23 Sacrum
25 Erector spinae muscle
29 Piriform muscle
31 Ilium
33 Gluteus maximus muscle
34 Gluteus minimus muscle
44 Ileum

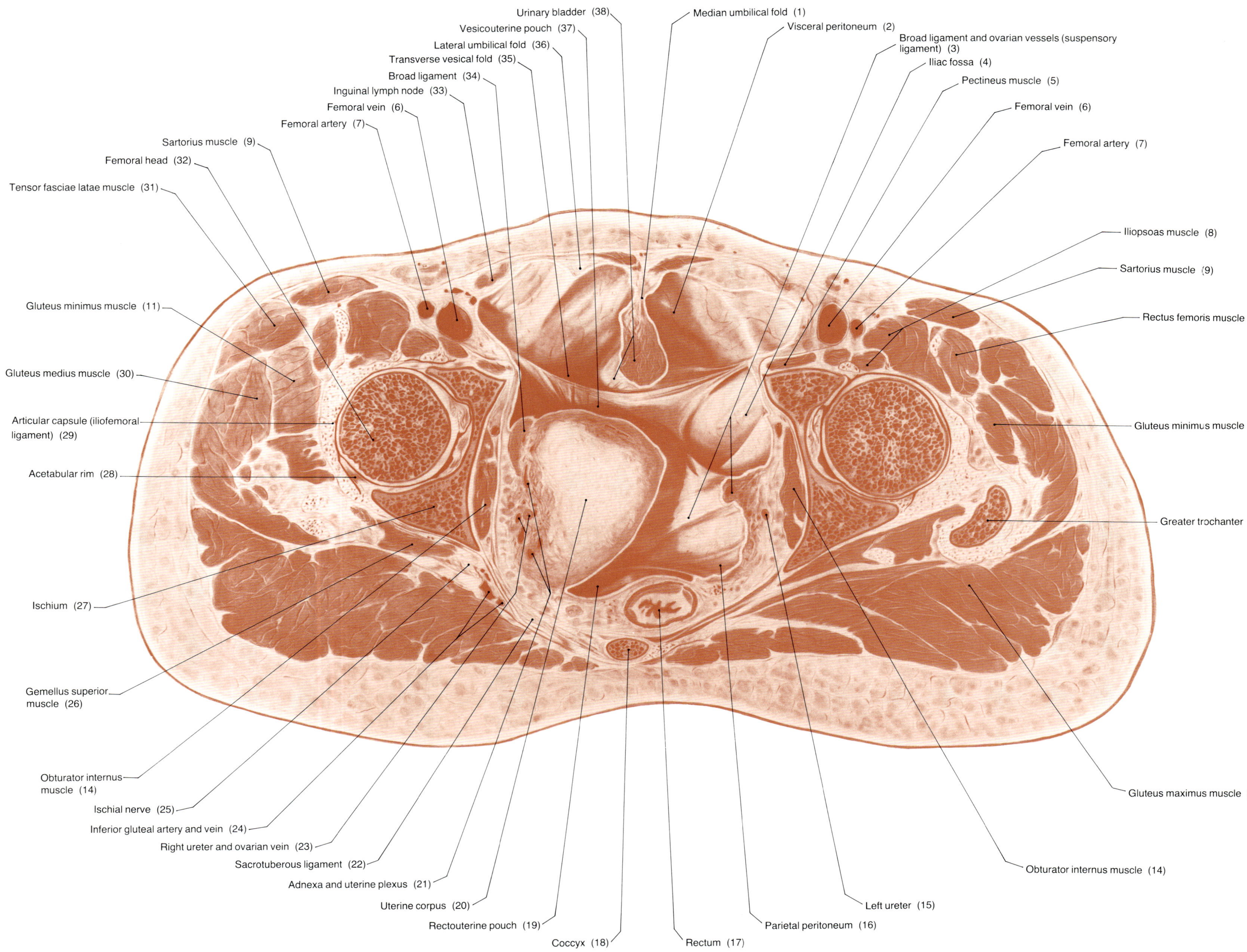

1 Plica umbilicalis mediana
2 Peritoneum viscerale
3 Lig. latum et Vasa ovarica (Lig. suspensorium)
4 Fossa iliaca
5 M. pectineus
6 V. femoralis
7 A. femoralis
8 M. iliopsoas
8.1 Fossa acetabuli
9 M. sartorius
10 M. rectus femoris
11 M. glutaeus minimus
12 Trochanter major
13 M. glutaeus maximus
14 M. obturatorius internus
15 Ureter sinister
16 Peritoneum parietale
17 Rectum
18 Os coccygis
19 Excavatio rectouterina
20 Corpus uteri
20.1 Colon sigmoideum
21 Adnexa et plexus uteri
22 Lig. sacrotuberale
23 Ureter dexter et V. ovarica
24 A. et V. glutaea inferior
25 N. ischiadicus
26 M. gemellus superior
27 Os ischii
28 Labrum acetabulare
29 Capsula articularis (Lig. iliofemorale)
30 M. glutaeus medius
31 M. tensor fasciae latae
32 Caput femoris
32.1 Os pubis
33 Lymphonodus inguinalis
34 Lig. latum
35 Plica vesicalis transversa
36 Plica umbilicalis lateralis
37 Excavatio vesicouterina
38 Vesica urinaria
38.1 Ileum

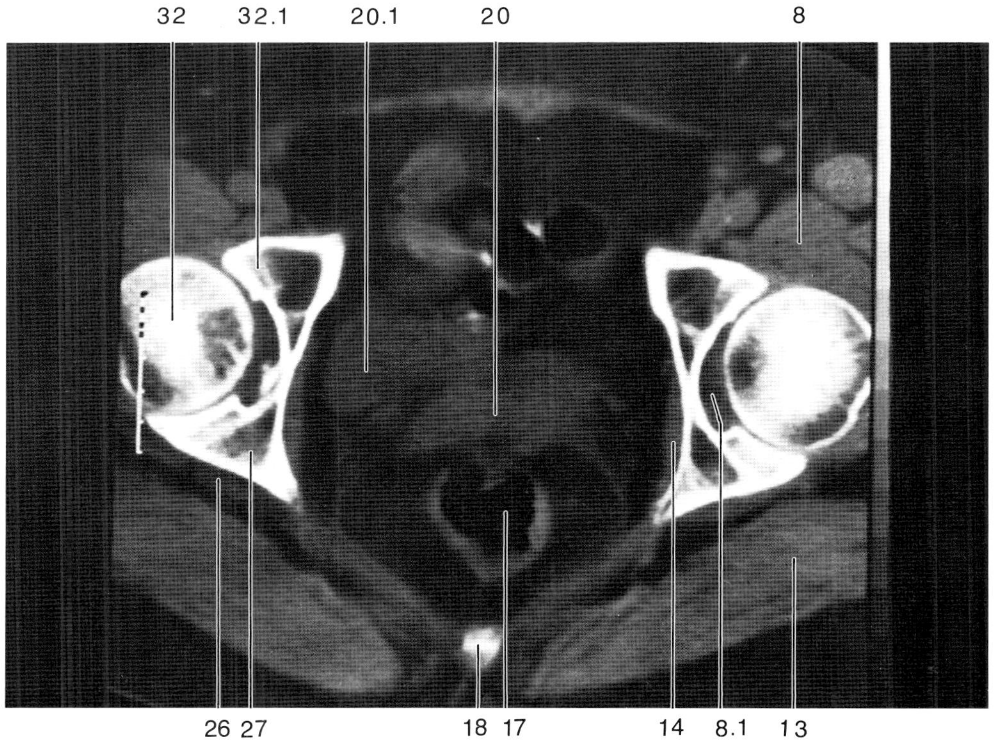

CT scan, unenhanced

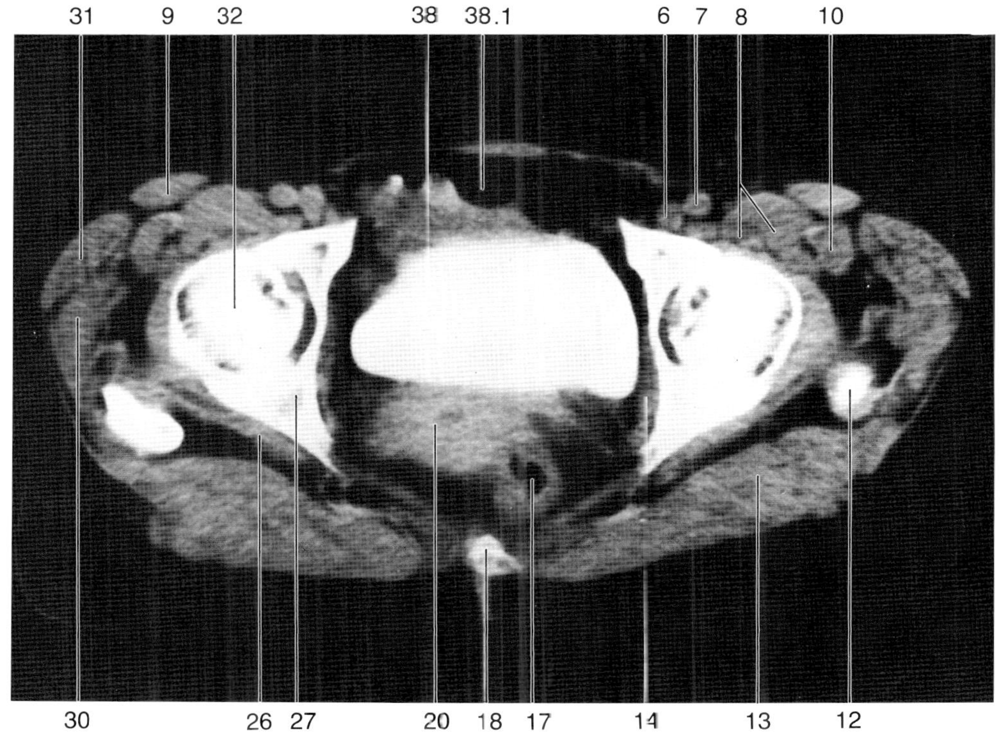

CT, enhanced after injection of contrast medium

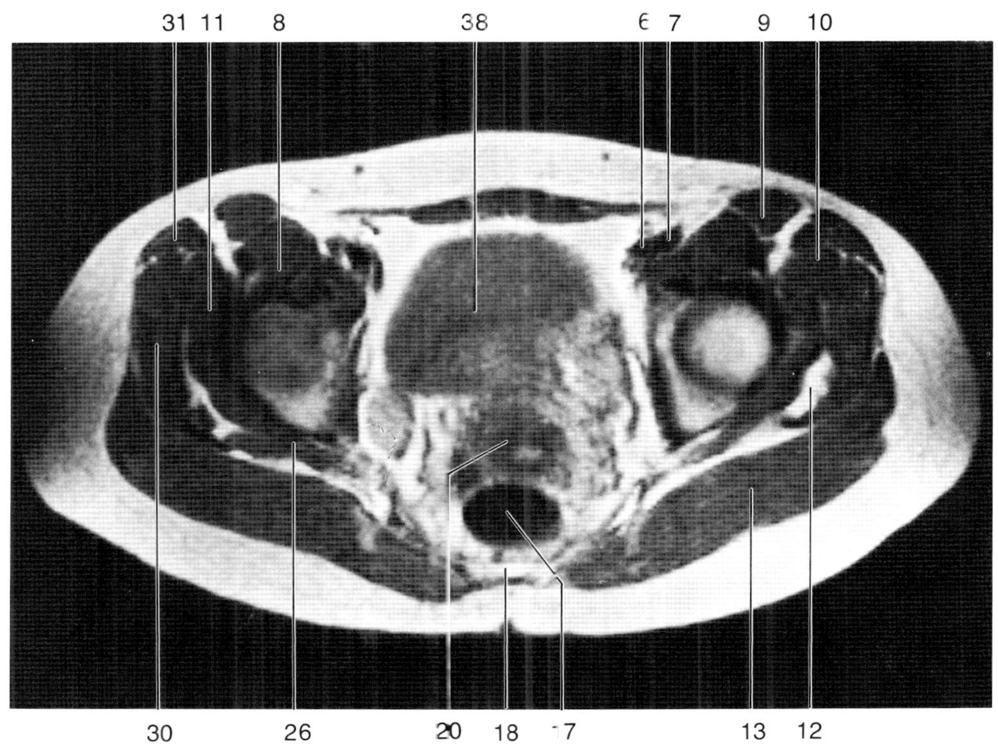

MRI, SE 500/50

6 Femoral vein
7 Femoral artery
8 Iliopsoas muscle
8.1 Acetabular fossa
9 Sartorius muscle
10 Rectus femoris muscle
11 Gluteus minimus muscle
12 Greater trochanter
13 Gluteus maximus muscle
14 Obturator internus muscle
17 Rectum
18 Coccyx
20 Uterine corpus
20.1 Sigmoid colon
26 Gemellus superior muscle
27 Ischium
30 Gluteus medius muscle
31 Tensor fasciae latae muscle
32 Femoral head
32.1 Pubic bone
38 Urinary bladder
38.1 Ileum

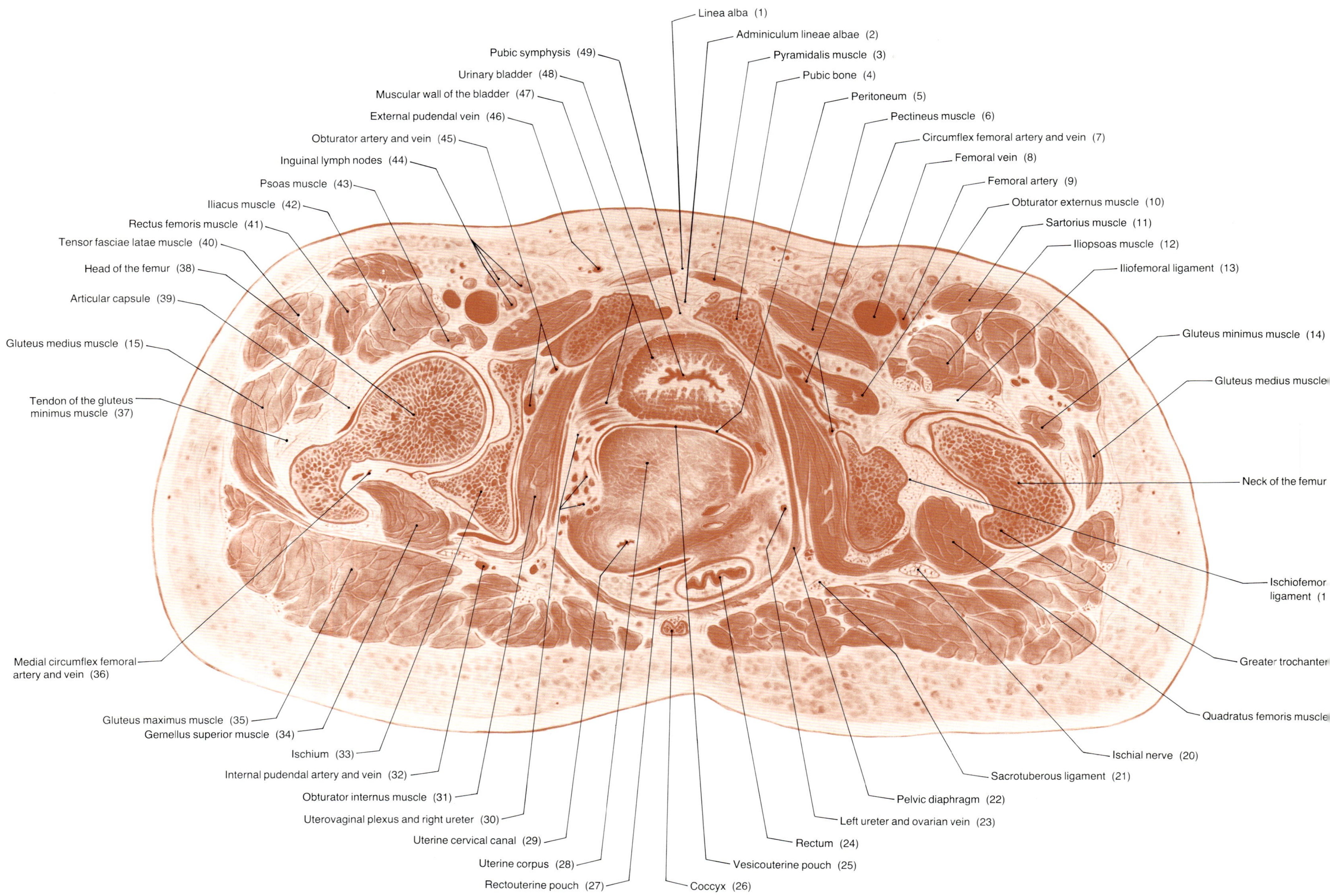

1 Linea alba
2 Adminiculum lineae albae
3 M. pyramidalis
4 Os pubis
5 Peritoneum
6 M. pectineus
7 A. et V. circumflexa femoris
8 V. femoralis
9 A. femoralis
10 M. obturatorius externus
11 M. sartorius
12 M. iliopsoas
13 Lig. iliofemorale
14 M. glutaeus minimus
15 M. glutaeus medius
16 Collum femoris
17 Lig. ischiofemorale
18 Trochanter major
19 M. quadratus femoris
20 N. ischiadicus
21 Lig. sacrotuberale
22 Diaphragma pelvis
23 Ureter sinister et V. ovarica
24 Rectum
25 Excavatio vesicouterina
26 Os coccygis
27 Excavatio rectouterina
28 Corpus uteri
29 Canalis cervicis uteri
30 Plexus uterovaginalis et Ureter dexter
31 M. obturatorius internus
32 A. et V. pudenda interna
33 Os ischii
34 M. gemellus superior
35 M. glutaeus maximus
36 A. et V. circumflexa femoris medialis
37 Tendo m. glutaei minimi
38 Caput femoris
39 Capsula articularis
40 M. tensor fasciae latae
41 M. rectus femoris
42 M. iliacus
43 M. psoas
44 Nodi lymphatici inguinales
45 A. et V. obturatoria
46 V. pudenda externa
47 Tunica muscularis vesicae
48 Vesica urinaria
49 Symphysis pubica

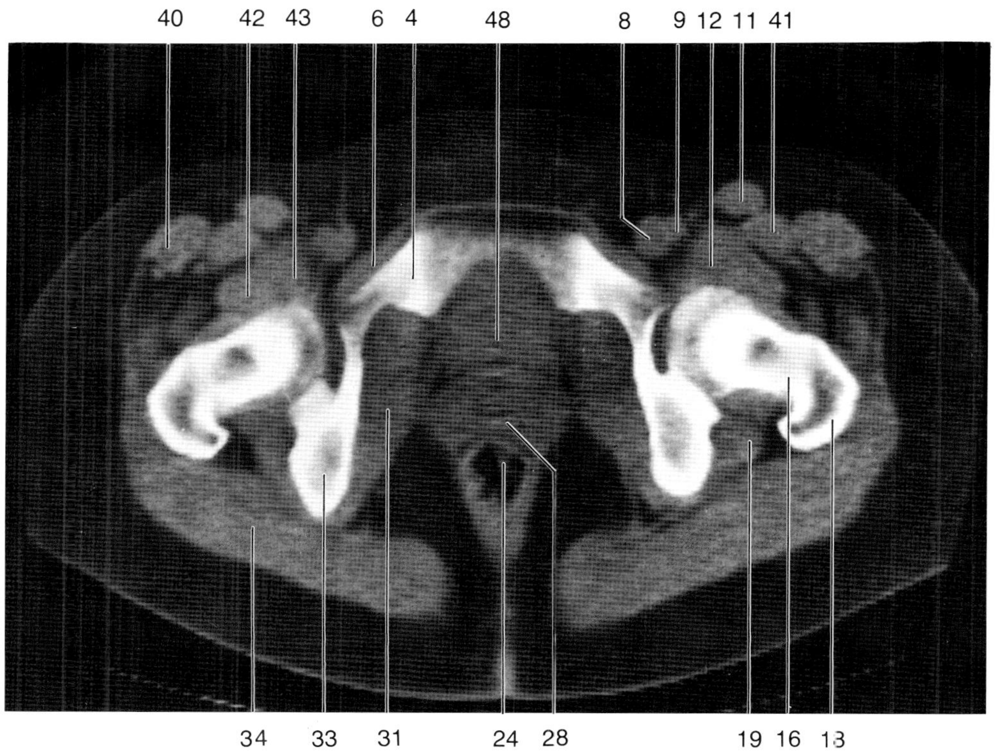

CT scan, unenhanced

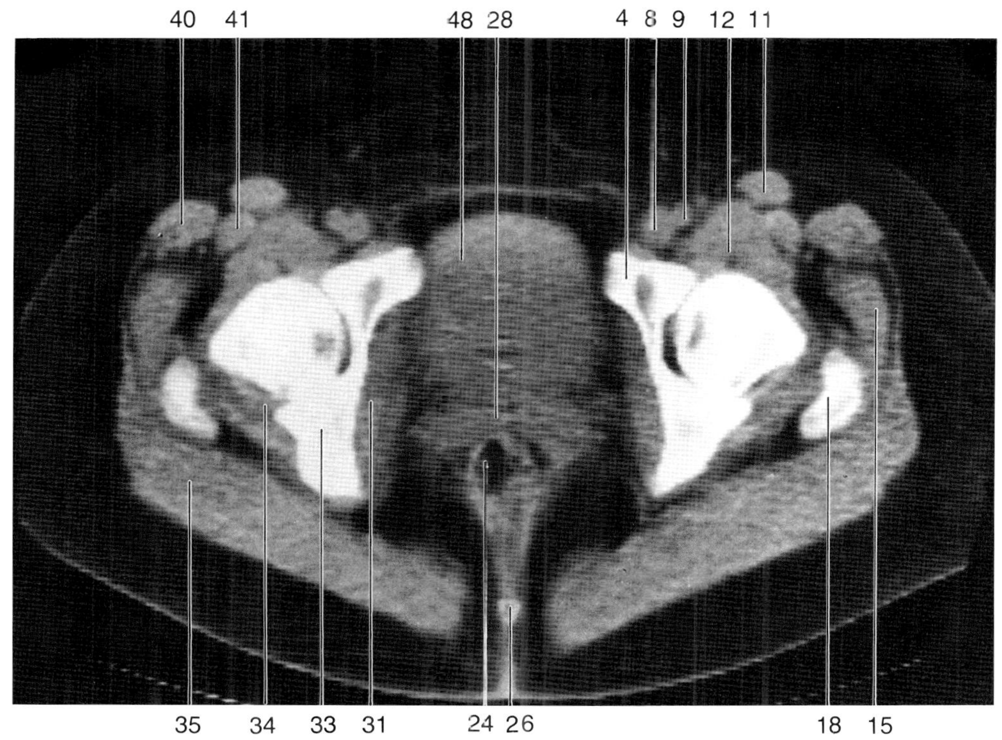

CT scan, unenhanced

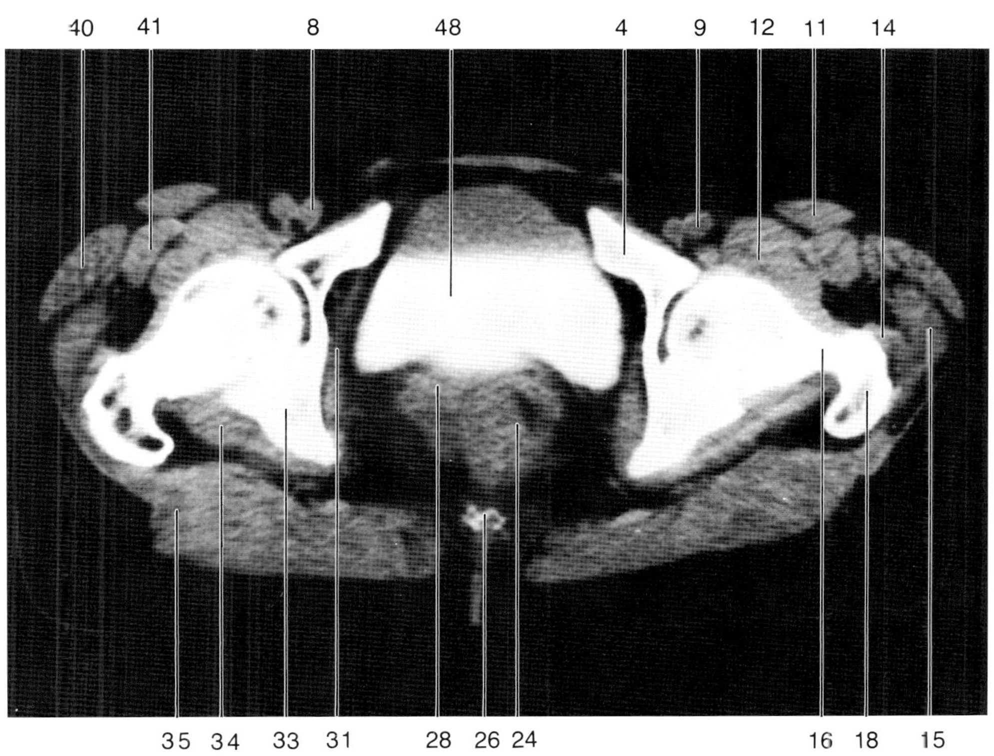

CT, enhanced after injection of contrast medium

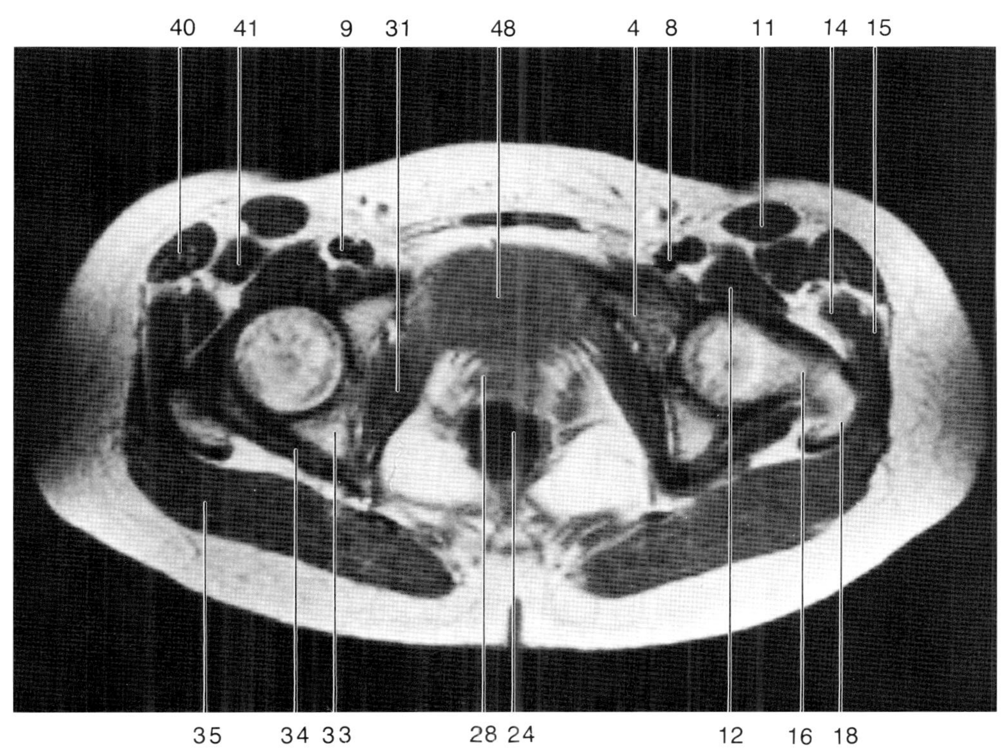

MRI, SE 500/50

4 Pubic bone
6 Pectineus muscle
8 Femoral vein
9 Femoral artery
11 Sartorius muscle
12 Iliopsoas muscle
14 Gluteus minimus muscle
15 Gluteus medius muscle
16 Neck of the femur
18 Greater trochanter
19 Quadratus femoris muscle
24 Rectum
26 Coccyx
28 Uterine corpus
31 Obturator internus muscle
33 Ischium
34 Gemellus superior muscle
35 Gluteus maximus muscle
40 Tensor fasciae latae muscle
41 Rectus femoris muscle
42 Iliacus muscle
43 Psoas muscle
48 Urinary bladder

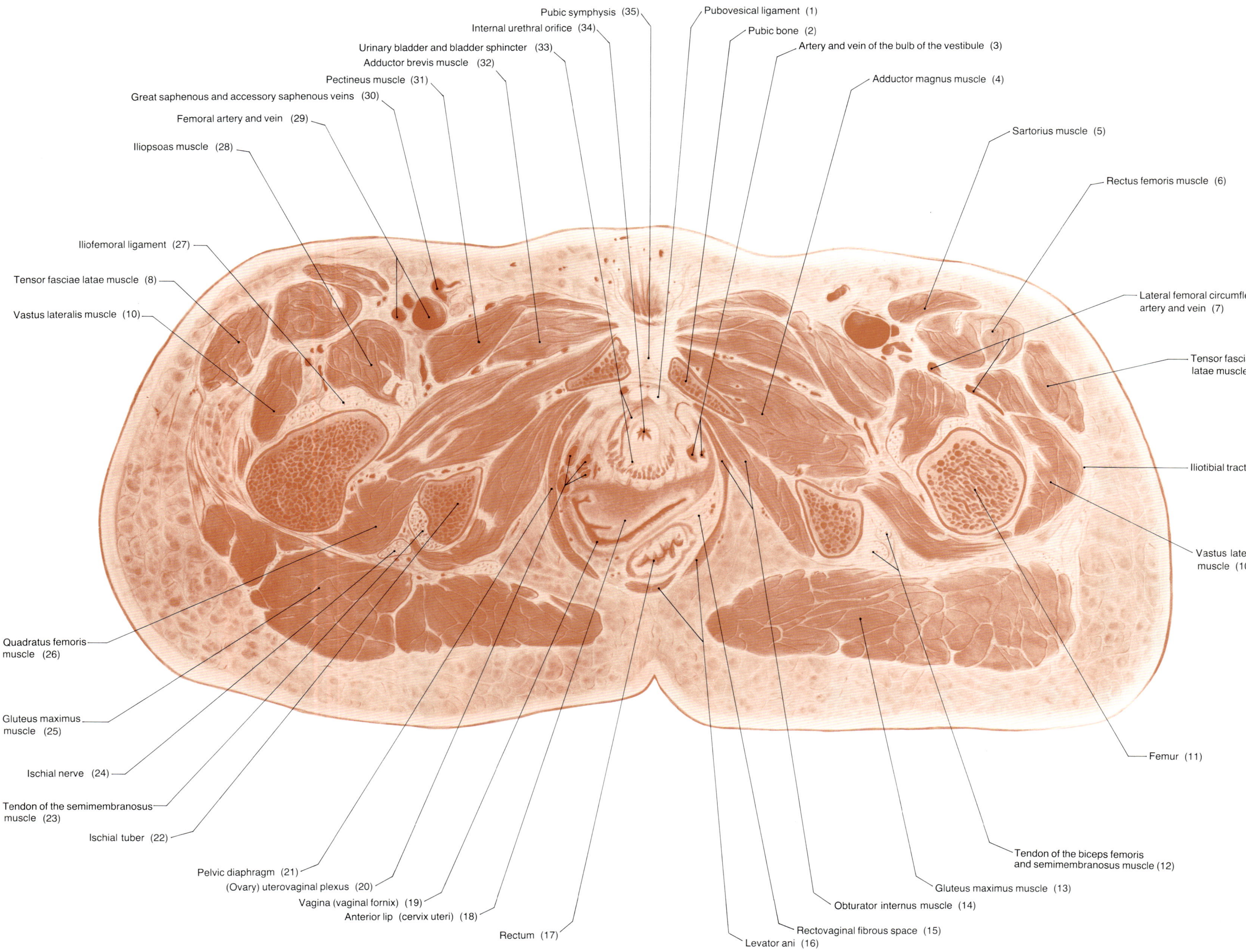

1 Lig. pubovesicale
2 Os pubis
3 A. et V. bulbi vestibuli
4 M. adductor magnus
5 M. sartorius
6 M. rectus femoris
7 A. et V. circumflexa femoris lateralis
8 M. tensor fasciae latae
9 Tractus iliotibialis
10 M. vastus lateralis
11 Femur
12 Tendo m. bicipitis femoris, Tendo m. semimembranosus
13 M. glutaeus maximus
14 M. obturatorius internus
15 Spatium fibrosum rectovaginale
16 Levator ani
17 Rectum
18 Cervix uteri
19 Vagina (Fornix vaginae)
20 Ovarium, Plexus uterovaginalis
21 Diaphragma pelvis
22 Tuber ischiadicum
23 Tendo m. semimembranosi
24 N. ischiadicus
25 M. glutaeus maximus
26 M. quadratus femoris
27 Lig. iliofemorale
28 M. iliopsoas
29 A. et V. femoralis
30 V. saphena magna et V. saphena accessoria
31 M. pectineus
32 M. adductor brevis
33 Vesica urinaria et Sphincter vesicae
34 Ostium urethrae internum
35 Symphysis pubica

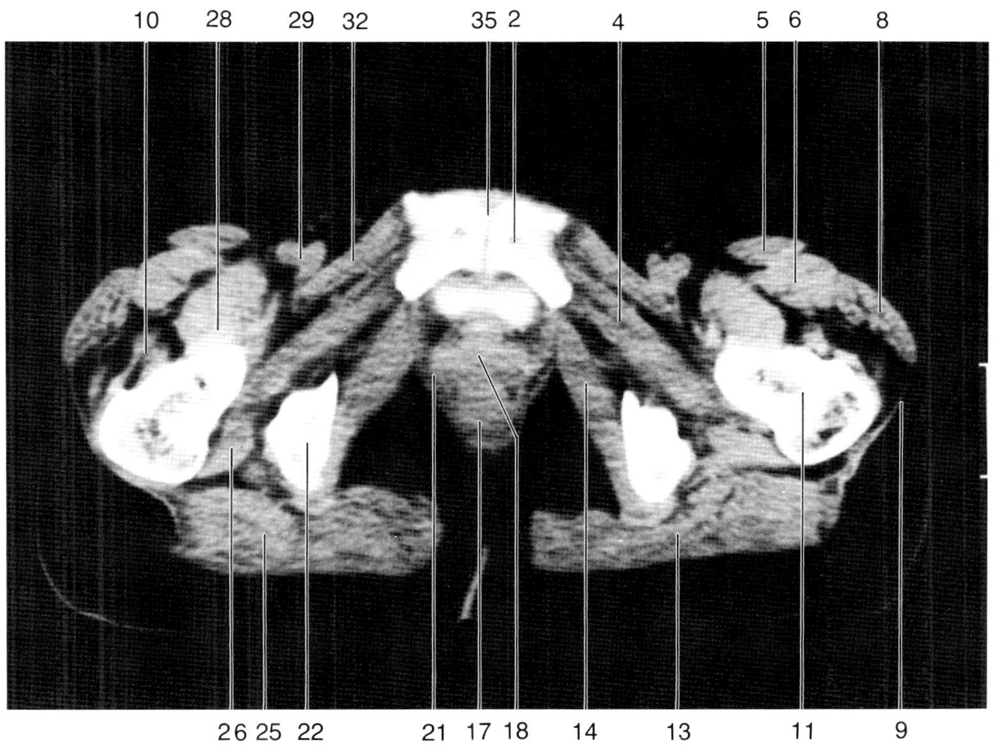

CT scan, unenhanced

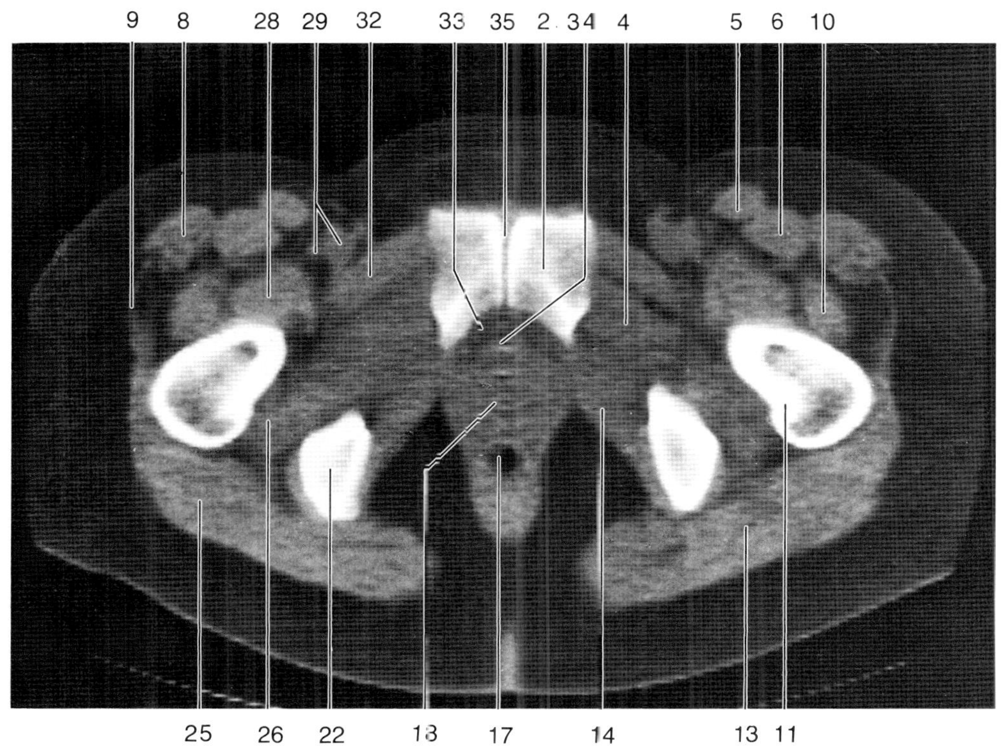

CT scan, unenhanced

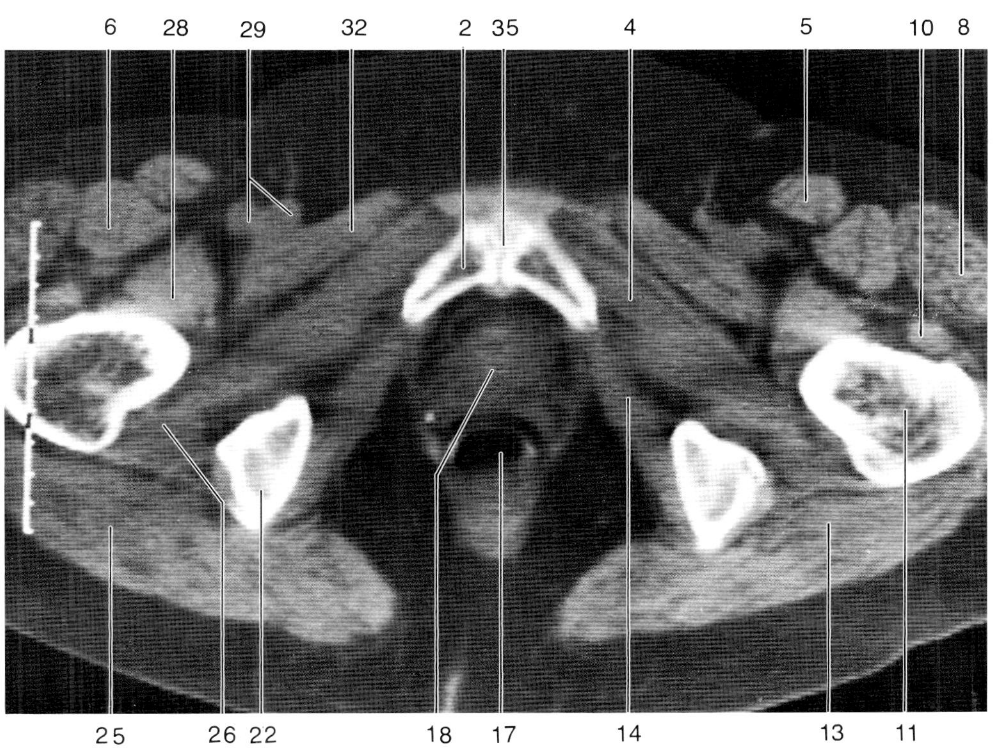

CT scan, unenhanced

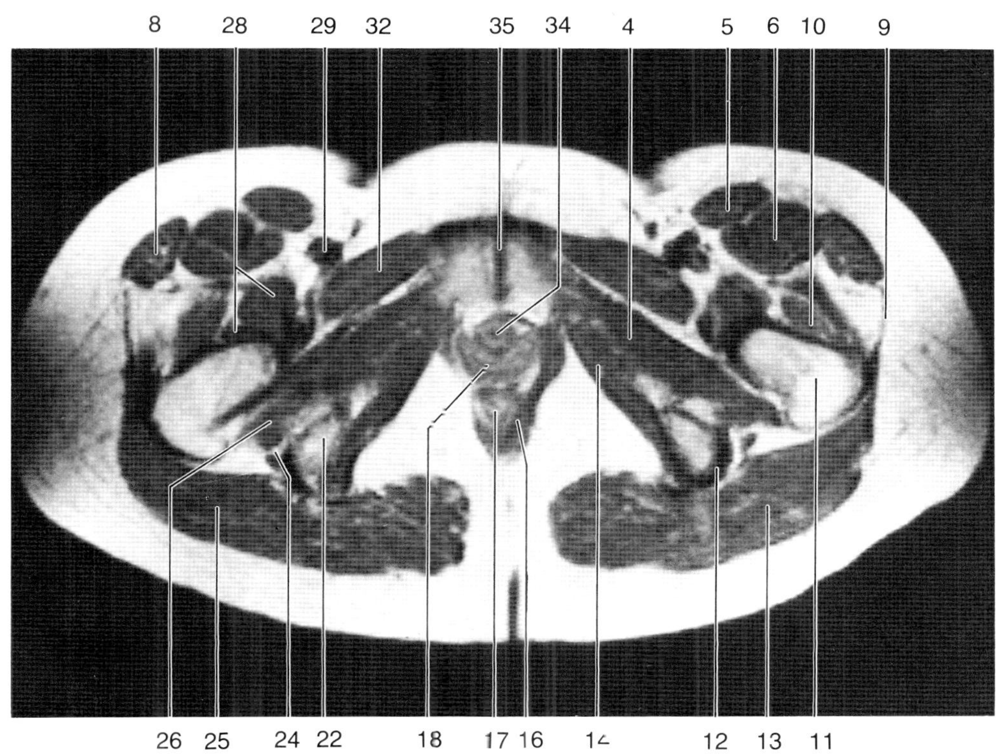

MRI, SE 500/50

2 Pubic bone
4 Adductor magnus muscle
5 Sartorius muscle
6 Rectus femoris muscle
8 Tensor fasciae latae muscle
9 Iliotibial tract
10 Vastus lateralis muscle
11 Femur
12 Tendon of the biceps femoris and semimembranosus muscle
13 Gluteus maximus muscle
14 Obturator internus muscle
16 Levator ani
17 Rectum
18 Anterior lip (cervix uteri)
21 Pelvic diaphragm
22 Ischial tuberosity
24 Ischial nerve
25 Gluteus maximus muscle
26 Quadratus femoris muscle
28 Iliopsoas muscle
29 Femoral artery and vein
32 Adductor brevis muscle
33 Urinary bladder and bladder sphincter
34 Internal urethral orifice
35 Pubis symphysis

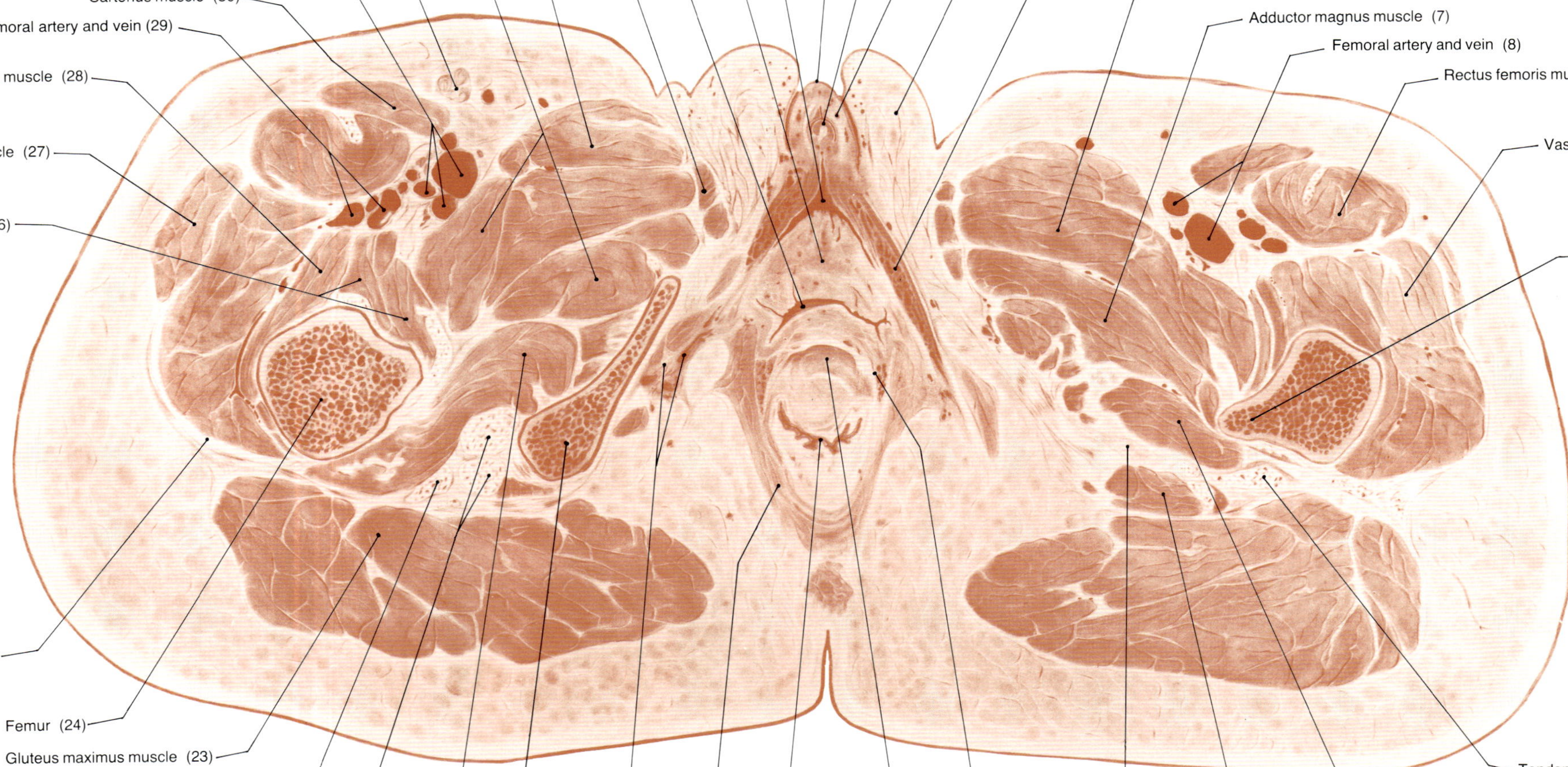

1 Praeputium clitoridis
2 Clitoris
3 Labium minus pudendi
4 Labium majus pudendi
5 Bulbus vestibuli
6 M. adductor brevis
7 M. adductor magnus
7.1 V. saphena magna
8 A. et V. femoralis
9 M. rectus femoris
10 M. vastus lateralis
11 Trochanter minor
12 Tendo m. semimembranosi
13 M. quadratus femoris
14 M. semitendineus
15 N. ischiadicus
16 Plexus uterovaginalis
17 Spatium fibrosum rectovaginale
18 Anus (Rectum)
19 M. sphincter ani
20 A. et V. pudenda interna
21 Os ischii
22 Tendo m. bicipitis femoris et Tendo m. semimembranosi
23 M. glutaeus maximus
24 Femur
25 Tractus iliotibialis
26 M. iliopsoas
27 M. tensor fasciae latae
28 M. vastus intermedius
29 A. et V. circumflexa femoris lateralis
30 M. sartorius
31 A. et V. femoralis et A. femoralis profunda
32 Nodus lymphaticus subinguinalis superficialis
33 M. pectineus et M. adductor magnus
34 M. adductor longus
35 M. gracillis
36 Vagina
36.1 Orificium urethrae internae
37 Spatium fibrosum vesicovaginale
38 Vagina (sinus paraurethralis)

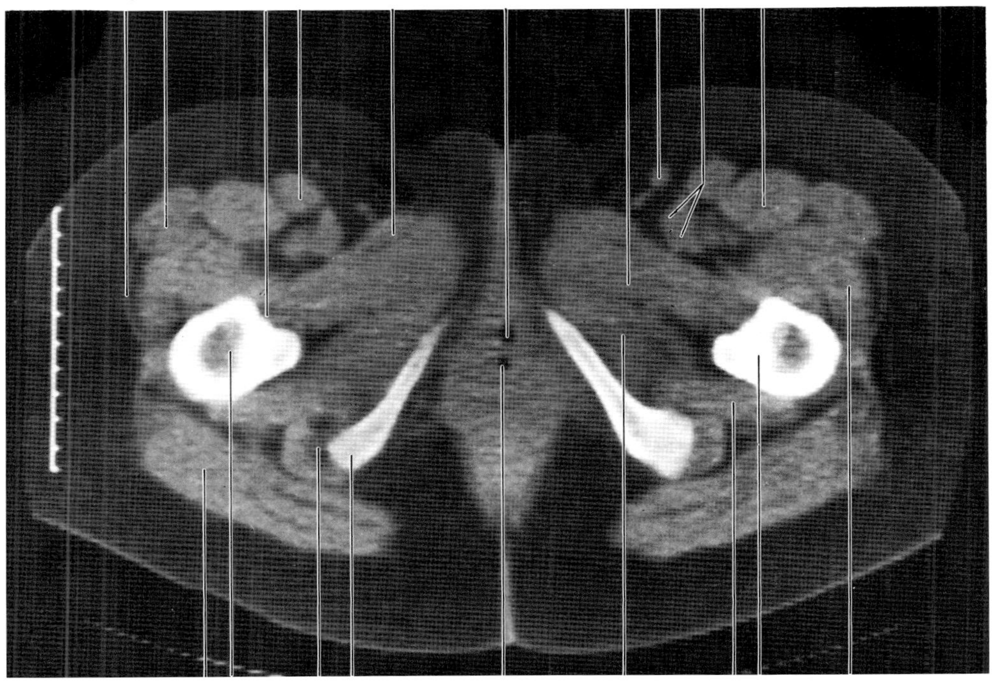

CT scan, unenhanced

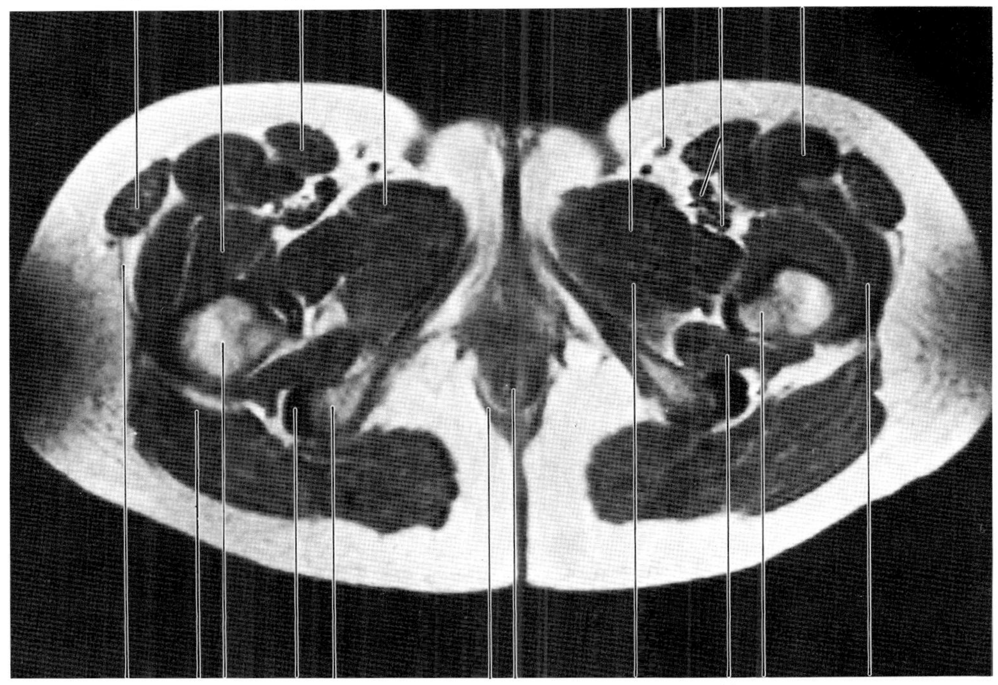

MRI, SE 500/50

6	Adductor brevis muscle
7	Adductor magnus muscle
7.1	Great saphenous vein
8	Femoral artery and vein
9	Rectus femoris muscle
10	Vastus lateralis muscle
11	Greater trochanter
13	Quadratus femoris muscle
18	Anus (rectum)
19	Sphincter ani muscle
21	Ischium
22	Tendon of the biceps femoris and semimembranosus muscle
23	Gluteus maximus muscle
24	Femur
25	Iliotibial tract
26	Iliopsoas muscle
27	Tensor fasciae latae muscle
30	Sartorius muscle
34	Adductor longus muscle
36	Vagina
36.1	Internal urethral orifice

Axial Sections of the Male Pelvis

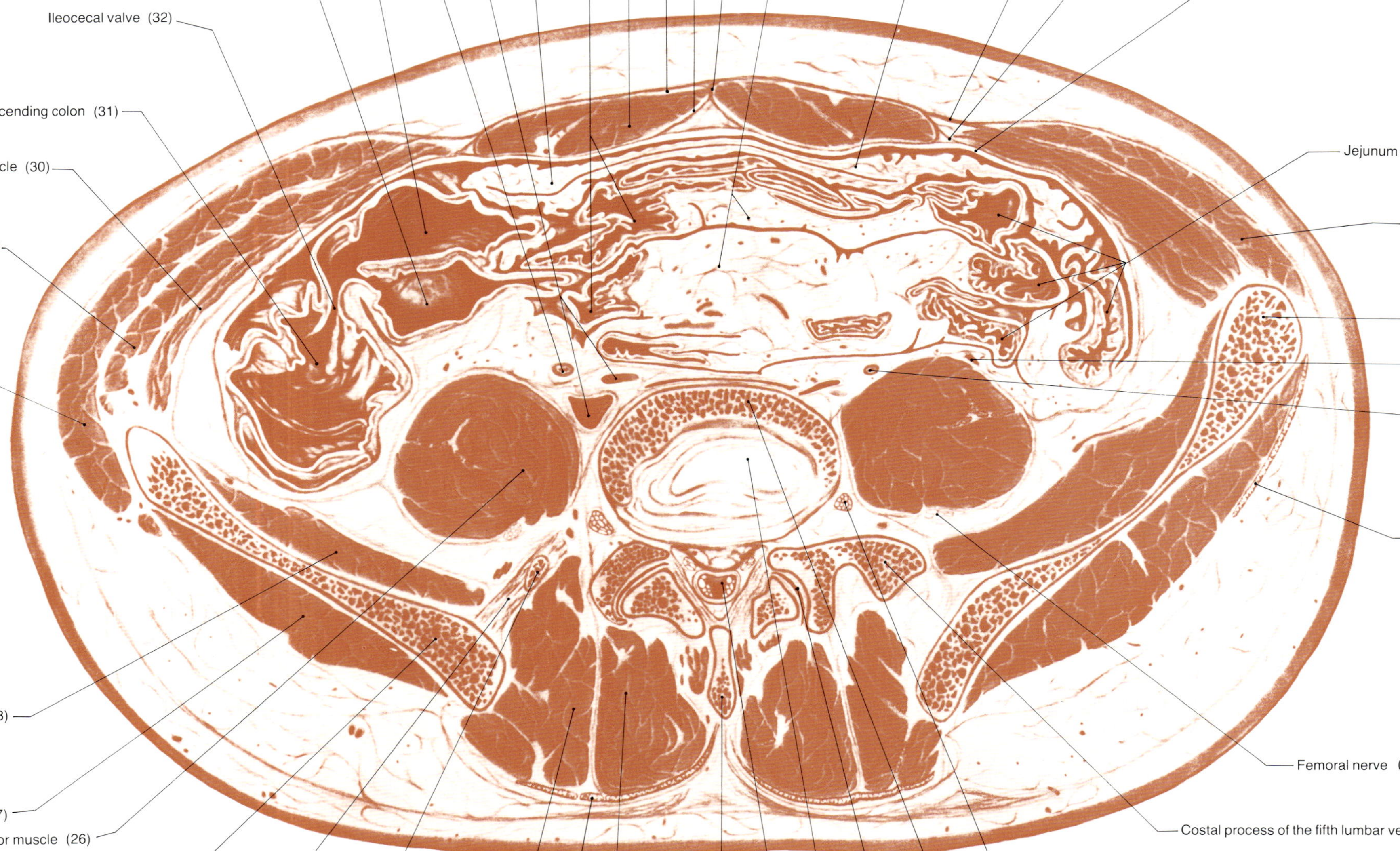

1 Linea alba
2 Mesenterium
3 Omentum majus
4 Aponeurosis m. obliqui externi
5 Fascia transversalis
6 Peritoneum
7 Jejunum
8 M. obliquus internus abdominis
9 Spina iliaca anterior superior
10 V. testicularis sinistra
11 Ureter sinister
12 Tractus iliotibialis
13 N. femoralis
14 Processus costarius lumbalis V
15 N. lumbalis IV
16 Vertebra lumbalis V
17 Articulatio intervertebralis
18 Discus intervertebralis
19 Spatium subdurale et Cauda equina
20 Processus spinosus vertebralis V
21 M. multifidus
22 Fascia thoracolumbalis
23 M. longissimus dorsi
24 Lig. iliolumbale
25 Os ilium
26 M. psoas major
27 M. glutaeus medius
28 M. iliacus
29 M. obliquus externus abdominis
30 M. transversus abdominis
31 Colon ascendens
32 Valva ileocaecalis
33 Ileum
34 Caecum
35 Ureter dexter
36 A. et V. iliaca communis
37 M. rectus abdominis
38 Lamina anterior fasciae m. recti abdominis
39 Lamina posterior fasciae m. recti abdominis

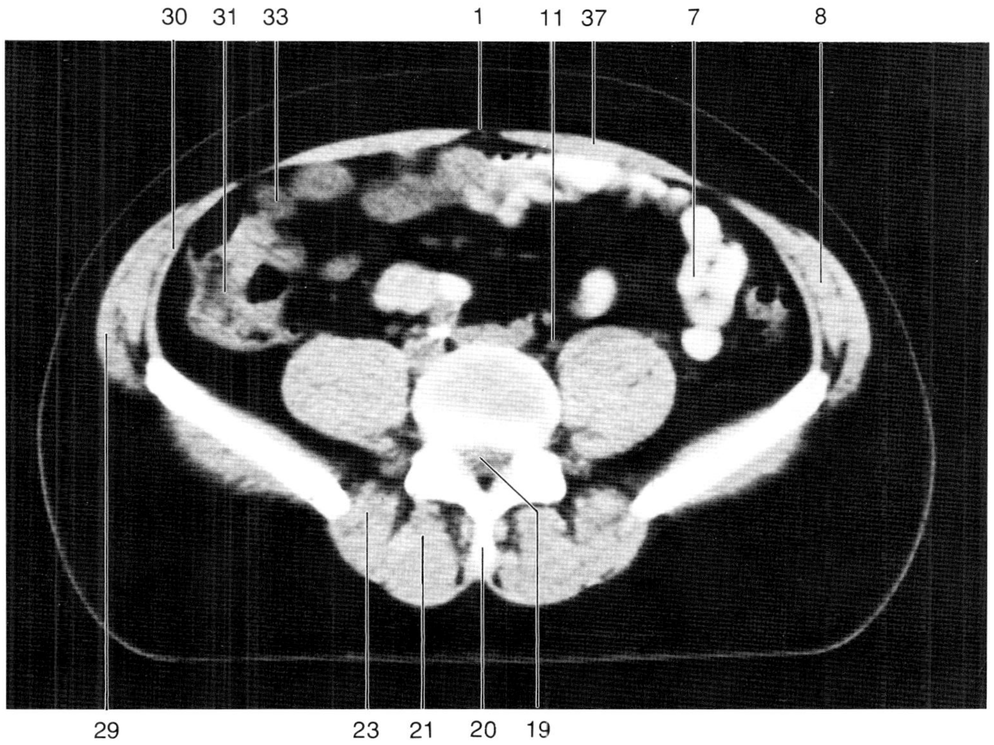

CT with contrast medium in the small bowel

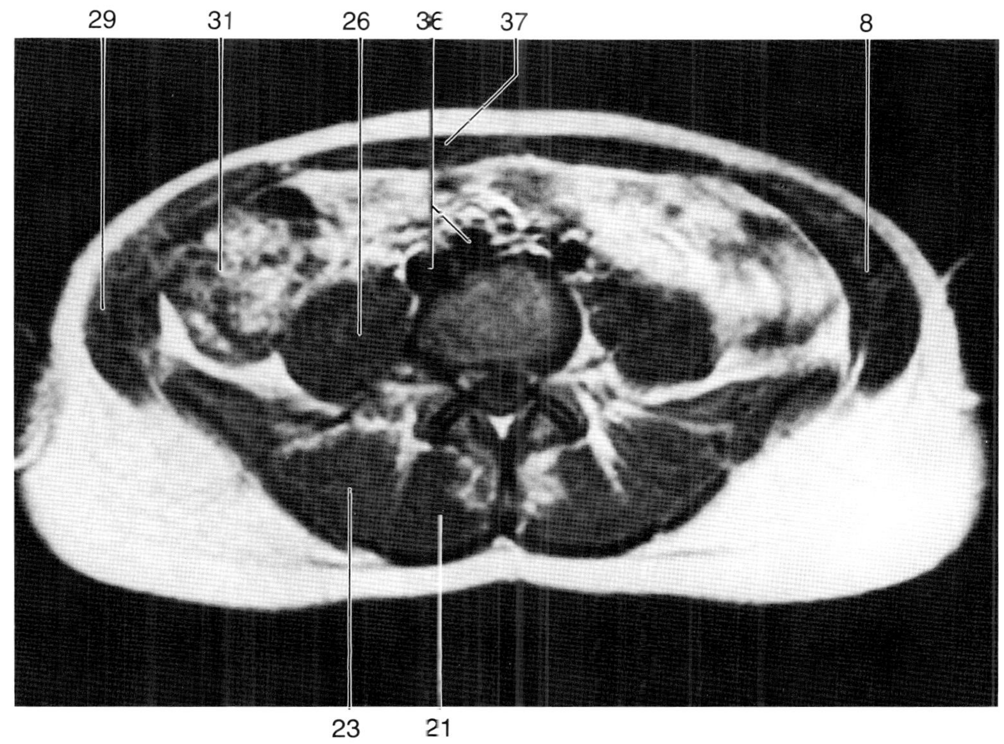

MRI, SE 700/30

1 Linea alba
7 Jejunum
8 Obliquus internus abdominis muscle
11 Left ureter
19 Dural sac with cauda equina
20 Spinous process of the fifth lumbar vertebra
21 Multifidus muscle
23 Longissimus dorsi muscle
26 Psoas major muscle
29 Obliquus externus abdominis muscle
30 Transversus abdominis muscle
31 Ascending colon
33 Ileum
36 Common iliac artery and vein
37 Rectus abdominis muscle

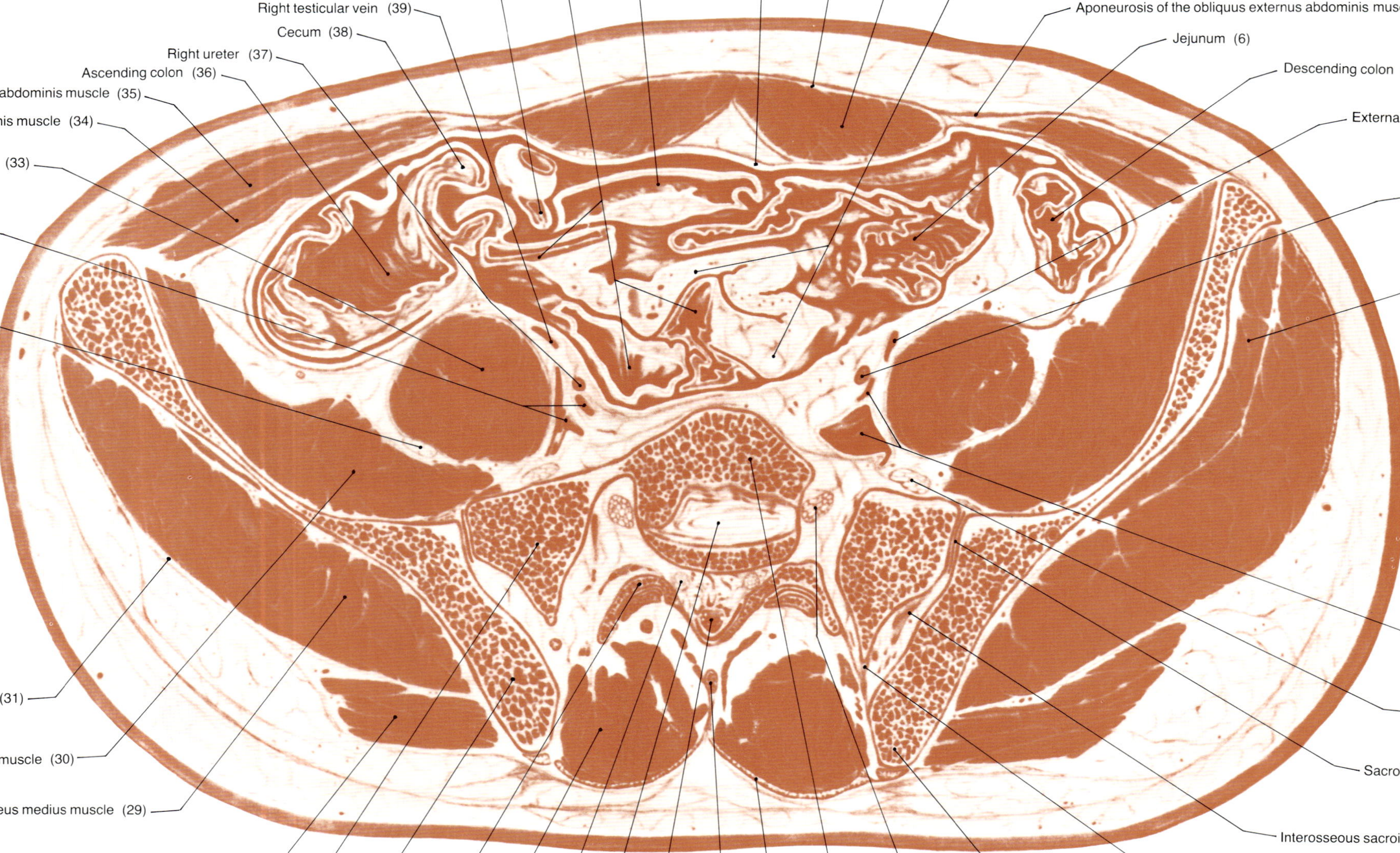

1 Fascia transversalis
2 Vagina m. recti abdominis, lamina anterior
3 M. rectus abdominis
4 Mesenterium
5 Aponeurosis m. obliqui externi abdominis
6 Jejunum
7 Colon descendens
8 A. iliaca externa
9 Ureter sinister
10 M. glutaeus minimus
11 A. et V. iliaca communis
12 N. lumbalis I
13 Articulatio sacroiliaca
14 Lig. sacroiliacum interosseum
15 Lig. sacroiliacum dorsale breve
16 Spina iliaca posterior superior
17 Truncus n. sacralis I
18 Vertebra sacralis I
19 Fascia thoracolumbalis
20 Crista sacralis mediana
21 Spatium subdurale et Cauda equina
22 Discus intervertebralis
23 Truncus n. sacralis II
24 M. erector spinae (Mm. longissimus dorsi et multifidus)
25 Processus articularis superior ossis sacrii
26 Os ilium
27 Pars lateralis ossis sacrii
28 M. glutaeus maximus
29 M. glutaeus medius
30 M. iliacus
31 Tractus iliotibialis
32 N. femoralis
33 M. psoas major
34 M. transversus abdominis
35 M. obliquus internus abdominis
36 Colon ascendens
37 Ureter dexter
38 Caecum
39 V. testicularis dextra
40 Appendix vermiformis
41 Ileum
42 Omentum majus

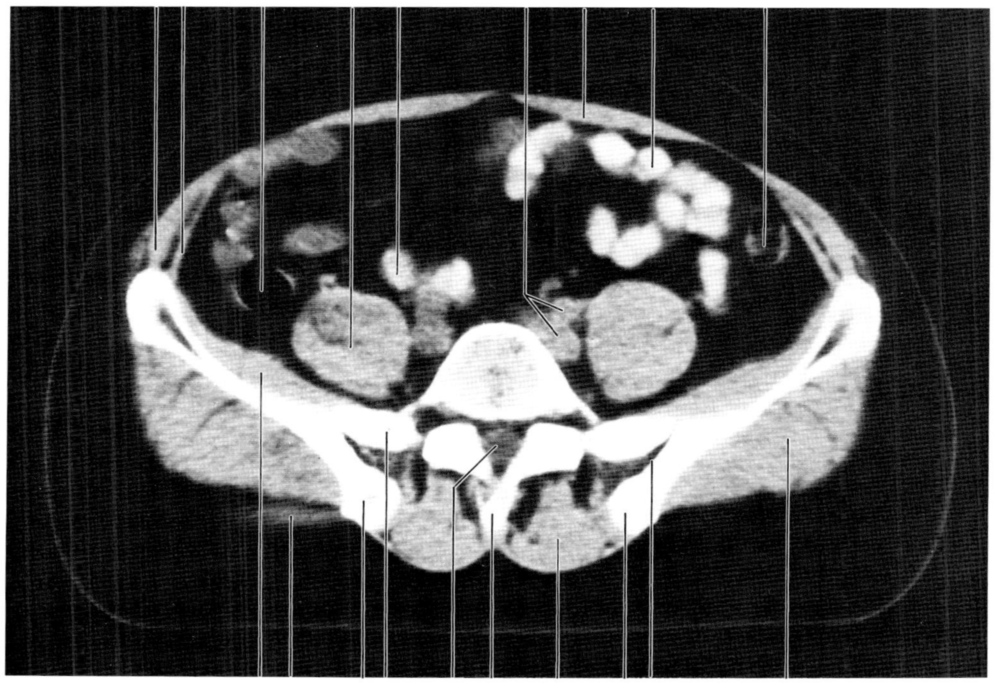

CT with contrast medium in the small bowel

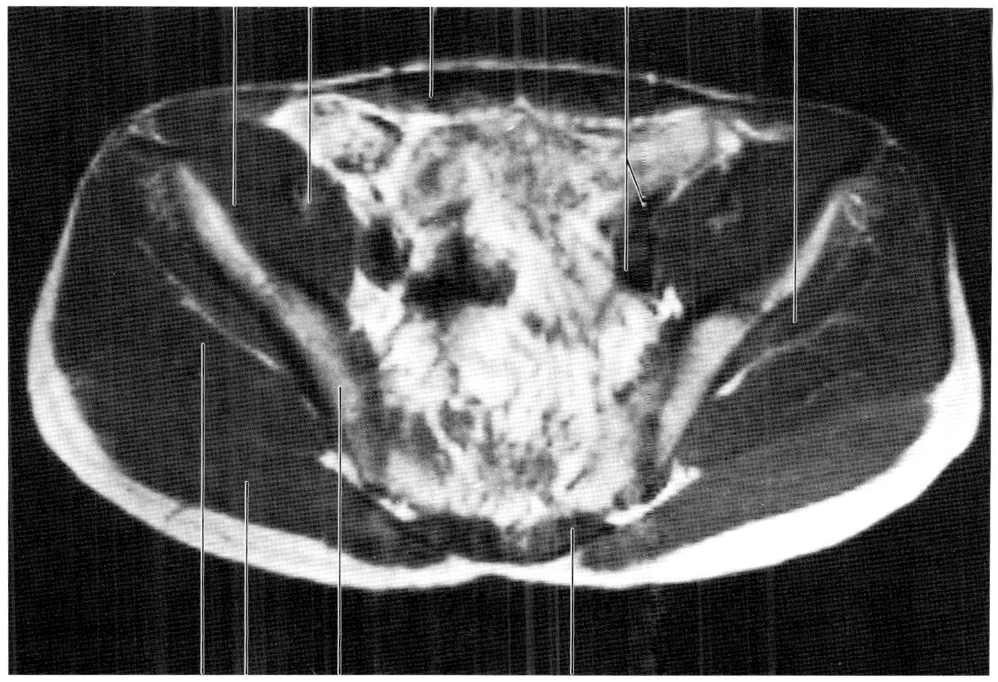

MRI, SE 1000/50

3 Rectus abdominis muscle
6 Jejunum
7 Descending colon
10 Gluteus minimus muscle
11 Common iliac artery and vein
13 Sacroiliac joint
16 Posterior superior iliac spine
20 Median sacral crest
21 Dural sac with cauda equina
24 Erector spinae muscle
26 Ilium
27 Lateral part of the sacral bone
28 Gluteus maximus muscle
29 Gluteus medius muscle
30 Iliacus muscle
32 Femoral nerve
33 Psoas major muscle
34 Transversus abdominis muscle
35 Obliquus internus abdominis muscle
36 Ascending colon
41 Ileum

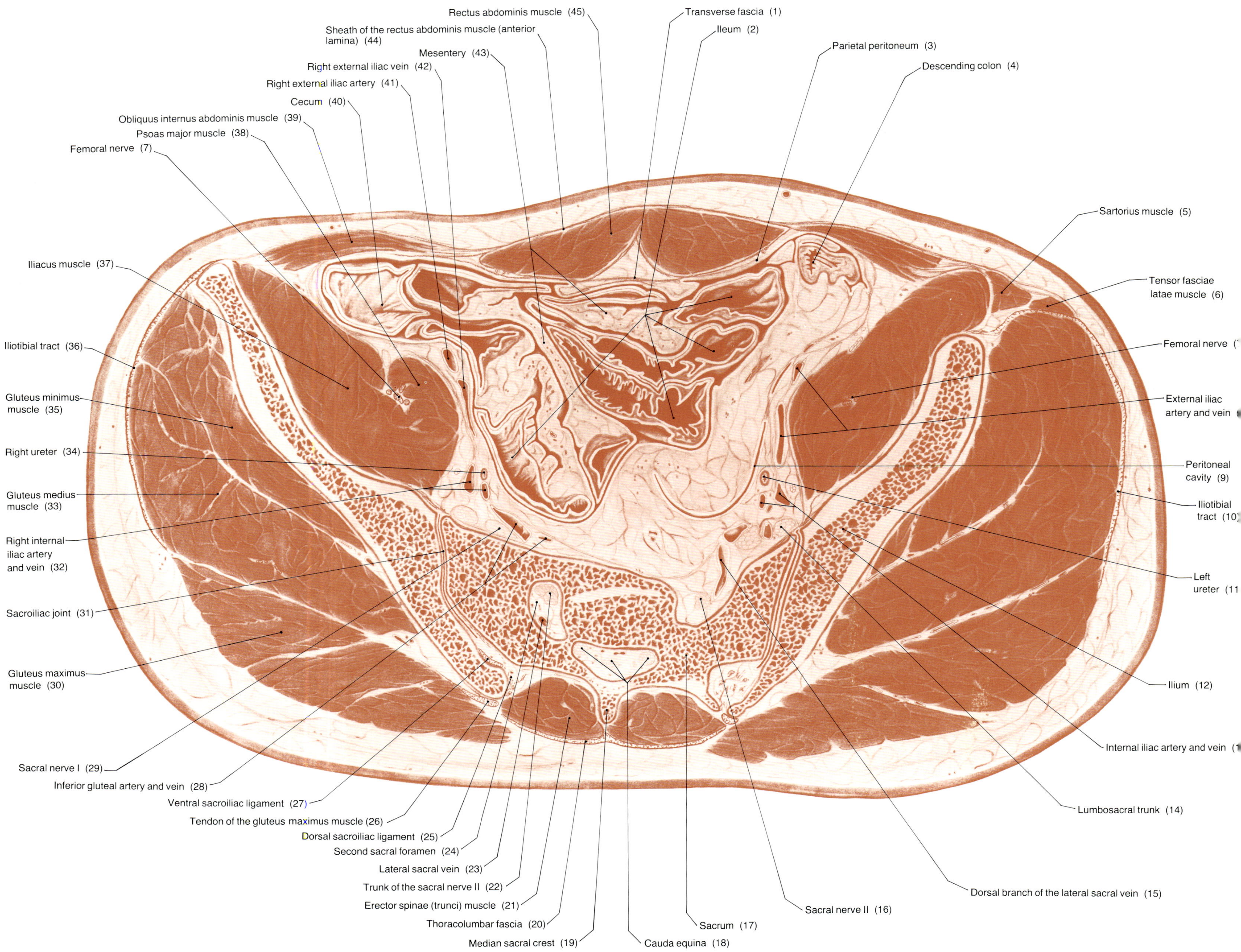

1 Fascia transversalis
2 Ileum
3 Peritoneum parietale
4 Colon descendens
5 M. sartorius
6 M. tensor fasciae latae
7 N. femoralis
8 A. et V. iliaca externa
9 Cavitas peritonealis
10 Tractus iliotibialis
11 Ureter sinister
12 Os ilium
12.1 Rectum
13 A. et V. iliaca interna
14 Truncus lumbosacralis
15 R. dorsalis v. sacralis lateralis
16 N. sacralis II
17 Os sacrum
18 Cauda equina
19 Crista sacralis mediana
20 Fascia thoracolumbalis
21 M. erector spinae
22 Truncus n. sacralis II
23 V. sacralis lateralis
24 Foramen sacrale II
25 Lig. sacroiliacum dorsale
26 Tendo m. glutaei maximi
27 Lig. sacroiliacum ventrale
28 A. et V. glutaea inferior
29 N. sacralis I
30 M. glutaeus maximus
31 Articulatio sacroiliaca
32 A. et V. iliaca interna dextra
33 M. glutaeus medius
34 Ureter dexter
35 M. glutaeus minimus
36 Tractus iliotibialis
37 M. iliacus
38 M. psoas major
39 M. obliquus internus abdominis
40 Caecum
41 A. iliaca externa dextra
42 V. iliaca externa dextra
43 Mesenterium
44 Vagina m. recti abdominis (Lamina anterior)
45 M. rectus abdominis

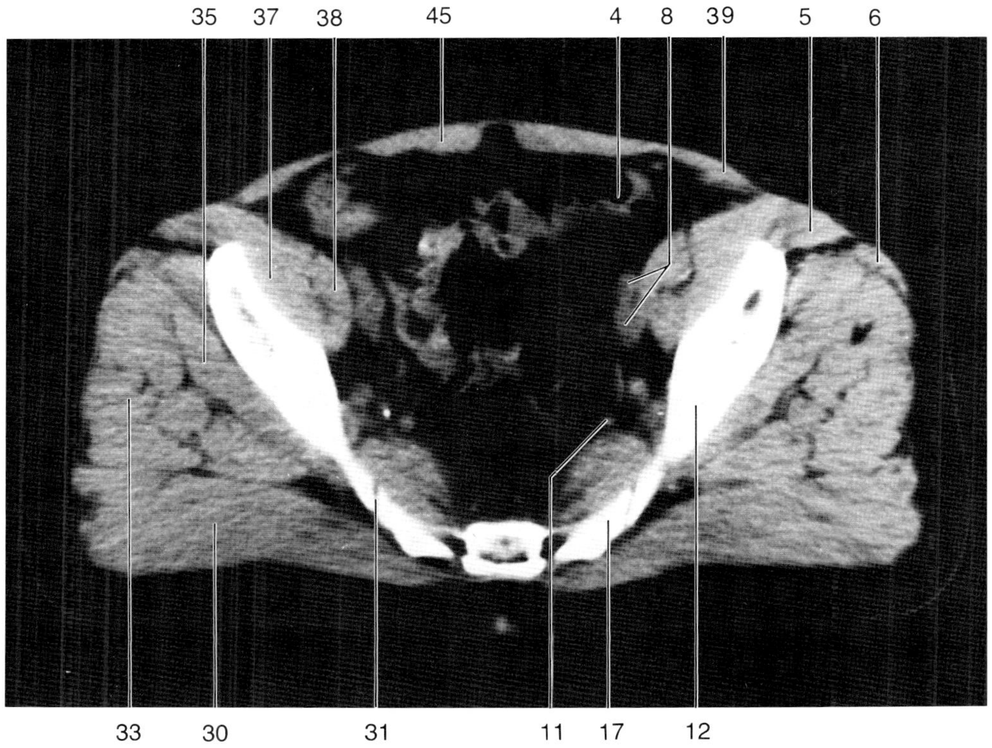

CT scan, unenhanced

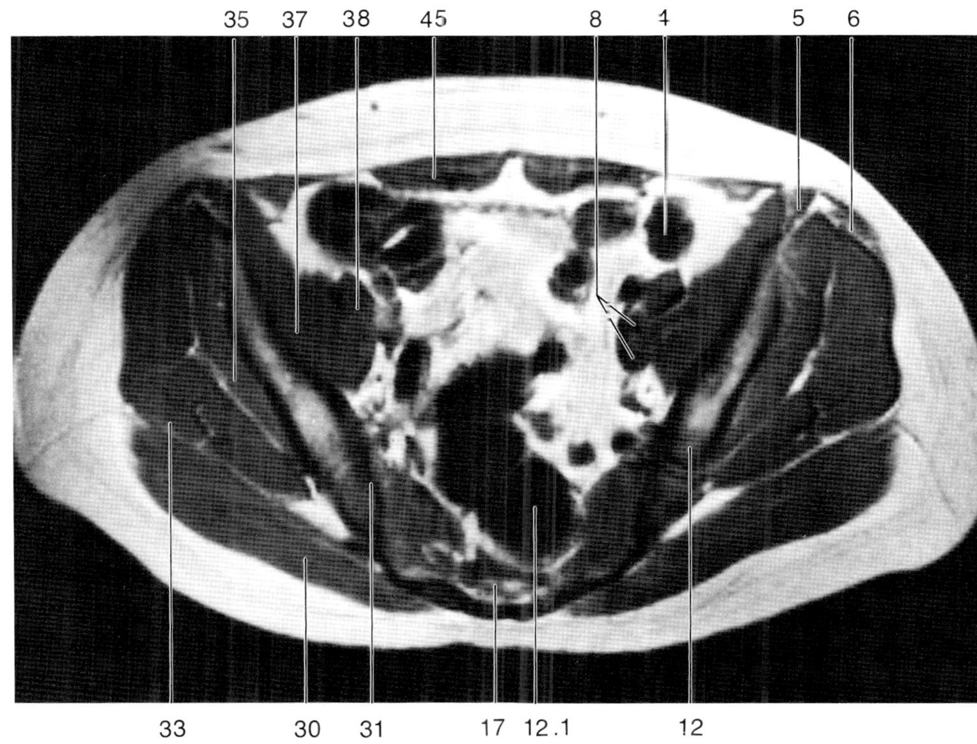

MRI, SE 500/30

4 Descending colon
5 Sartorius muscle
6 Tensor fasciae latae muscle
8 External iliac artery and vein
11 Left ureter
12 Ilium
12.1 Rectum
17 Sacrum
30 Gluteus maximus muscle
31 Sacroiliac joint
33 Gluteus medius muscle
35 Gluteus minimus muscle
37 Iliacus muscle
38 Psoas major muscle
39 Obliquus internus abdominis muscle
45 Rectus abdominis muscle

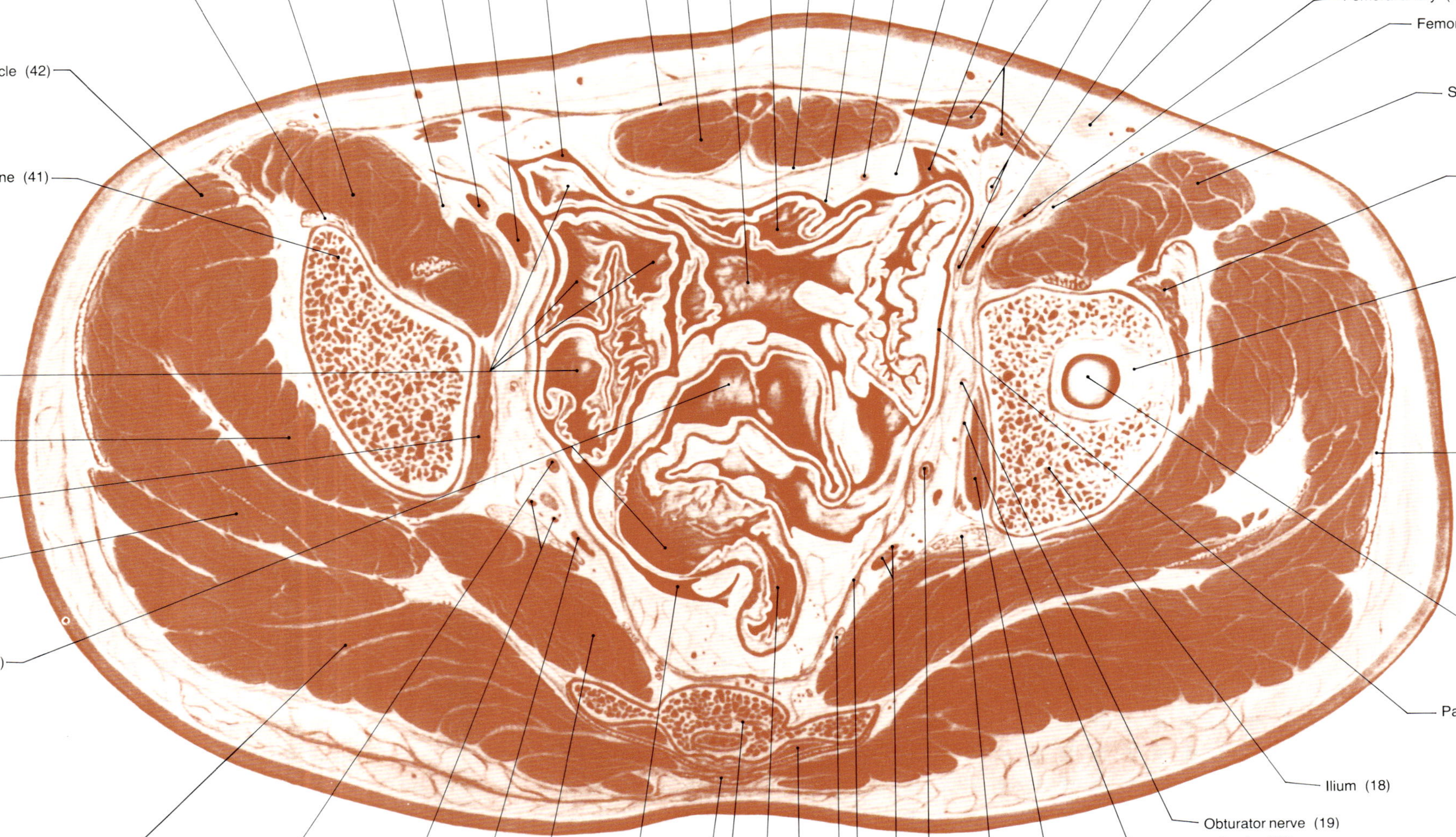

1 Fascia transversalis
2 Plica umbilicalis medialis
3 A. et V. epigastrica inferior
4 Plica umbilicalis lateralis
5 Fossa inguinalis lateralis
6 M. cremaster
7 Ductus deferens
8 V. femoralis
9 Nodus lymphaticus inguinalis
10 A. femoralis
11 N. femoralis
12 M. sartorius
13 M. rectus femoris
14 Capsula articularis
15 Tractus iliotibialis
16 Caput femoris
17 Peritoneum parietale
18 Os ilium
19 N. obturatorius
20 Fascia obturatoria
21 M. obturatorius internus
22 N. ischiadicus
23 Ureter sinister
24 A. et V. pudenda
25 Fascia pelvis interna
26 N. pudendus
27 Lig. sacrotuberale
28 Rectum
29 Os sacrum
30 Lig. sacrococcygeum dorsale
31 Peritoneum viscerale
32 M. piriformis
33 A. et V. pudenda interna
34 A. et V. glutaea inferior
35 Ureter dexter
36 M. glutaeus maximus
37 Colon sigmoideum
38 M. glutaeus medius
39 M. glutaeus minimus
40 Ileum
41 Spina iliaca anterior inferior
42 M. tensor fasciae latae
43 M. iliopsoas
44 Fossa inguinalis medialis
45 Vagina m. recti abdominis (Lamina anterior)
46 M. rectus abdominis
47 Vesica urinaria

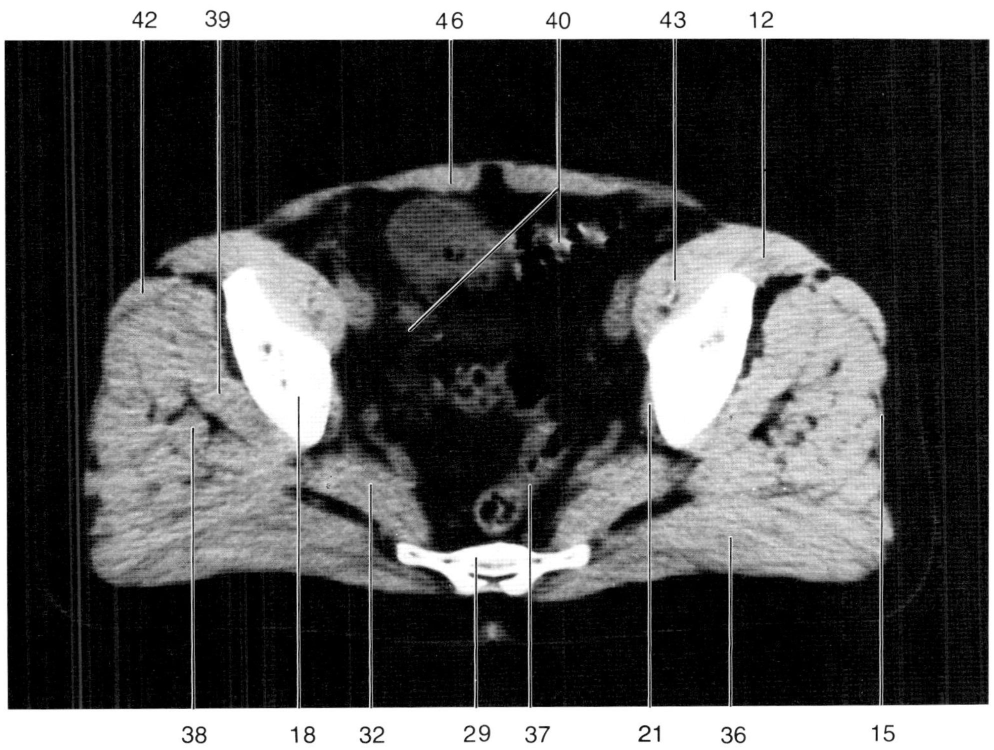

CT scan, unenhanced

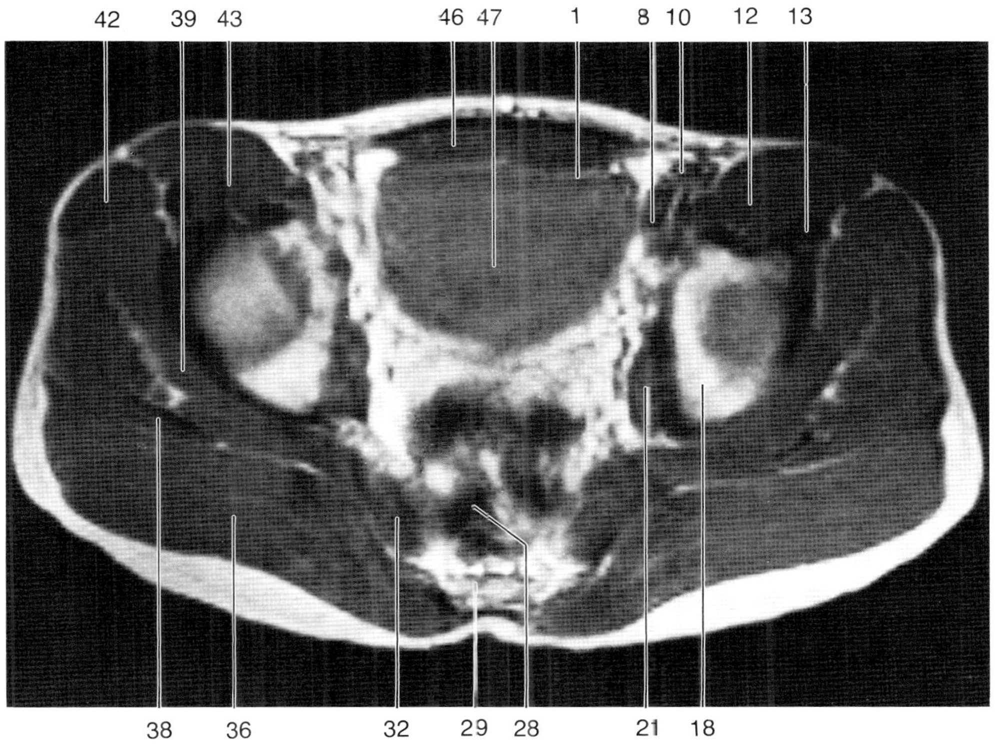

MRI, SE 500/50

1 Fascia transversalis
8 Femoral vein
10 Femoral artery
12 Sartorius muscle
13 Rectus femoris muscle
15 Iliotibial tract
18 Ilium
21 Obturator internus muscle
28 Beginning of the rectum
29 Sacrum
32 Piriformis muscle
36 Gluteus maximus muscle
37 Sigmoid colon
38 Gluteus medius muscle
39 Gluteus minimus muscle
40 Ileum
42 Tensor fasciae latae muscle
43 Iliopsoas muscle
46 Rectus abdominis muscle
47 Urinary bladder

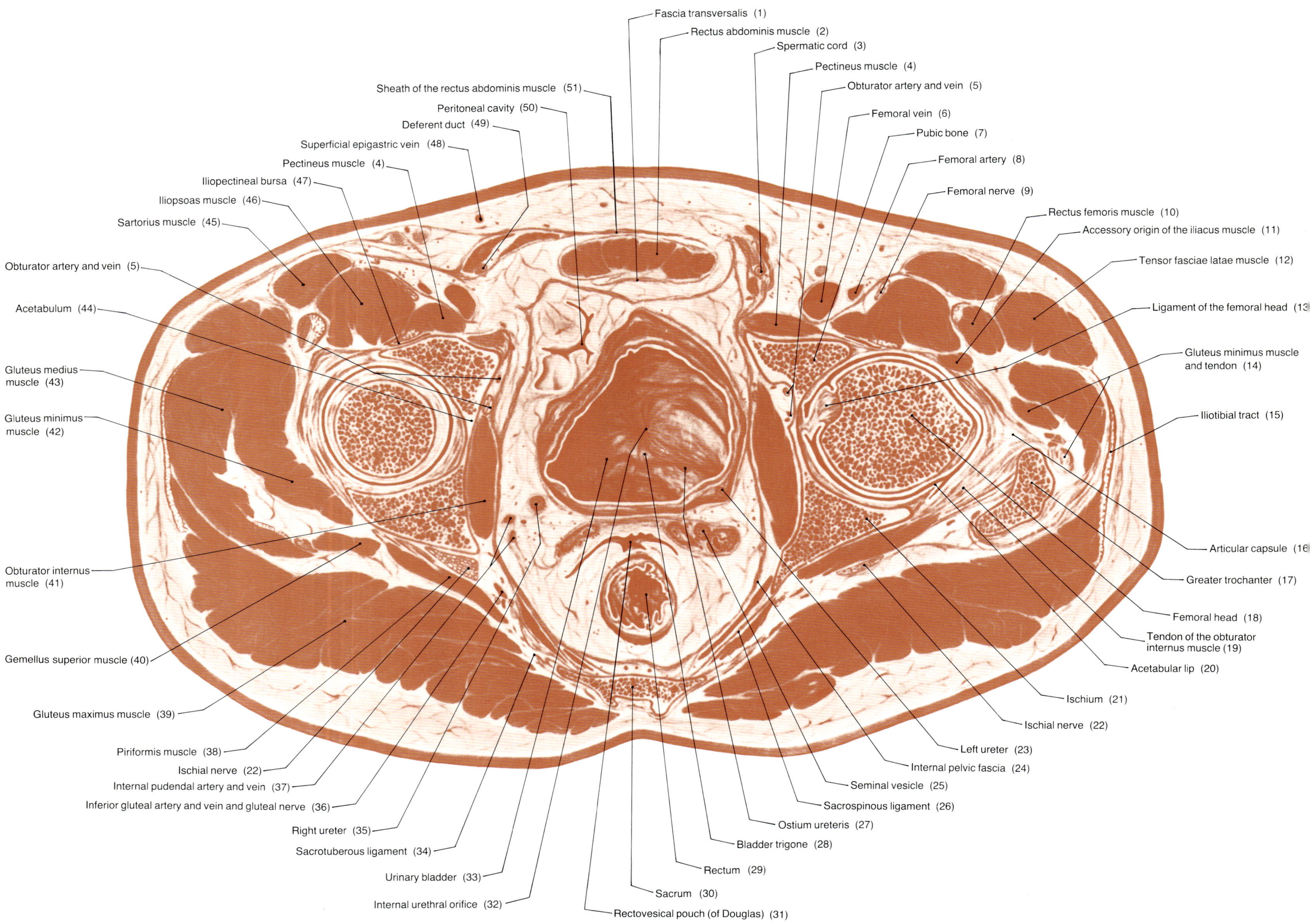

1 Fascia transversalis
2 M. rectus abdominis
3 Funiculus spermaticus
4 M. pectineus
5 A. et V. obturatoria
6 V. femoralis
7 Os pubis
8 A. femoralis
9 N. femoralis
10 M. rectus femoris
11 Origo accessorius m. iliaci
12 M. tensor fasciae latae
13 Lig. capitis femoris
14 M. glutaeus minimus et Tendo
15 Tractus iliotibialis
16 Capsula articularis
17 Trochanter major
18 Caput femoris
19 Tendo m. obturatorii interni
20 Labrum acetabulare
21 Os ischii
22 N. ischiadicus
23 Ureter sinister
24 Fascia pelvis interna
25 Vesicula seminalis
26 Lig. sacrospinale
27 Ostium ureteris
28 Trigonum vesicae
29 Rectum
30 Os sacrum
31 Excavatio rectovesicalis (Cavum Douglasi)
32 Ostium urethrae internum
33 Vesica urinaria
34 Lig. sacrotuberale
35 Ureter dexter
36 A. et V. glutaea inferior et N. glutaeus
37 A. et V. pudenda interna
38 M. piriformis
39 M. glutaeus maximus
40 M. gemellus spinalis
41 M. obturatorius internus
42 M. glutaeus minimus
43 M. glutaeus medius
44 Os acetabuli
45 M. sartorius
46 M. iliopsoas
47 Bursa iliopectinea
48 V. epigastrica superficialis
49 Ductus deferens
50 Cavum peritonaei
51 Vagina m. recti abdominis

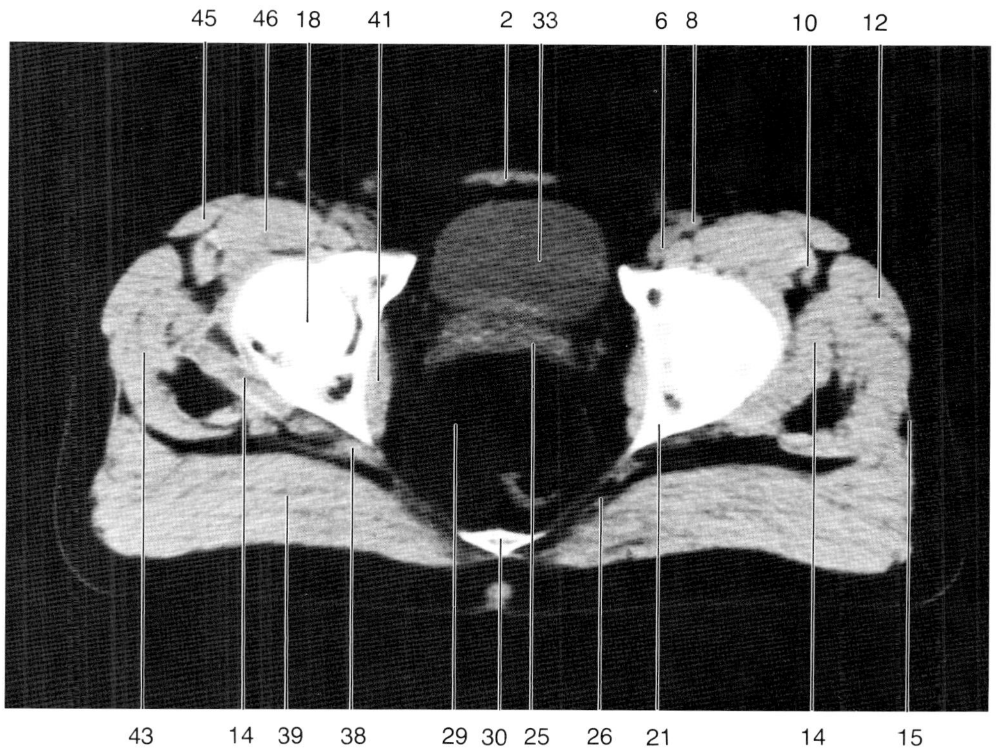

CT scan, unenhanced

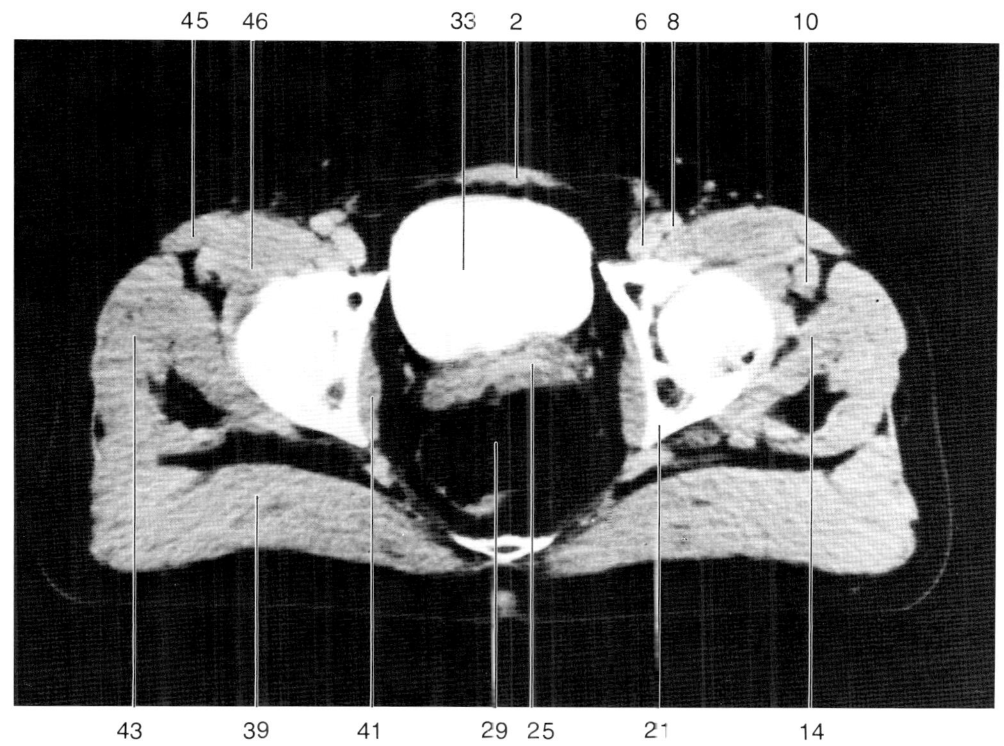

CT, enhanced after injection of contrast medium

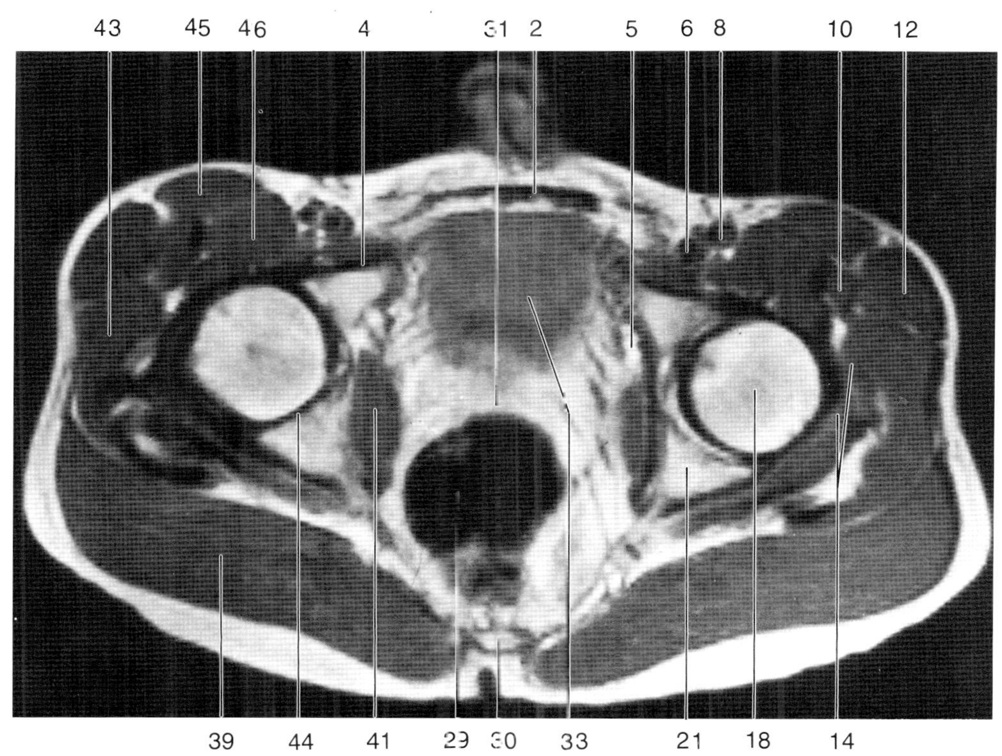

MRI, SE 500/50

2 Rectus abdominis muscle
4 Pectineus muscle
5 Obturator artery and vein
6 Femoral vein
8 Femoral artery
10 Rectus femoris muscle
12 Tensor fasciae latae muscle
14 Gluteus minimus muscle and tendon
15 Iliotibial tract
18 Femoral head
21 Ischium
25 Seminal vesicle
26 Sacrospinous ligament
29 Rectum
30 Sacrum
31 Rectovesical pouch (of Douglas)
33 Urinary bladder
38 Piriformis muscle
39 Gluteus maximus muscle
41 Obturator internus muscle
43 Gluteus medius muscle
44 Acetabulum
45 Sartorius muscle
46 Iliopsoas muscle

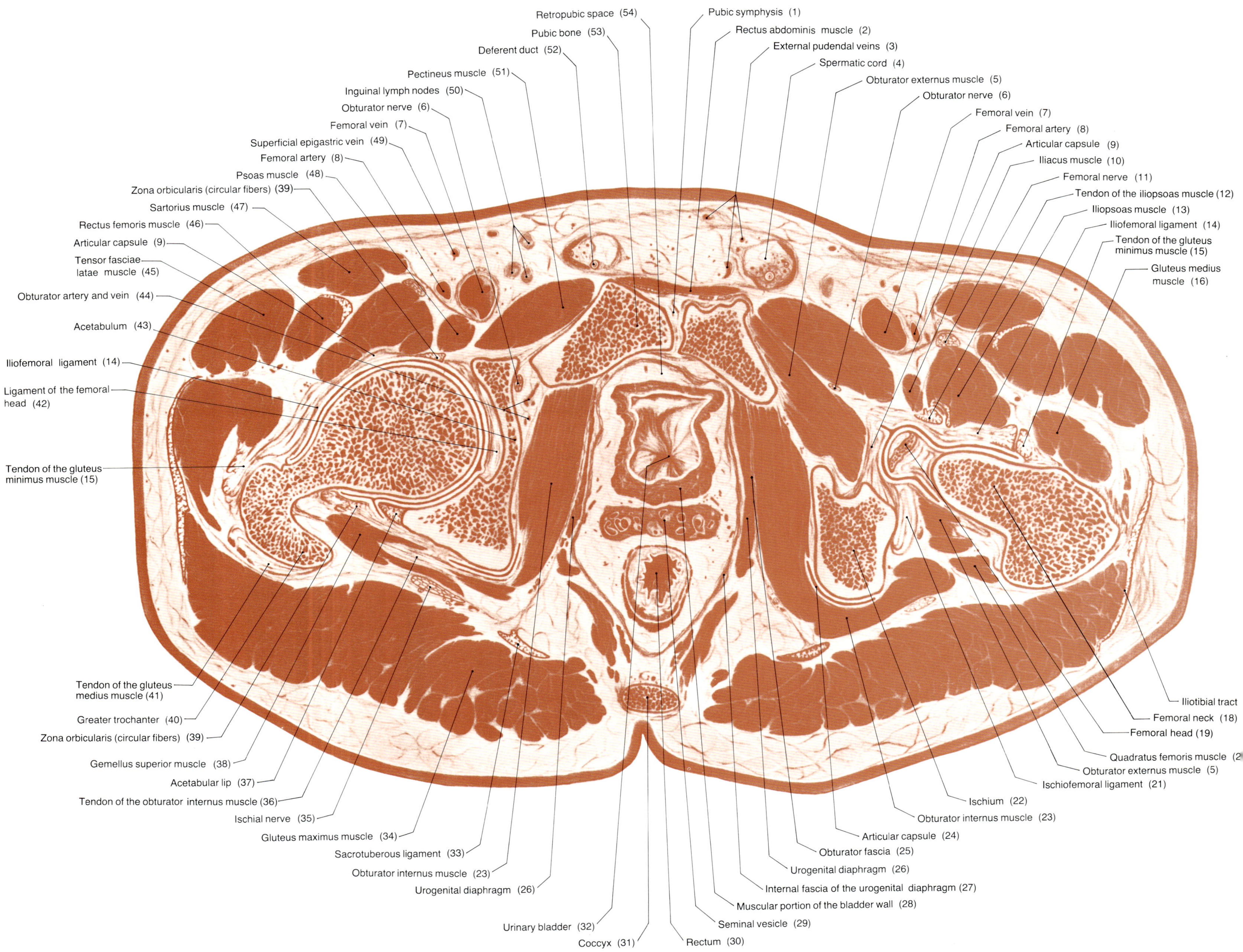

1 Symphysis pubica
2 M. rectus abdominis
3 Vv. pudendae externae
4 Funiculus spermaticus
5 M. obturatorius externus
6 N. obturatorius
7 V. femoralis
8 A. femoralis
9 Capsula articularis
10 M. iliacus
11 N. femoralis
12 Tendo m. iliopsoas
13 M. iliopsoas
14 Lig. iliofemorale
15 Tendo m. glutaei minimi
16 M. glutaeus medius
17 Tractus iliotibialis
18 Collum femoris
19 Caput femoris
20 M. quadratus femoris
21 Lig. ischiofemorale
22 Os ischii
23 M. obturatorius internus
24 Capsula articularis
25 Fascia obturatoria
26 Diaphragma urogenitale
27 Fascia diaphragmatis urogenitalis inferior
28 Tunica muscularis (Vesica urinaria)
29 Vesicula seminalis
30 Rectum
30.1 Prostata
31 Os coccygis
32 Vesica urinaria
32.1 M. pubococcygeus
33 Lig. sacrotuberale
34 M. glutaeus maximus
35 N. ischiadicus
36 Tendo m. obturatorii interni
37 Labrum acetabulare
38 M. gemellus superior
39 Zona orbicularis
40 Trochanter major
41 Tendo m. glutaei medii
42 Lig. capitis femoris
43 Os acetabuli
44 A. et V. obturatoria
45 M. tensor fasciae latae
46 M. rectus femoris
47 M. sartorius
48 M. psoas major
49 V. epigastrica superficialis
50 Nodi lymphatici inguinales
51 M. pectineus
52 Ductus deferens
53 Os pubis
54 Spatium retropubicum

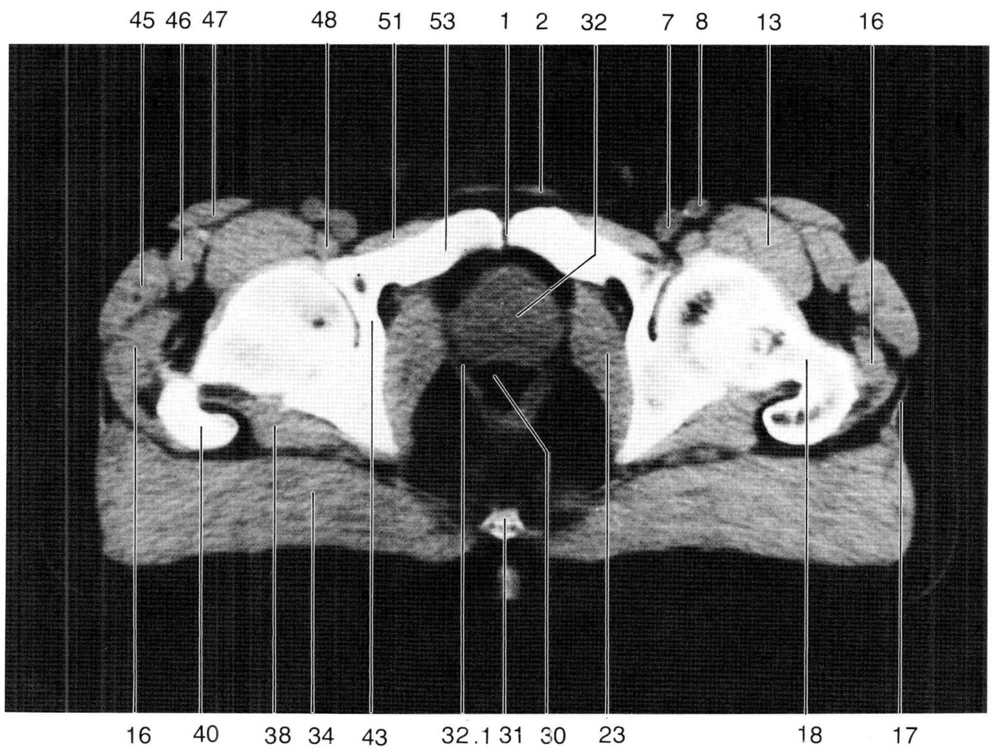

CT scan, unenhanced

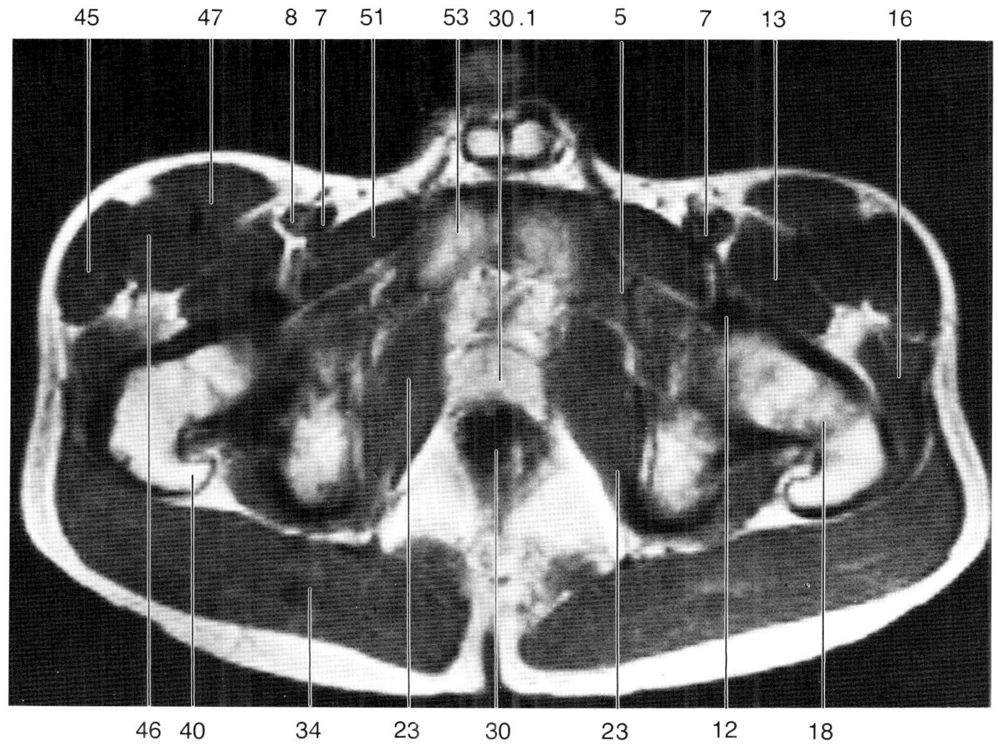

MRI, SE 500/50

- 1 Pubic symphysis
- 2 Rectus abdominis muscle
- 5 Obturator externus muscle
- 7 Femoral vein
- 8 Femoral artery
- 12 Tendon of the iliopsoas muscle
- 13 Iliopsoas muscle
- 16 Gluteus medius muscle
- 17 Iliotibial tract
- 18 Femoral neck
- 23 Obturator internus muscle
- 30 Rectum
- 30.1 Prostate
- 31 Coccyx
- 32 Urinary bladder
- 32.1 Pubococcygeus muscle
- 34 Gluteus maximus muscle
- 38 Gemellus superior muscle
- 40 Greater trochanter
- 43 Acetabulum
- 45 Tensor fasciae latae muscle
- 46 Rectus femoris muscle
- 47 Sartorius muscle
- 48 Psoas muscle
- 51 Pectineus muscle
- 53 Pubic bone

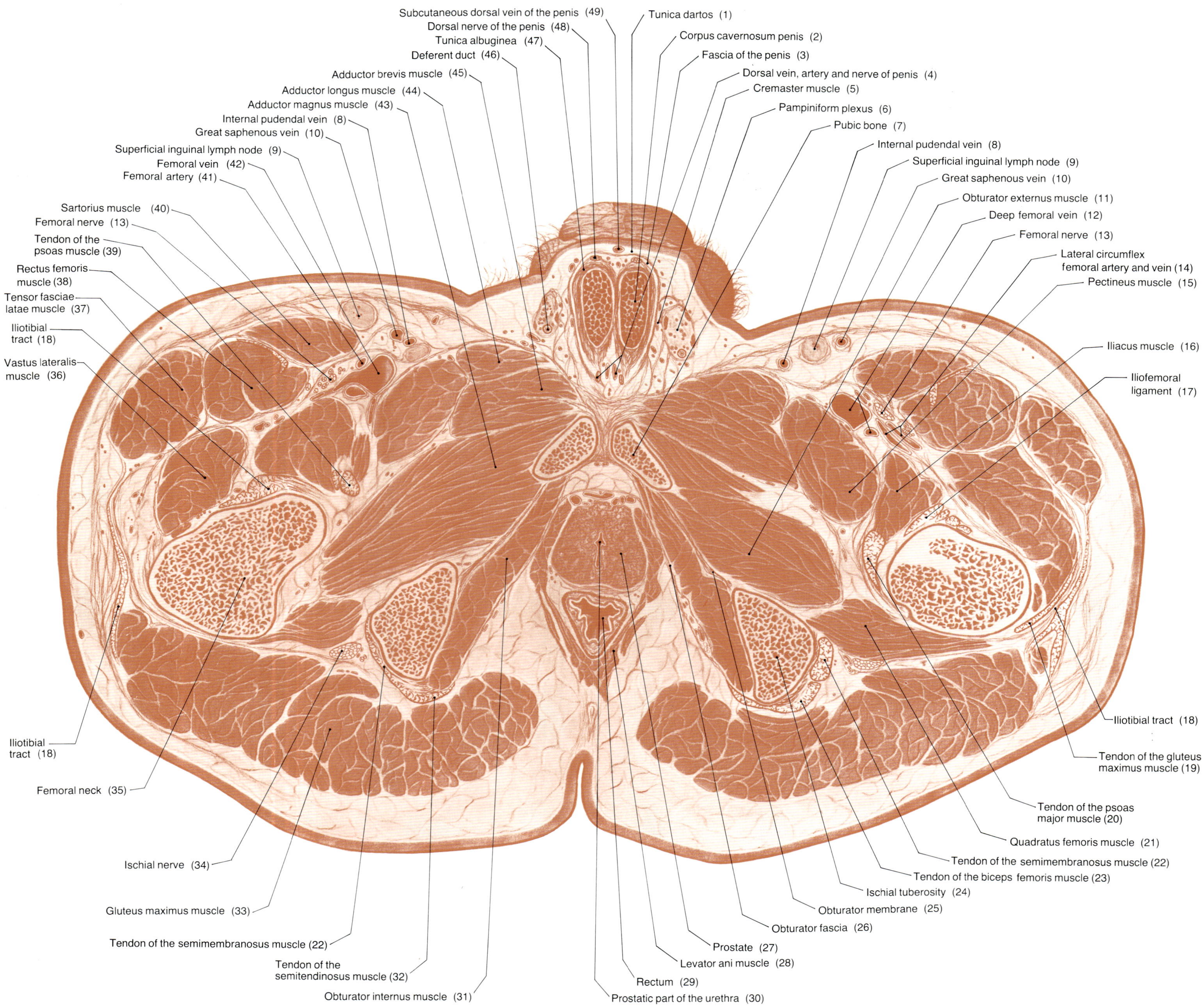

1 Tunica dartos
2 Corpus cavernosum penis
3 Fascia penis
4 V. et A. et N. dorsalis penis
5 M. cremaster
6 Plexus pampiniformis
7 Os pubis
8 V. pudenda interna
9 Nodus lymphaticus inguinalis superficialis
10 V. saphena magna
11 M. obturatorius externus
12 V. et A. femoralis
13 N. femoralis
14 A. et V. circumflexa femoris lateralis
15 M. pectineus
16 M. iliacus
17 Lig. iliofemorale
18 Tractus iliotibialis
19 Tendo m. glutaei maximi
20 Tendo m. psoas majoris
21 M. quadratus femoris
22 Tendo m. semimembranosi
23 Tendo m. bicipitis femoris
24 Tuber ischiadicum
25 Membrana obturatoria
26 Fascia obturatoria
27 Prostata
28 M. levator ani
29 Rectum
30 Pars prostatica urethrae
31 M. obturatorius internus
32 Tendo m. semitendinosi
33 M. glutaeus maximus
34 N. ischiadicus
35 Collum femoris
36 M. vastus lateralis
37 M. tensor fasciae latae
38 M. rectus femoris
39 Tendo m. psoas
40 M. sartorius
41 A. femoralis
42 V. femoralis
43 M. adductor magnus
44 M. adductor longus
45 M. adductor brevis
46 Ductus deferens
47 Tunica albuginea
48 N. dorsalis penis
49 V. dorsalis penis subcutanea

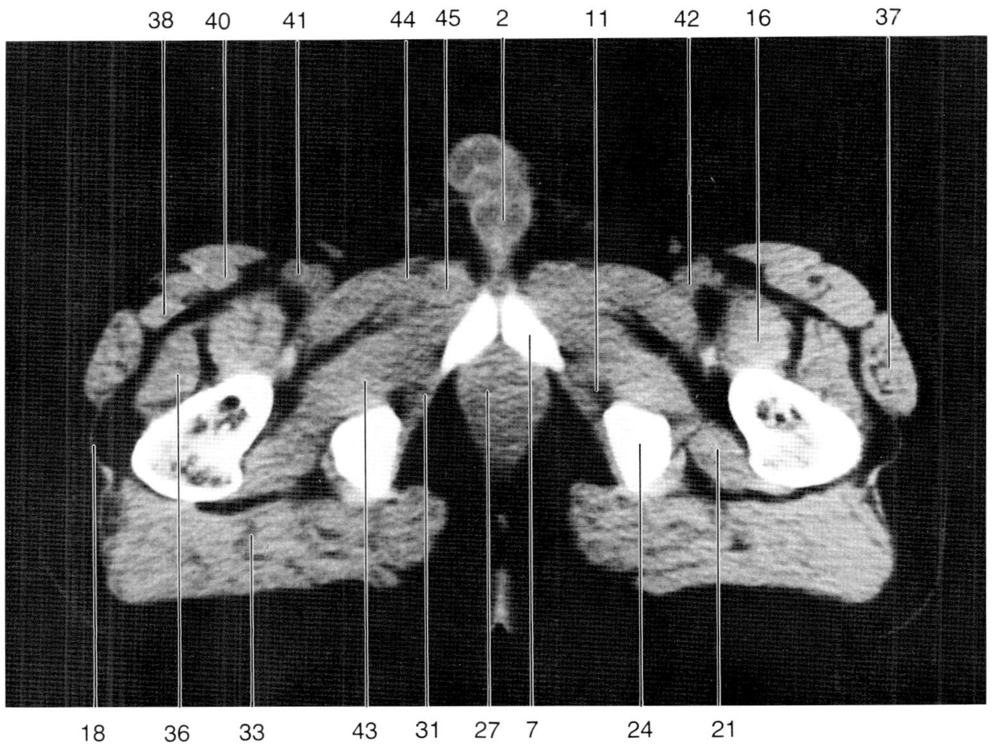

CT scan, unenhanced

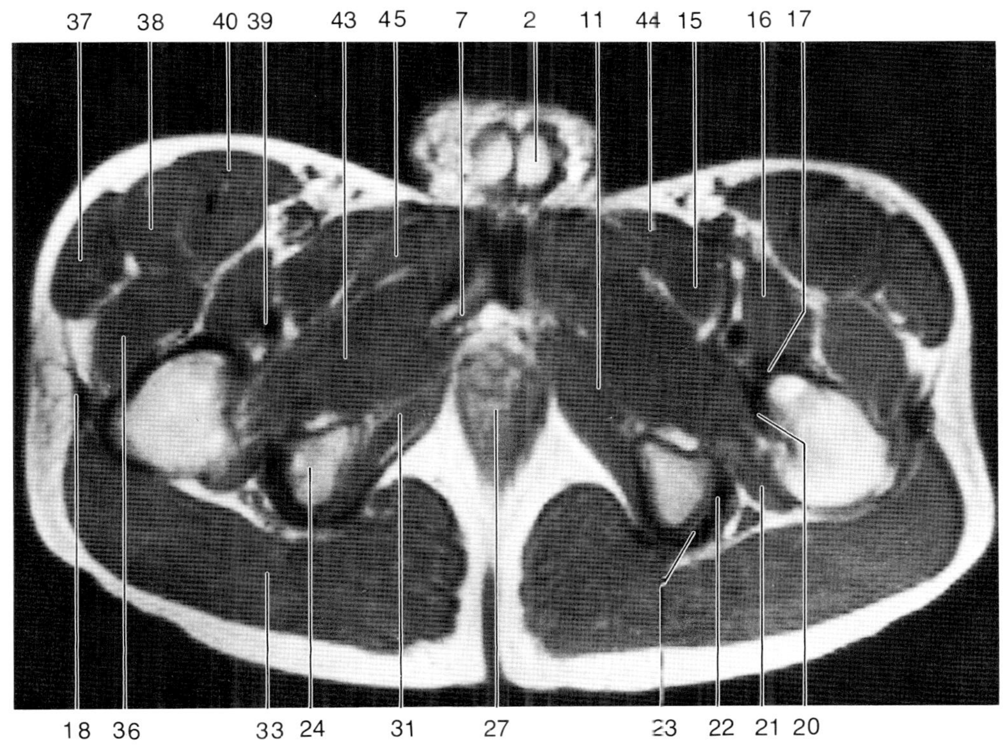

MRI, SE 500/50

2 Corpus cavernosum penis
7 Pubic bone
11 Obturator externus muscle
15 Pectineus muscle
16 Iliacus muscle
17 Iliofemoral ligament
18 Iliotibial tract
20 Tendon of psoas major muscle
21 Quadratus femoris muscle
22 Tendon of the semimembranosus muscle
23 Tendon of the biceps femoris muscle
24 Ischial tuberosity
27 Prostate
31 Obturator internus muscle
33 Gluteus maximus muscle
36 Vastus lateralis muscle
37 Tensor fasciae latae muscle
38 Rectus femoris muscle
39 Tendon of the psoas muscle
40 Sartorius muscle
41 Femoral artery
42 Femoral vein
43 Adductor magnus muscle
44 Adductor longus muscle
45 Adductor brevis muscle

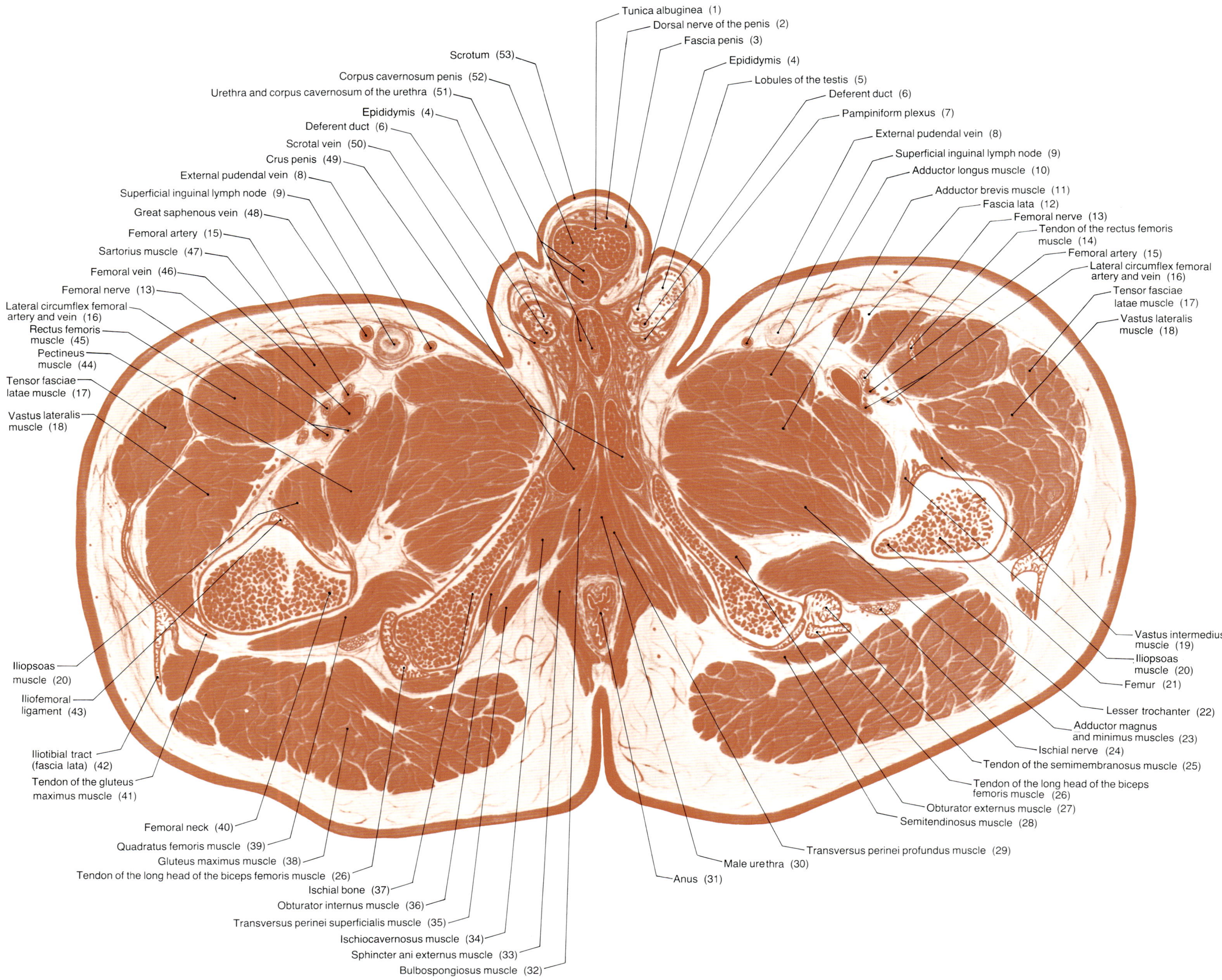

1 Tunica albuginea
2 N. dorsalis penis
3 Fascia penis
4 Epididymis
5 Lobuli testis
6 Ductus deferens
7 Plexus pampiniformis
8 V. pudenda externa
9 Nodus lymphaticus inguinalis superficialis
10 M. adductor longus
11 M. adductor brevis
12 Fascia lata
13 N. femoralis
14 Tendo m. recti femoris
15 A. femoralis
16 A. et V. circumflexa femoris lateralis
17 M. tensor fasciae latae
18 M. vastus lateralis
19 M. vastus intermedius
20 M. iliopsoas
21 Femur
22 Trochanter minor
23 M. adductor magnus et minimus
24 N. ischiadicus
25 Tendo m. semimembranosi
26 Tendo capitis longi (M. biceps femoris)
27 M. obturatorius externus
28 M. semitendinosus
29 M. transversus perinei profundus
30 Urethra masculina
31 Anus
32 M. bulbospongiosus
33 M. sphincter ani externus
34 M. ischiocavernosus
35 M. transversus perinei superficialis
36 M. obturatorius internus
37 Os ischii
38 M. glutaeus maximus
39 M. quadratus femoris
40 Collum femoris
41 Tendo m. glutaei maximi
42 Tractus iliotibialis (Fascia latae)
43 Lig. iliofemorale
44 M. pectineus
45 M. rectus femoris
46 V. femoralis
47 M. sartorius
48 V. saphena magna
49 Crus penis
50 V. scrotalis
51 Urethra et Corpus cavernosum urethrae
52 Corpus cavernosum penis
53 Scrotum

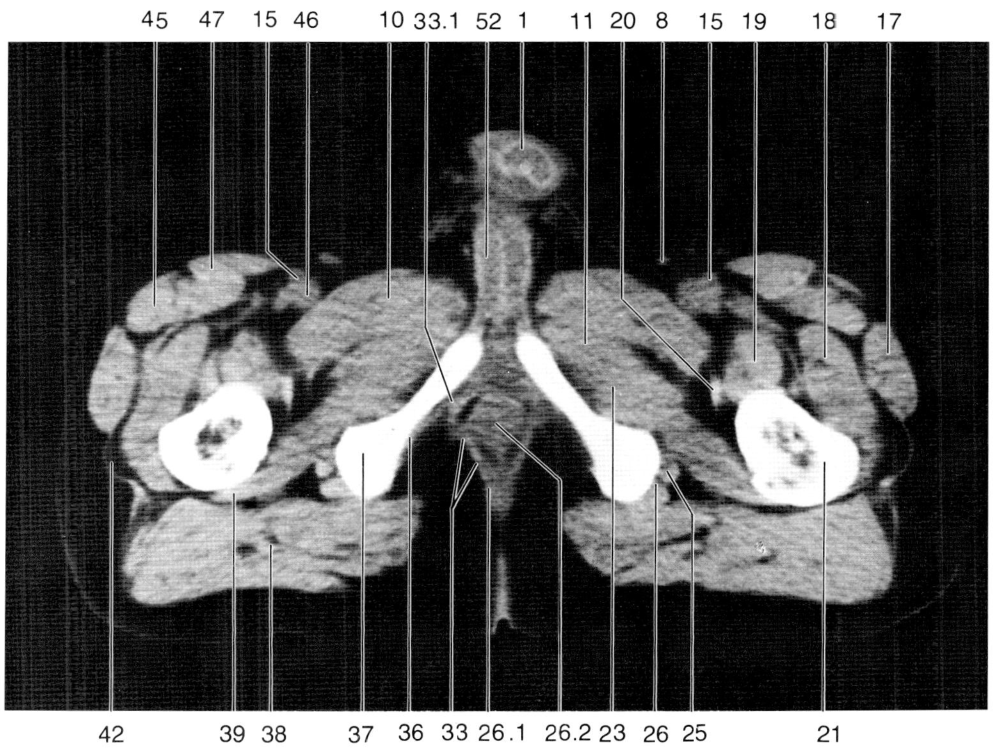

CT scan, unenhanced

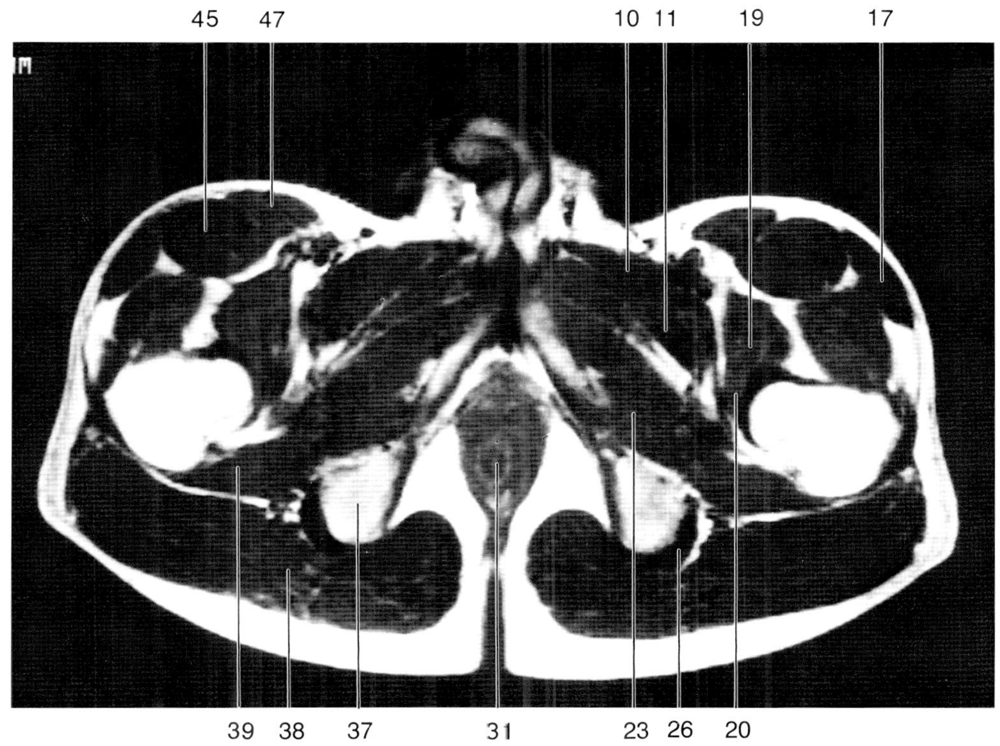

MRI, SE 1000/30

- 1 Tunica albuginea
- 8 External pudendal vein
- 10 Adductor longus muscle
- 11 Adductor brevis muscle
- 15 Femoral artery
- 17 Tensor fasciae latae muscle
- 18 Vastus lateralis muscle
- 19 Vastus intermedius muscle
- 20 Iliopsoas muscle
- 21 Femur
- 23 Adductor magnus and minimus muscles
- 25 Tendon of the semimembranosus muscle
- 26 Tendon of the long head of the biceps femoris muscle
- 26.1 Levator ani muscle
- 26.2 Prostate
- 31 Anus
- 33 Sphincter ani externus muscle
- 33.1 Pubococcygeus muscle
- 36 Obturator internus muscle
- 37 Ischial bone
- 38 Gluteus maximus muscle
- 39 Quadratus femoris muscle
- 42 Iliotibial tract (fascia lata)
- 45 Rectus femoris muscle
- 46 Femoral vein
- 47 Sartorius muscle
- 52 Corpus cavernosum penis

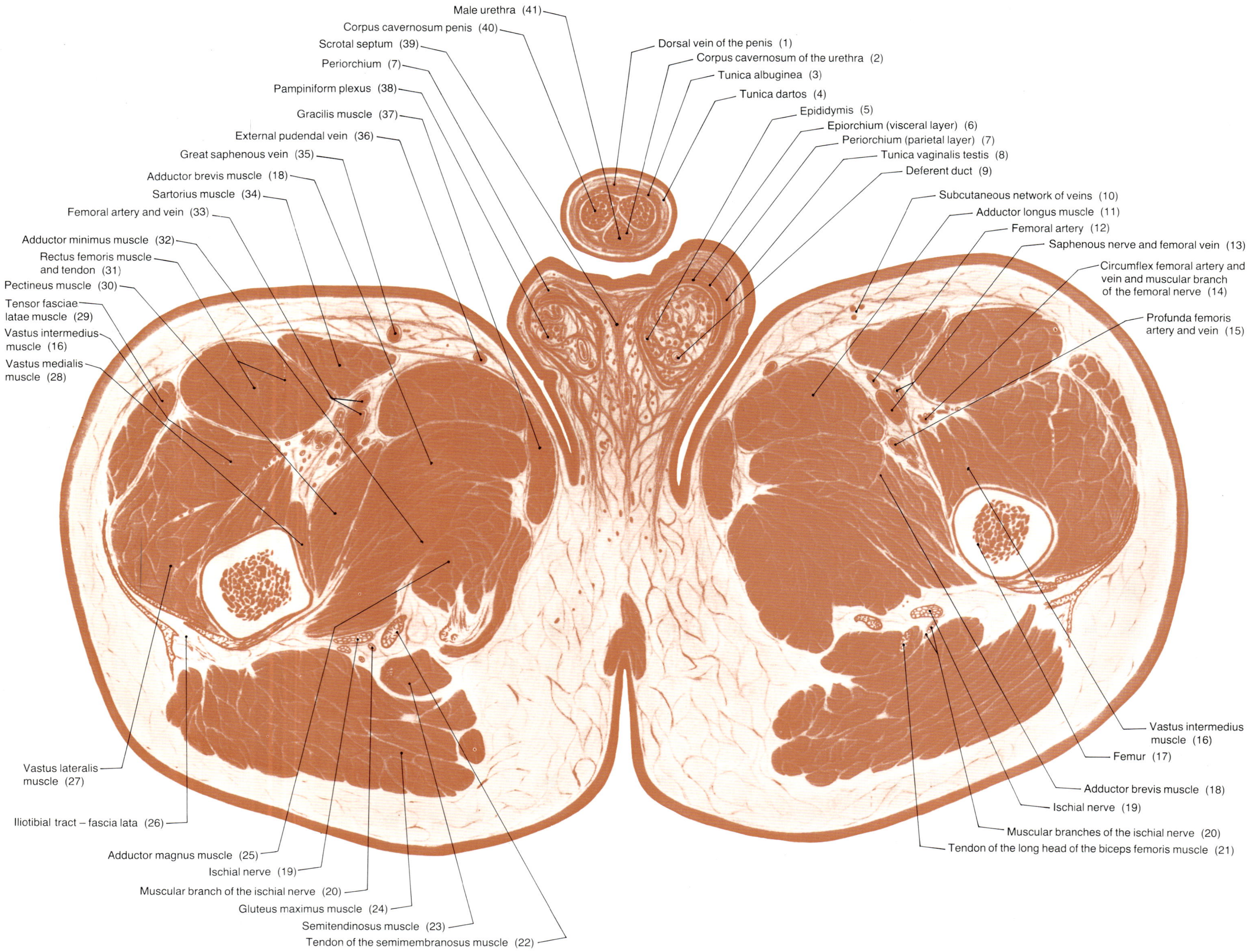

1 V. dorsalis penis
2 Corpus cavernosum urethrae
3 Tunica albuginea
4 Tunica dartos
5 Epididymis
6 Epiorchium (Lamina visceralis)
7 Periorchium (Lamina parietalis)
8 Tunica vaginalis testis
9 Ductus deferens
10 Vv. subcutaneae
11 M. adductor longus
12 A. femoralis
13 N. saphenus et V. femoralis
14 A. et V. circumflexa femoris et R. muscularis (N. fem.)
15 A. et V. profunda femoris
16 M. vastus intermedius
17 Femur
18 M. adductor brevis
19 N. ischiadicus
20 Rr. musculares (N. ischii)
21 Tendo capitis longi (M. biceps femoris)
22 Tendo m. semimenbranosi
23 M. semitendinosus
24 M. glutaeus maximus
25 M. adductor magnus
26 Tractus iliotibialis (Fascia lata)
27 M. vastus lateralis
28 M. vastus medialis
29 M. tensor fasciae latae
30 M. pectineus
31 M. rectus femoris et Tendo
32 M. adductor minimus
33 A. et V. femoralis
34 M. sartorius
35 V. saphena magna
36 V. pudenda externa
37 M. gracilis
38 Plexus pampiniformis
39 Septum scroti
40 Corpus cavernosum penis
41 Urethra masculina

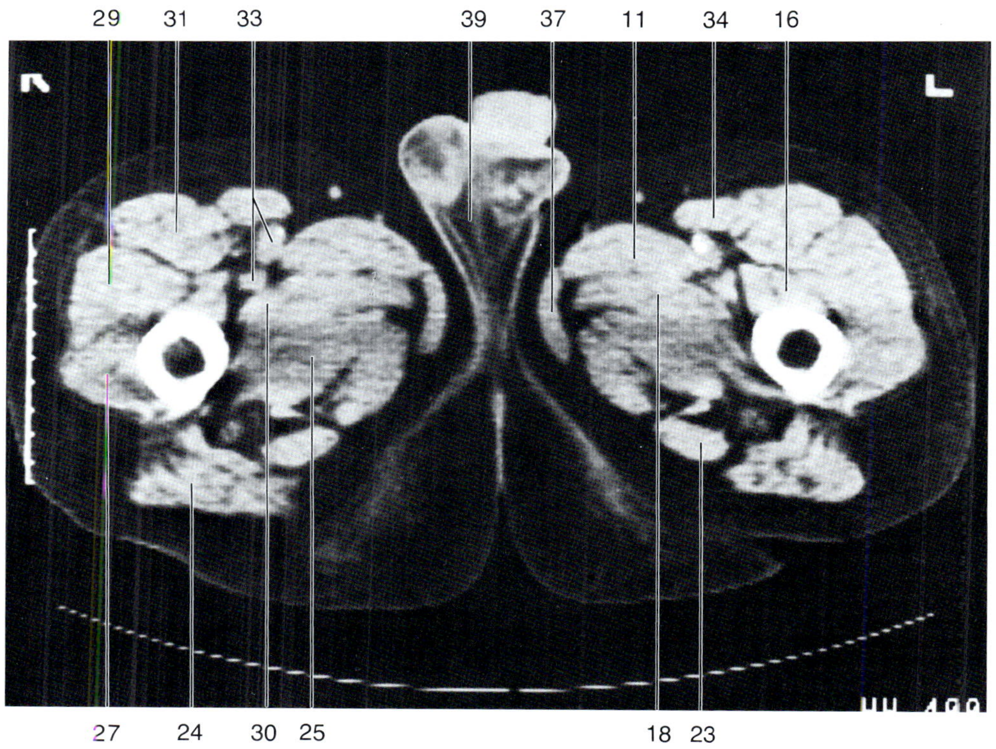

CT scan, unenhanced

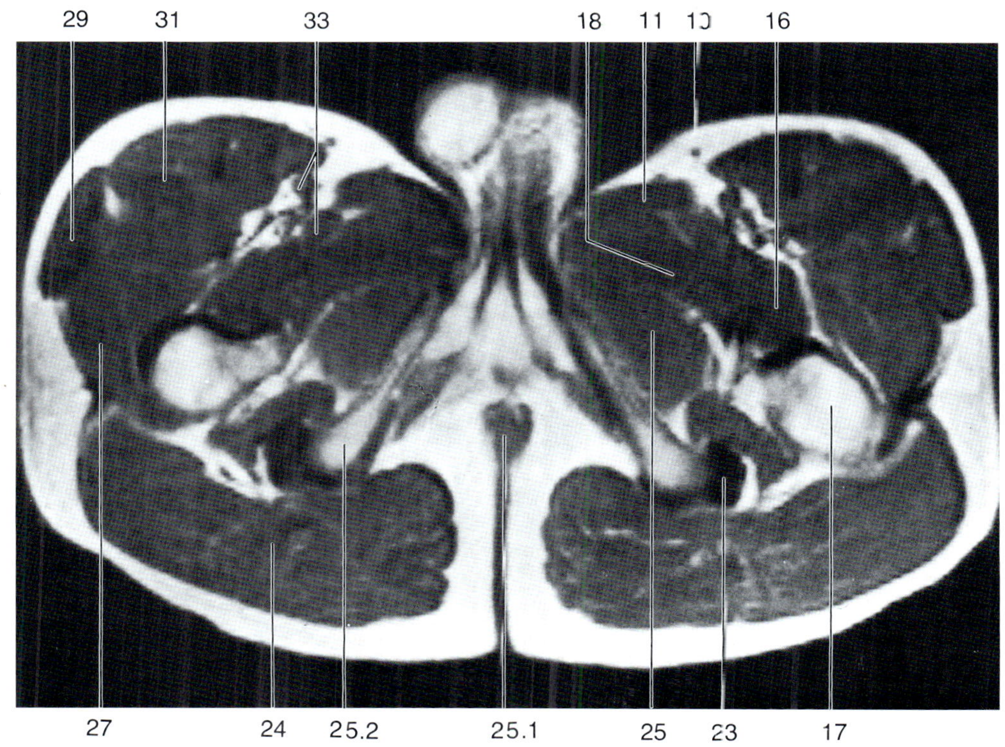

MRI, SE 500/50

10 Subcutaneous network of veins
11 Adductor longus muscle
16 Vastus intermedius muscle
17 Femur
18 Adductor brevis muscle
23 Semitendinosus muscle
24 Gluteus maximus muscle
25 Adductor magnus muscle
25.1 Anus
25.2 Ischial bone
27 Vastus lateralis muscle
29 Tensor fasciae latae muscle
30 Pectineus muscle
31 Rectus femoris muscle and tendon
33 Femoral artery and vein
34 Sartorius muscle
37 Gracilis muscle
39 Scrotal septum